Clinical Case Studies in Home Health Care

D0921953

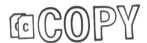

Clinical Case Studies in Home Health Care

Edited by

Leslie Neal-Boylan, PhD, RN, CRRN, APRN-BC, FNP

Professor and Graduate Program Coordinator
Southern Connecticut State University
New Haven, CT

WILEY-BLACKWELL

A John Wiley & Sons, Inc., Publication

Contents

Contributors

EDITOR

Leslie Neal-Boylan, PhD, RN, CRRN, APRN-BC, FNP
Professor and Graduate Program Coordinator
Southern Connecticut State University
New Haven, CT

CONTRIBUTORS

Susan Breakwell, APHN-BC, DNP
Associate Professor
Department of Community, Systems and Mental Health
College of Nursing
Rush University
Chicago, IL

Kathleen Francis, RN, MSN, CWOCN
Clinical Nurse Specialist
The Brooklyn Hospital Center
Brooklyn, NY

Lisa A. Gorski, MS, HHCNS, BC, CRNI, FAAN
Clinical Nurse Specialist
Wheaton Franciscan Home Health & Hospice
Milwaukee, WI

Sharron E. Guillett, PhD, RN
Director of Nursing
Stratford University
Falls Church, VA

Leigh Ann Howard, RN, MSN
VNA Home Health and Hospice
South Portland, ME

Joanne DeSanto Iennaco, PhD, PMHCNS-BC, APRN
Assistant Professor
School of Nursing
Yale University
New Haven, CT

Lannette Johnston, RN, BSN, MS, CPST
Pediatric Private Duty Patient Care Supervisor
Home Nursing Agency
Altoona, PA

Teresa LaMonica, PhD, MSN, RN, CPNP
Assistant Professor of Nursing
School of Health Professions
Marymount University
Arlington, VA

Sharon D. Martin, RN, MSN, PhD(c)
Associate Professor of Nursing
Department of Nursing
Saint Joseph's College of Maine
Standish, ME

Lelah R. Marzi, RN, MBA, BSN, COS-C, HCS-D
Branch Director
Gentiva Health Services
Ocala, FL

Mary Curry Narayan, MSN, RN, HHCNS-BC, COS-C
Intermittent Adjunct Faculty/Clinical Instructor
College of Health and Human Services
George Mason University
Fairfax, VA
Staff Orientation and Development Specialist
Professional Healthcare Resources Home Health and Hospice Agency
Annandale, VA
Consultant
Narayan Associates
Vienna, VA

Caryl Ann O'Reilly, CNS, CDE, MBA
Center of Excellence
Visiting Nurse Service of New York
New York, NY

Debra Riendeau, MN, APRN, BC, PMHNP-BC
Assistant Professor of Nursing
Department of Nursing
Saint Joseph's College of Maine
Standish, ME

Linda Royer, PhD, RN
School of Nursing
Florida Hospital College of Health Sciences
Orlando, FL

Ruth Smillie, RN, MSN
Assistant Professor of Nursing
Department of Nursing
Saint Joseph's College of Maine
Standish, ME

Sheila Spurlock-White, MSN, RN
Associate Professor
Department of Nursing
Stratford University
Vienna, VA

Jeanie Stoker, MPA, RN, BC
Director of Home Care
AnMed Health
Anderson, SC

Pamela Teenier, RN, BSN, MBA, CHCE, HCS-D, COS-C
AVP, Medicare Operations
Gentiva Health Services
Corpus Christi, TX

Preface

This book has been a long time coming. Having worked in home care for many years, taught about home care both in agency and in university settings, and written extensively about home care, I have been consistently dismayed and amazed that there appear to be no case study books specific to home care. When I taught home health, I'd have to adapt inpatient cases to suit my needs. I continue to see a lack of understanding about what home care is or an appreciation for its value and the tremendous work that home care clinicians perform. The skill that is required of all of the home care disciplines has for too long gone under-acknowledged. I hope that this book will help to demonstrate the kind of work they do and how vital they are to the health care of patients everywhere.

Home care is unique. There is nothing to compare with giving care to someone in his or her own surroundings. The challenge of adapting care to the home is both awe inspiring and gratifying. This is not to diminish inpatient care in any way. However, as Florence Nightingale so aptly put it: "Hospitals are but an intermediate stage of civilisation [sic] . . . the ultimate objective is to nurse all sick at home." (*The Times*, London, April 14, 1876). The nurse in the inpatient setting typically has equipment and personnel at hand to assist him/her. The nurse in the home can call with questions but is largely on his/her own.

Not all nurses can function effectively in the home setting because of this lack of available resources or a structured setting in which to work. Those of us who love home care love the autonomy it gives us. We love the challenges we face when trying to work with each patient and caregiver to assist the patient in staying in his/her own home.

The patient and the patient's significant others are part of our plan of care. The environment, both physical and intangible, must play a role in our planning. Our care is truly holistic in every sense of the word. Many of our patients tend to see us many times and get to know us. We often have more than one visit to teach them self-care and to get to know them as people. If they are rehospitalized, we try very hard to take care of them on their return if we were the clinicians who cared for them before they left home. We embody the "continuity-of-care" principle.

The primary care provider tends to trust our judgments because WE are their eyes and ears in the home. It is clear that home health clinicians must be very knowledgeable, skilled, and comfortable working in unstructured settings, as well as flexible, adaptable, and able to roll with the punches.

The purpose of this book, then, is to introduce students and other clinicians who are not familiar with home care to its many wonders. It is hoped that students will dog-ear its pages, carry it with them to home visits, and refer to it often. If one student or nurse who otherwise did not previously see home care as a possible career choice changes his/her mind because of this book, then it will have been worthwhile. However, what is more important is that students and nurses should learn how exciting and rewarding home care can be; and, even if they don't see it in their future, they should at least appreciate their colleagues who devote their professional lives to their home care patients.

Staff educators and academic instructors are encouraged to use the cases to teach nurses and students how clinicians manage health care in the home setting. Although, the book is geared toward registered nurses and students, the importance of the interdisciplinary team is woven throughout the pages of the book so that clinicians in other disciplines will find these cases helpful as well.

Editor's note: As this book goes to press, it is important to acknowledge that the ability of nurse practitioners to write orders for home health care and hospice appears imminent. The term "physician" is used in the book. However, the reader is asked to substitute "nurse practitioner" once this legislation passes.

HOW TO USE THIS BOOK

Chapter 1 introduces the theoretical frameworks that support home care. The chapter does not cover every theoretical framework that might apply to home care but attempts to address those to which students and nurses can best relate and with which they may be most familiar. The Neal Theory of Home Health Nursing Practice is woven throughout this book. The theory is explained in Chapter 1, but each case includes an explanation of how a nurse in each stage of the theory's model might view the case. The Neal Theory is a research-based theory that contends that nurses move through stages and have/

develop certain characteristics required to become autonomous home health nurses.

Chapter 2 addresses the complexities of home care. Relevant health care policy, reimbursement practices, and standards and guidelines for home care are discussed.

Chapter 3 describes how patients are transitioned into home care from other settings. The chapter identifies the types of settings from which one might be admitted to home care and how that process occurs.

Chapter 4 discusses the steps of preparing for and making the home visit. It also describes the post-visit tasks that are involved.

The remaining sections in the book are divided using a systems approach. Each case is organized in a readable, consistent manner to enable the student and clinician to easily follow the patient's presentation, the relevant data about the patient and caregivers, and the approach to patient care. Each case includes information regarding relevant reimbursement practices, the stages of the Neal Theory, the role of cultural competence, relevant community resources, and rehabilitation needs. An interdisciplinary care plan concludes each case and demonstrates how the team works to care for the patient.

Acknowledgments

I would like to acknowledge and sincerely thank the contributors to this book. These nurses are dedicated to home care, and I have known many of them for years as we have all worked hard to bring recognition to the specialty and to help it to grow. This book was completed ahead of schedule because these authors are fine writers and their expertise is vast. They are exemplars of nursing in general, and of home health nursing, in particular. I am honored to work with them on our various home care projects.

I would also like to acknowledge Tina Marrelli, the editor of *Home Healthcare Nurse*. While she was not a contributor to this project, she has been a very staunch supporter of all things home care and is a very prolific author in her own right. She has offered me kindness, as well as personal and professional support. I so admire her for all that she has done to advance home care.

There are many other devoted home health care clinicians (of all disciplines), researchers, teachers, and administrators. Thank you all for your tremendous contributions.

Finally, thank you to my editor, Shelby Allen, for being so supportive, dependable, responsive, and very easy to work with.

Clinical Case Studies in Home Health Care

Section 1

Introduction

Theoretical Frameworks That Support Home Care

By Leslie Neal-Boylan, PhD, RN, CRRN, APRN-BC, FNP

Several theoretical frameworks provide the foundation for home health practice. This chapter will describe those frameworks and lay the foundation for the rest of this book. It is important that home health clinicians use theory to guide their practice so that home care can continue to distinguish itself as a setting of care that is quite different from inpatient settings. Clinicians considering a move into home care should understand that clinical expertise is not automatically transferred to the home care setting. Rather, the clinician must be able to work in an unstructured setting and be confident enough to practice autonomously.

REHABILITATION THEORY

Rehabilitation theory revolves around the concept of self-care management. That is, the patient is encouraged toward maximal self-care. Rehabilitation professionals strive to assist the patient to regain functional independence, if possible. If independence is not possible, then the patient is assisted to do as much as she/he can for her/himself without pain, loss of quality of life, or the progression of disability. Patients are assisted to adapt to the alterations that may be imposed by their disability or illness.

Orem's (1995) [10] theory of self-care management is one of the theories that are used to support the rehabilitation and restoration of the

Clinical Case Studies in Home Health Care, First Edition. Edited by Leslie Neal-Boylan.
© 2011 John Wiley & Sons, Inc. Published 2011 by John Wiley & Sons, Inc.

patient. Orem suggests that the nurse offers wholly compensatory, partly compensatory, or supportive-educative care to the patient. The patient who must have total care because she/he is unable to participate in self-care receives wholly compensatory care, while the patient who can do some things for her/himself receives partly compensatory care. The clinician compensates for the things that the patient cannot do. Supportive-educative care is the ideal. This involves supporting and educating the patient who is able to provide self-care but needs to be taught how and to be supported in efforts to do so.

Henderson's (1978) [7] theory also revolves around the concept of self-care. The home health clinician stands in or substitutes for those activities or functions that the patient is unable to complete alone. As the patient gets better, the clinician helps the patient convalesce and works in partnership with the patient toward progressing through the plan of care. The clinician also works on the environment to make it malleable to the patient's needs and abilities. In the case of projected death due to the illness, the clinician assists the patient to make it peaceful and dignified.

Roy's adaptation model [13] focuses on the adaptation of the patient to the alteration in lifestyle caused by the illness or disability. The clinician's role is to encourage adaptation and to help the patient channel his/her resources toward adaptation.

THEORIES OF CHRONIC ILLNESS MANAGEMENT

Home care patients are often chronically ill. Consequently, home care clinicians must understand concepts of chronic illness since caring for those who are chronically ill is inherently different from caring for acutely ill patients. The Commission on Chronic Illness (1957) [2] originally outlined certain characteristics that describe someone who has a chronic illness. The illness or impairment caused by the illness:

- Is permanent
- Leaves a residual disability
- Is caused by a nonreversible pathologic condition
- Requires special training of the patient for rehabilitation
- Requires a long period of supervision, observation, or care [2, 6]

Patients with chronic illnesses often gain experience with aspects of their illness such as wound care, procedures, or medications. It is important that the home health clinician respect that knowledge and the routine with which the patient has become comfortable. That is not to say that the clinician (and the ordering provider) will not have better methods. However, if a method needs to be altered, the patient should be taught the reasoning behind the need for change and the patient should be made a partner in the plan of care.

Patients with chronic illnesses live with the consequences of their illnesses all of the time, such as pain, possible disfigurement, reduced function, dependence on others, and the inability to participate in everything they'd like to do. These patients often experience a lack of patience with their symptoms on the part of health care providers, friends, and family. They are often not taken seriously and may tell people they feel well when they don't so that they don't disappoint others. They may worry that others will tire of hearing about how they feel or what they cannot do.

Home care clinicians are likely to achieve a rapport and cooperation from chronically ill patients if they allow time to listen to patient concerns and show respect and empathy for what these patients know about how they feel and how they want to be cared for. Patients in home care (as should all patients regardless of setting) should be made to feel that they are equal partners in care particularly because care takes place in the patients' homes and the patients must be willing to allow the care to be provided. Family members and other caregivers must be recruited to "buy into" the plans for home care so that they can encourage and assist patients to participate.

Some patients with chronic illness may blame others for their misfortune, and other patients may feel that they have done something wrong, such as smoking or gaining weight, to cause their illness. The truth is probably a combination of both, but it is helpful for the clinician to assess the patient's perspective regarding the illness so the clinician will be able to know how to approach the patient as they work together to proceed through the plan of care.

In order to effect changes in health behaviors to move toward the restoration of function, it is helpful to understand how people perceive health behaviors. This understanding can enable the home care clinician to identify and begin with the patient's perception so that interventions can be realistic and doable. It is unrealistic to expect a patient to change behavior when they are not ready and willing. However, the clinician can help the patient reach a point of readiness to accept change.

One model of health behavior change is the Health Belief Model (HBM) [3, 12]. The patient must accept that he/she has or can get the disease or condition (perceived susceptibility), then must recognize that the condition is serious and that it has serious consequences (perceived severity). Once the patient has accepted these concepts, he/she must accept that the recommended intervention or treatment can work to reduce the risk of acquiring the disease or reduce its impact. However, the patient must then recognize the perceived barriers (tangible and intangible) that can prevent changing the behavior and be ready to learn about how those barriers can be reduced or eliminated. Cues to action are useful to clinicians to remind patients of the need to change, and self-efficacy is ultimately the confidence one has to take action.

The Shifting Perspectives Model [4] explains how patients switch the perspectives of their illness at any given time. When the patient views wellness as in the foreground, the illness is viewed as an opportunity for growth and for meeting people the patient might otherwise not have met. The person who is thinking this way seems able to separate his/her sense of self from the illness and does not allow the illness to define them. During this time, the person may also neglect to seek health care when they need services because they may avoid allowing themselves to focus on their symptoms.

When illness is in the foreground, the patient's illness may be tied up with their identity. They may appreciate the secondary gain from having an illness, such as getting attention from others, being excused from activities or responsibilities they do not want to be part of, and avoiding other painful aspects of their lives by dwelling on their illness. This perspective allows clinicians to feel needed by their patients but also fosters patient dependence when the patient should be achieving optimal and maximal self-care management.

HOME HEALTH NURSING THEORY

There are three major theories or conceptual frameworks in home care. The first two are based on the theorists' experience, anecdotal experience, and reviews of the literature. The last theory is based on a research study of home health nurses.

The Rice Model of Dynamic Self-Determination (1996) [11]

This framework is patient focused and incorporates the patient's perceptions, motivations, health beliefs, sociocultural influences, support systems, and disease process. As the title suggests, the goal is for the patient to be able to manage their own health care needs and in so doing, achieve personal harmony. The nurse's role is to facilitate patient independence by educating, advocating, and case managing. The patient and caregiver form a unit and should be cared for in a holistic manner. The nurse, patient, and caregiver move through stages of dependence, interdependence, and independence. They work together in partnership to achieve independence in the home.

The Albrecht Model for Home Health Care (1990) [1]

Albrecht used a review of the literature and her own experience to identify 18 concepts that are interrelated and reflect the dynamic relationships and complex processes of home care. Like the other models

Table 1.1.1. Albrecht's 18 Concepts.

Accessibility	Accountability
Availability	Comprehensiveness
Continuity	Coordination
Cost-effectiveness	Client/consumer
Demand	Efficiency
Intervention	Nurse
Client classification	Productivity
Provider	Quality of care
Satisfaction	Use of home care

used in home care, Albrecht describes the primary goal of home care as patient self-care. (Table 1.1.1)

The Neal Theory of Home Healthcare Nursing Practice [8, 9]

The Neal theory is based on a study of practicing home health nurses. Nurses were asked to define their practice. From the research evolved a model consisting of 3 stages: dependence, moderate dependence, and autonomy. The ability to adapt to an unstructured setting enables the clinician to move through the stages toward autonomy. Once the clinician has achieved stage 3, autonomy, it is possible to fall back briefly to stages 2 or 1, because of role changes, process changes, the physician-nurse relationship, reimbursement factors, office procedures, unfamiliar clinical situations, or the influence of anyone or anything that has an influence or potential impact on the patient's care (patient entity).

The theory is helpful to home health care clinicians because certain characteristics define a clinician who can function effectively in home care, and the theory helps clinicians to see that not everyone can function effectively in the home setting. The ability to adapt is key to being able to move through the stages. Clinicians in different stages will likely handle patient cases differently, and home health agencies can help clinicians to move more quickly through the stages to reach their optimal effectiveness. Each case discussed in this book will further highlight how a nurse in each stage, according to the theory, would act and perform (Figure 1.1.1).

Family Theory

Home health is holistic and very frequently involves the family as the unit of care. Caregivers may or may not be relatives of the patient. Regardless, the people who informally care for the patient, whether related by blood or not, are often the patient's family for the purposes of home care.

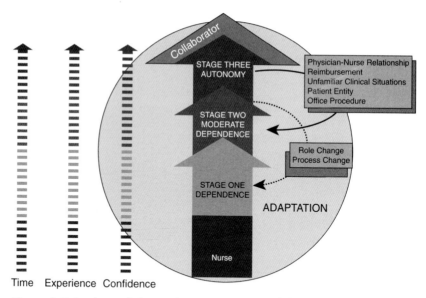

Figure 1.1.1. The Neal Theory of Home Health Nursing Practice.

It is important that clinicians in home care understand family theory so that the power and influence of the "family" is not underestimated. A thorough understanding by the clinician can help him/her work with the family in order to attain patient-centered goals.

One family theory is Duvall's Family Development Theory [5]. Duvall identified 8 stages through which the family proceeds, beginning with the couple separating from their families of origin and ending with the aging family. While, Duvall's theory needs some updating to reflect families who are not always made up of the traditional heterosexual married couple, the stages through which a couple and, later, a family progress remain largely unchanged. Certain fundamental principles underlie Duvall's family theory:

- Families progress through predictable stages.
- There are different expectations of the family in each stage.
- The relationships and interactions among family members change as the expectations change.
- Roles change as family members try to fulfill their roles in each stage.
- The family has its tasks to accomplish in each stage, as does each individual.
- The family as a whole must help the family and the individuals accomplish their tasks in order to function effectively as family unit.
- Conflict can result between the tasks of the family and the tasks of the individual.

THE PHILOSOPHY OF HOME CARE

The theoretical foundation of home care rests solidly on a core of patient self-care, functional restoration or substitution, and chronic illness management. The setting of care is in the patient's home, whether that is the street, a homeless shelter, or a mansion. The environment of the patient's home influences patient care and the role of the nurse. The environment has both tangible and intangible qualities. The tangible environment includes the building or street, the rooms, the furniture, the hallways, the presence or lack thereof of food or refrigeration, heat, or air-conditioning.

The intangible aspects of the environment are just as important. They include, but are not limited to, the dynamics between the patient and the family and/or caregivers, the knowledge and/or educational level of the patient, the perceptions of the patient and caregivers regarding receiving care in the home and their ability to comply with recommended treatment. Often the environment outside of the home filters inside, such as in the case of an unsafe neighborhood or the lack of neighbor support, community resources, or transportation. However, the environment outside of the home can have positive effects, such as a spiritual community that helps the patient and offers support.

The home setting is inherently different from the inpatient setting. The clinician must be comfortable working in an unstructured setting and in making many autonomous decisions, often without assistance or guidance. The clinician must have excellent communication skills, not only to communicate with the patient and the caregivers but to report efficiently and accurately to the primary care provider and other health care professionals who are involved with the case. Interdisciplinary conferencing and collaboration are even more vital when working in home care than in other settings, because other professionals are not as readily available. Communication must be regular and goal-oriented so that all team members work toward the same goals and reinforce each other's plans of treatment.

Since care occurs in the patient's home, the clinician must be certain to partner with the patient and caregivers and make the effort to understand the patient's routine, what is realistic within the patient's environment, and what is not possible to accomplish. The clinician becomes very creative and flexible as he/she works with the patient and caregiver to find ways to achieve goals and objectives.

The following 3 chapters will further enlighten the reader regarding the processes of home care and the details that make it so different and so rewarding for both patients and clinicians. The cases that follow these chapters will further illustrate how the home health clinician works to care for patients who have specific needs, conditions, and treatment goals in their home.

REFERENCES & RESOURCES

[1] M.N. Albrecht, "The Albrecht nursing model for home health care: Implications for research, practice, and education," *Public Health Nursing*, 7(2):118–126, 1990.

[2] Commission on Chronic Illness, *Chronic Illness in the United States*, Vol. 1, L. Braslow (ed.), Harvard University Press, 1957.

[3] M. Conner and P. Norman, *Predicting Health Behavior: Search and Practice with Social Recognition Models*, Open University Press, 1996.

[4] R. Davis and J.K. Magilvy, "Quiet pride: The experience of chronic illness by rural older Americans," *Image Journal of Nursing Scholarship*, 32(4):385–390, 2000.

[5] E.M. Duvall and B.C. Miller, *Marriage and Family Development* (6th ed.), Harper & Row, 1990.

[6] S.E. Guillett, "Understanding chronic illness and disability," *Care of the Adult with a Chronic Illness or Disability*, L.J. Neal and S.E. Guillett (eds.), pp. 1–10, Mosby, 2004.

[7] V. Henderson, "The concept of nursing," *Journal of Advances in Nursing*, 3(2):113–130, 1978.

[8] L.J. Neal (ed.), *Rehabilitation Nursing in the Home Health Setting*, Association of Rehabilitation Nurses, 1998.

[9] L. Neal-Boylan, *On Becoming a Home Health Nurse: Practice Meets Theory in Home Care Nursing*, National Association for Home Care, 2009.

[10] D.E. Orem, *Nursing Concepts of Practice* (5th ed.), Mosby, 1995.

[11] R. Rice, *Home Health Nursing Practice: Concepts and Application*, Mosby, 1996.

[12] I. Rosenstock, "Historical origins of the Health Belief Model," *Health Education Monographs*, 2(4):328–335, 1974.

[13] C. Roy and H.A. Andrews, *The Roy Adaptation Model* (2nd ed.), Prentice Hall, 1999.

Managing the Complexities of Home Health Care

By Mary Curry Narayan, MSN, RN, HHCNS-BC, COS-C

Home health care nursing is a highly complicated field of nursing practice. Its complexity frequently astounds nurses when they first step into patients' homes to provide patient care. Even nurses who come to home health from intensive care units, critical care units, and emergency rooms frequently find home health nursing to be quite challenging and overwhelmingly complex. To become autonomous home health nurses—confident, proficient and highly effective at helping patients achieve optimal health and well-being and maximal independence—requires time and experience in the distinct nursing field of home health nursing [1].

Yet despite its challenges and complexities, many nurses in home care say they love home health nursing and would never return to facility-based care. They emphasize that home health nursing is a particularly rewarding type of practice despite its challenges and complexities. They value the opportunity they have to use all their nursing assessment and care planning skills to help patients with multiple diagnoses from AIDS to wounds. They enjoy home health nursing, because it gives them the opportunity to care for patients at all stages across the life spectrum from prenatal patients on bedrest to palliative care patients who choose to die at home.

Clinical Case Studies in Home Health Care, First Edition. Edited by Leslie Neal-Boylan.
© 2011 John Wiley & Sons, Inc. Published 2011 by John Wiley & Sons, Inc.

Home health nurses talk about the satisfaction they get from using their creative talents to adapt care to meet the needs of patients in diverse home environments, from mansions to homeless shelters. They report that they enjoy teaching patients in their homes, adapting educational plans to unique patient needs and unique home situations and settings, and enabling optimal self-care and maximal independence. Although home health nurses complain about the difficulty in keeping up with productivity standards, regulatory and payers' requirements, and the massive documentation burden in home care (which shocks and, at first, overwhelms most nurses new to home health nursing), they quickly tell you that the independence, autonomy, flexibility, and daily challenges that occur in home care keep home health nursing interesting and rewarding.

This chapter provides an overview of the characteristics that make home health nursing a distinct and complex field of nursing practice, including the roles home health nurses undertake and the way they use the nursing process. It outlines the structure of a typical home health agency and the typical course of care home health nurses provide to patients in their homes.

DEFINITION OF HOME HEALTH NURSING

Home health nursing is defined by the American Nurses Association's (ANA) *Scope and Standards of Home Health Nursing Practice* (2008) [2]. Home health nurses provide care to patients in their homes, wherever patients live, including assisted living facilities and even sometimes, though rarely, in unconventional residences, such as shacks under bridges. Home health nurses provide care to patients of all ages, to anyone who needs nursing care within their homes. Thus, they provide care for patients with diagnoses that occur across the life spectrum.

Home health nurses focus not only on the needs of the patient, but on the needs of the family and others caring for the patient, to achieve optimal health and well-being for the patient. The goals of home health nursing are to help patients achieve optimal health, well-being, function, and self-care and to support patients and families at the end of life. "Nursing activities necessary to achieve this . . . may include preventive, maintenance, restorative, and rehabilitative interventions to manage existing health problems and prevent potential problems" [1]. Nurses assess the needs of patients and their families within the home environment, including assessments of the patient's physical, mental, spiritual, cultural, social, functional, safety, medication, and equipment needs and the needs of the family/caregivers which impact the patient's health and well-being.

DISTINGUISHING CHARACTERISTICS OF HOME HEALTH NURSES

By examining the definition of home health nursing, it becomes obvious that the complexity of home health nursing includes the scope of its practice—all ages, all diagnoses, every type of dwelling. Another level of complexity is the independence of the home health nursing practice.

Independence and Autonomy

Since nurses provide care in patients' homes, they practice independently (by themselves). When they are in a patient's home, everything the patient needs is up to them. There are no colleagues to confirm assessment findings, no doctor who will make rounds, no second shift to pick up any missed pieces. (Of course new home health nurses will have preceptors and mentors, and supervisors should always be available to provide support when requested.) The home health nurse may be the only health professional that the patient sees for months.

Thus home health nurses not only assess the patient, they develop a plan of care for the patient, essentially writing the orders for the patient's stay in home care and making those recommendations to the physician. If the physician agrees with the plan of care, the physician authorizes and signs the nurse's plan of care for the patient. Home health nurses update the orders as the patient's needs change based on their ongoing patient assessments.

In addition, home health nurses generally determine their patients' schedules. They determine, along with the patient, caregiver, physician, and other interdisciplinary team members, when the patient will be seen, how often, and at what time of the day. "When considering the professional autonomy of the nurse, it is helpful to remember that the nurse is no less autonomous than is the physician.... The nurse assesses the patient's needs, develops a plan to meet those needs, and recommends interventions to the physician who then gives the orders" [1].

Adaptability, Flexibility and Creativity

Home health nurses must adapt care to the patient's unique home situation. Without the supplies and resources available in facilities, home health nurses frequently must use their adaptation skills to "make things work" in the home setting. According to the *Scope and Standards of Home Health Nursing Practice* [2], "competent home health nursing practice requires flexibility, creativity and innovative approaches to situations and problems in the context of individual environmental differences and widely varying resource availability." And Neal-Boylan states:

> The nurse adapts to logistical and clinical aspects of home health, to each patient's home, to the patient's ability to learn, resources, and needs, and to change. The nurse adapts procedures, equipment, him or herself, and his/her own resources (both tangible and intangible) to provide patient care. To be adaptable, the nurse must be creative, innovative, and flexible (2008, p. 22).

Highly Developed Clinical Assessment Skills

Since many home health patients are homebound, unable to see their physicians except with great difficulty, home health nurses are the "eyes and ears" of patients' physicians, reporting their assessment findings to the physicians. Thus, home health nurses must have expert physical assessment skills. They need to be able to perform complete physical assessments (as appropriate for nursing practice), hone in on signs and symptoms, and be able to relate normal and abnormal findings to the physician.

In addition, home health nurses need to develop several assessment skills not ordinarily needed by nurses in other settings or, at least, in as much depth, as they are needed within home health nursing. For instance, home health nurses must be able to perform a functional assessment, identifying abnormalities in the patient's strength, balance, gait, ambulation, ability to do activities of daily living, and ability to live independently. Related to the functional assessment is the safety assessment, as nurses need to assess the home for all kinds of safety hazards from fire to infestations. They must assess the patient's ability to access basic needs, such as adequate food and shelter (e.g., heat in winter) and to avoid injuries such as those caused by medication errors or by falls in the bathroom.

Medication assessment is one of the most important parts of home health nursing practice. Home health nurses assess the effectiveness of medications in achieving their desired goals, the presence or risk of adverse effects and side effects, and the ability and compliance of the patient to take medications as prescribed.

Psychosocial assessment is another area of importance. Patients are unable to meet the home care goals of self-care and independence unless they have mental health and social support. In addition to assessing the patient, home health nurses must assess the family's and caregiver's knowledge and skills to assist and cope with the patient's care needs. Cultural norms and spiritual needs must also be assessed, and care must be adapted to the patient's and family's cultural/spiritual needs and preferences. In other words, excellent holistic assessment skills are crucial to home health nursing practice.

Highly Developed Care Coordination and Care Management Skills

Holistic comprehensive assessments demand holistic and comprehensive care planning. In home health, the "leader" of the interdisciplinary team is usually the nurse. The nurse's responsibility is not only to identify the patient's nursing needs, but the nurse must also coordinate the care of all the other members of the patient's team—physicians, rehabilitation therapists, home health aides, volunteers, family members, caregivers, and, of course, the patient—to achieve the patient's optimal health, well-being, self-care, and interdependence goals. If the physician did not order services the patient needs during the referral to home care, it is the nurse's responsibility to identify the need for those services, discuss the need with the physician, write the order (which the physician will sign), and secure those services.

If the nurse's home health agency does not provide a particular service or resource that the patient needs, the nurse needs to identify where and how the patient can obtain the service. The depth and breadth of the services that the patient might need are practically infinite, but include things like medical equipment (e.g., oxygen, wound vac); equipment to promote safety (e.g., shower seats, raised toilet seats, grab bars); supplies needed for nursing care (e.g., wound care dressings, catheter kits, venipuncture and laboratory tubes); services of additional disciplines (e.g., dietician, chaplain, clinical nurse specialists), services to meet psychological, social, spiritual, functional, and financial needs (e.g., counseling, socialization opportunities, respite services, homemaker services, medication assistance programs); and all of the other unique needs patients have in the home environment if they are to achieve health and well-being.

Home health nurses need to provide this type of care coordination and management throughout the patient's stay in home care, evaluating effectiveness of each service and discipline in meeting the patient's expected outcomes, always evaluating, reassessing, and updating the care plan. In order to achieve expert care coordination and management, home health nurses need to communicate concisely yet comprehensively, in a way that is organized and timely.

Teaching and Consulting Skills

One of the main duties of a home health nurse is patient education because patient self-care and independence are among home health nursing's primary objectives. The first step in achieving this goal is to determine *with the patient and family/caregivers* what the education goals are. Home health nurses cannot tell the patient what they need to know, as they are "guests" in the patient's home and serve more as "consultant coordinators" rather than as "directors" or as "the person in charge." The patient (or the family/caregiver) is "in charge." The nurse must be a motivator and learn to relinquish control while maintaining responsibility [1].

From the moment patients are admitted to home care, the nurse needs to begin assessing their learning needs and needs to begin planning education interventions that will enable patients to be safe at home; to be able to manage independently within the home situation; and to be able to manage signs, symptoms, and chronic illnesses without needing rehospitalization. According to the *Scope and Standards of Home Health Nursing Practice* [2]:

> A major responsibility of home health nurses is to provide instruction to patients, families and other care providers on acute and chronic disease processes, and to help patients develop other self management skills and abilities. In this role, nurses provide information, demonstrate techniques, and evaluate performance of procedures by patients, families, and other caregivers. Nurses must be able to identify barriers to learning, provide instructions using a variety of methods, and incorporate health beliefs and cultural and religious practices into the process of patient education.

Reimbursement Knowledge and Skills

The primary payer for home health care is Medicare, which is administered under the Medicare Home Health Benefit established by Congress in 1965. The Centers for Medicare and Medicaid Services (CMS) prescribes and manages these systems.

The amount an agency is paid for a patient's care varies depending on the patient's status and needs *as assessed by the nurse* at the admission to home care (and every 60 days after that if the patient continues to need home care services). The nurse admitting the patient completes a demanding Medicare document called the OASIS (Outcomes and Assessment Information Set) assessment, which is used to calculate the payment the agency will receive for 60 days of care. In many home health agencies, in order to complete the OASIS, the nurse also needs to have a working knowledge of how the international classification of diagnoses (ICD) coding system applies to the diagnoses their home care patients have.

The nurse must also determine if the patient meets Medicare's stringent criteria for home care. The patient must be "homebound" and need "skilled and intermittent" nursing or rehabilitation services. The services must be administered "under the care of a physician," and they must be "reasonable and necessary." The CMS defines each one of these criteria in detail, sometimes in surprising ways (http://www.cms.gov). Mastering this body of knowledge can be quite daunting, yet it is a necessity for home health practice.

Although Medicare is the major payer, it is not the only home care payer; and so, in addition to Medicare criteria for home care, home health nurses also need to master or know how to access, information about other payers' criteria for home care. These payers include other government programs—Medicaid, Veterans Administration, and Title programs—and many different private insurance companies and health maintenance organizations. Each has their own criteria for when the program or insurance carrier will pay for home care and when it will not pay. The admitting nurse needs to discuss these criteria with the patient and determine if the patient meets these criteria before admitting the patient for home health services. Once admitted, many private insurance companies and health maintenance organizations (HMO) require the nurse case manager to obtain authorization for each visit before the visit is performed. This may require the nurse to justify the reason the patient needs home care services, negotiating with the insurance case manager to obtain those authorizations.

Tolerance for Documentation

Since home health nursing is such an independent nursing practice, it is nonetheless, highly regulated. In addition, agency reimbursement is directly related to how well the nurse's documentation addresses the patient's fit into the payer's criteria for home care reimbursement. Therefore, home health documentation is notoriously demanding.

To meet regulatory standards, documentation for each visit needs to clearly demonstrate that the nurse followed the nursing process including assessment, identification of diagnoses and expected outcomes, care planning, implementation and evaluation. Paradoxically, despite the autonomy of home health nursing practice, anything and everything the nurse assesses, plans, or implements must be included within the plan of care. Even basic nursing care, which does not need a physician's order in other settings, requires a physician's order in home care. (This serves as a checks-and-balances system to assure that all of the care that agencies provide, and for which they bill, is necessary service). Remembering to obtain such orders and completing the documentation for those orders is one of home health nursing's great challenges.

Organization and Time Management Skills

Home health nurses usually carry a "caseload" of patients; these are the patients for whom they are directly responsible for as long as each patient requires nursing services. Caseload size varies depending on the acuity of the patients and the geographic area each nurse covers, but it is typically about 20–30 patients. In addition, home health nurses typically make 5–8 visits per eight-hour day. Managing a caseload, while meeting each patient's multiple needs, requires advanced organization and time management.

Home health nurses need to plan each day to assure that each patient is home for scheduled visits and that the nurse has all the telephone numbers, directions, teaching resources, and supplies needed for the day's care. Many nurses keep a "car office" and a "car supply closet," which they must keep stocked and organized in way that doesn't case waste from expirations, yet enables the nurse to always have what is needed for patients' unplanned needs.

WORKING FOR A HOME HEALTH AGENCY

Home health agencies, whether they are large or small, generally have a similar organizational structure. If the agency is large, it may have many offices with many people required to fulfill the responsibilities of each department within each office. If the agency is small, one person may be responsible for multiple responsibilities within the agency.

The basic "working unit" of an agency is the interdisciplinary clinical team. The team is usually coordinated by a clinical manager (sometimes called a coordinator or supervisor) who frequently works primarily in the office coordinating the interdisciplinary clinical team members who see the team's patients. Within the team are nurses, physical therapists (PTs), occupational therapists (OTs), speech language pathologists (SLPs), medical social workers (MSWs) and home health aides (HHAs). Most teams have several nurses and PTs and perhaps only one OT, SLP and MSW.

- **Nurses** coordinate and deliver patient care, working closely with the patient, family, physician, interdisciplinary team and community resource agencies. Nurses provide comprehensive patient assessments and skilled nursing care procedures. They teach patients and their families to become independent in meeting self-care needs, and they manage patients who have complex care needs. Usually, one nurse is responsible for a patient's care from admission to discharge from the agency, coordinating the care of the interdisciplinary team to achieve the patient's expected outcomes and the patient-determined goals.
- **Physical Therapists (PTs)** provide therapy exercises to improve patients' physical strength, balance, and ability to ambulate and transfer. They determine the best assistive devices to assure safe ambulation and safety in the home.
- **Speech-Language Pathologists (SLPs)** specialize in communication and swallowing problems. They help patients with speech, hearing, or comprehension problems. SLPs also assess and make recommendations for patients who are having difficulty with swallowing or who have tracheostomies.
- **Occupational Therapists (OT)** assist patients in meeting their optimal ability to perform their activities of daily living (ADL) and

other physical, mental, and social activities that make life meaningful. They also specialize in fine motor skills needed to perform ADL and instrumental activities of daily living (IADL).

- **Medical Social Workers (MSWs)** help patients and their families identify needs and community resources that can help meet those needs. MSWs also help patients develop solutions to long-term social/living problems. They are experts in the local, state, and federal assistance programs, and help find financial assistance for medications, safe housing, adequate nutrition, and so forth.
- **Home Health Aides (HHAs)** are also known as home care aides (HCAs). They provide personal care, such as bathing, dressing, and grooming. They may also perform some basic nursing tasks (e.g., vital signs) and homemaking tasks (e.g., change bed linens).

Very small agencies may contract for some of the less frequently used rehabilitation or social services. Larger agencies may have additional staff who can help the interdisciplinary team meet the patients' needs, including clinical nurse specialists (e.g., Certified Diabetic Educators, Wound-Ostomy-Continence Nurses, and Psych-Mental Health Nurses), Licensed practical Nurses (LPNs), Licensed Physical Therapy Assistants (LPTAs), Certified Occupational Therapy Assistants (COTAs), dieticians, chaplains, and volunteers who serve as friendly visitors. When working for smaller agencies that do not have these staff resources, nurses need to know how to obtain these services from other community-based agencies and resources if their patients need these services.

Supporting the clinical team are other agency employees and departments, such as **administration** (e.g., CEO or Executive Director, and Quality Director); **administrative support** (e.g., staff who help with telephone calls, data entry, and scheduling); **human resources** (who help with hiring, benefit programs, maintaining mandatory employee records, etc.); and the **financial department** (who send bills to Medicare and the patients' other insurance providers, pay the staff for the patient visits they make, etc.). Each agency also has a person or department in charge of **intake/referrals**, which takes the referrals made by hospital discharge planners, physicians, and other referral sources and obtains the initial information about patients that the agency will admit for home health care services.

REFERENCES & RESOURCES

[1] L. Neal-Boylan, *On Becoming a Home Health Nurse: Practice Meets Theory in Home Care Nursing* (2nd ed.), Association for Home Care and Hospice, 2009.
[2] American Nurses Association, *Scope and Standards of Home Health Nursing*, Author, 2008.

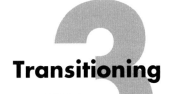

Transitioning

By Jeanie Stoker, MPA, RN, BC

The *Wall Street Journal* reported in December of 2007 [6] that nearly 18% of Medicare patients admitted to the hospital were readmitted within 30 days of discharge accounting for $15 billion in health care spending. It was also reported by the Institute for Healthcare Improvement that as many as 46% of the admissions could have been prevented. It is articles like these, as well as findings from the Medicare Payment Advisory Commission (MedPac), that have pushed rehospitalization to the forefront of healthcare reform. This single item has shifted the acute care mind set to see beyond "getting them out of the hospital" to a true care transitions model.

Beginning in October, 2011, hospitals will receive a reduction in all Diagnostic Related Groups (DRGs) if their readmission rates exceed the defined bar. While inpatient organizations have attempted to reduce length of stay and rehospitalization, the loss of funding in an already scaled back reimbursement model forces this issue to become a key priority. Enter post acute care providers.

While home health providers have seen the value of this model, we are now at the dawn of new opportunities that will not only provide significant cost savings, but improved clinical outcomes and improve the quality of life for chronic care patients.

"Transitional care" is defined by Mary Naylor, PhD, RN as "a range of time limited services and environments designed to ensure health care continuity and avoid preventable poor outcomes among at risk populations as they move from one level of care to another, among multiple providers and/or across settings" [9].

Key roles have been developed across all continuums of care to assess chronic care needs as well as alternative service providers. The Care Manager/Coordinator of Care (Case Manager) is often the one who leads the acute care discharge planning process. Some of his/her duties include:

- Coordination and collaboration of services by all disciplines
- Performance of a comprehensive, holistic assessment
- Development of a plan of care based on each patient's needs and unique situation
- Collaboration with each patient to develop mutual goals
- Completion of thorough and precise documentation
- Delegation of care, education, and discharge planning to other staff
- Evaluation of services and goals for outcomes [1]

The discharge planner is an RN or social worker who is responsible for arranging for post acute care needs based on an established plan of care. Medicare requires a participating hospital to complete a discharge evaluation and discharge plans developed by or under the supervision of an RN, social worker, or other qualified individual.

Discharge Planning Services provided by the hospital discharge planner include:

- Identifying those in need of post acute care services
- Completing an evaluation on all patients based on a physician's order or the discharge planning evaluation
- Documenting the evaluation and ensuring that it is part of the medical record
- Discussing alternatives with the patient and family or representative
- Developing and completing the discharge plan

The National Alliance for Caregiving states "Discharge Planning is a short term plan to get you out of the hospital. It is not a blueprint for the future." This organization encourages everyone to be proactive and participate in the discharge planning process. The National Alliance for Caregiving as well as the CMS website have good checklist for patients and caregivers so they can be part of this important process (National Alliance of Caregiving) [8].

The case manager and/or discharge planner will look at a variety of settings and services that will best meet the needs of the patient. While most patients want to go home, to do so often requires the support and services of many community providers. Community providers are organizations that provide medical and social support to the patient and family. Some examples include:

- Home health agency
- Home medical equipment
- Pharmacy

- Hospice
- Area agencies on aging
- Aging and disability resource centers
- Transportation services

Another key element in the discharge process is the "handoff". While the inpatient facility calls the transfer of care "a discharge," it is really a handoff from one health care provider to another. The Joint Commission requires that an organization have a process that addresses the patient's needs for continuing care or services after discharge or transfer. Additionally, when a patient is discharged or transferred, the organization is required to give information about the care, treatment, and services it provided to the patient to other service providers who will provide the patient with ongoing health care.

While there are many people involved in the process of handing off a patient from the acute care hospital to home care, more and more agencies are using a home care coordinator. The home care coordinator (HCC) may have a variety of titles (Liaison, Patient Care Coordinator, etc.) but serves as the transition coordinator from hospital to home care. Once the patient is given a choice of providers, the agency HCC may go to the hospital to gather data and provide information to the patient. The most common duties of this person include:

- Reviewing the medical record for continuing care needs
- Meeting with other providers to understand current treatment and goals
- Discussing orders and plans with the physician
- Beginning the teaching process
- Beginning the medication reconciliation process
- Initiating patient rights activities, including the review of the consent to treatment, HIPAA rights, advanced directives, financial responsibilities, and other similar items
- Interviewing the patient and caregivers to develop a rapport and define needs and expectations
- Assessing supply, equipment, and service needs for the patient at home

Another element in the transition of care is medication reconciliation. The Joint Commission has recognized the extreme importance of medication reconciliation at each point in transitioning the patient across the health care continuum. While the process and success has been a struggle for all areas, outcomes validate that this needs to be done.

Hospital 2 Home (H2H) is a joint initiative between the American Academy of Cardiology and the Institute for Healthcare Improvement with an overall objective to improve the transition from impatient to outpatient status for patients with cardiovascular disease. The stated goal is to reduce all cause readmission of heart failure patients by 20% in 2012. To achieve this, there are three action domains including medication management post hospital discharge. Home Care will play a vital role in this process.

ACUTE CARE TO HOME HEALTH

The discharge planning process begins at admission in the acute care setting when the nurse completes the admission assessment. As the patient progresses toward discharge, the staff will call in the discharge planner to provide additional direction and action as ordered by the physician. As previously discussed, a handoff must also occur between the hospital and home health agency. The Joint Commission recognizes that the process of transitioning the patient from one unit of health care to another is a critical opportunity to promote safety. Whether it is from the emergency department to the intensive care unit or from the medical floor to home health, a clean handoff promotes consistent and safe patient care across the continuum.

The Joint Commission had previously deemed patient handoffs as a serious issue. In March 2009 it was reported from The Joint Commission's Sentinel Event Database that communications break-downs were the root cause of more than 65% of 3811 sentinel events with 75% resulting in the patient's death. Many home health agencies still get limited information about the patient coming home, as the discharge practice of "the easiest referral gets the business" remains. This leads to poor transitions and challenging home care admissions. The patient expects that the home health agency will come to their home with the knowledge and details of the acute care stay so that care is not compromised and their rehabilitation period continues in a positive direction.

HOME HEALTH TO ACUTE CARE

A hand-off is required when a patient is admitted to an acute care setting. This is often done with a phone call or transfer summary. The transfer summary provides basic medical information including the reason for the transfer, a summary of the care and services provided by home health, the patient's progress towards goals, and any additional referrals made. A phone call to the admitting floor is ideal, but this often goes undone. Several factors that prevent this from occurring include: lack of awareness by the agency of the admission, lack of awareness by the home health nurse regarding where the patient is, or failure of the staff on the inpatient floor to see the value in getting this information. While the two practice environments are very different, all parties have valuable information that will help care for the patient and improve overall health outcomes.

HOME HEALTH TO HOSPICE

Home Health is viewed as a provider that focuses on skilled care and assistance with activities of daily living (ADL) toward an overall objective of assisting the patient to return to his pre-event level of function. Hospice provides symptom management and holistic care to help a patient and support a family to a peaceful death. There are many times when home health providers recognize the need to transfer the patient to this type of care.

When transferring to hospice, the home health interdisciplinary team works together to ensure that all criteria are met and more importantly, that hospice care will better meet the needs of the patient and family. A referral is made: and at time of transfer, a call and transfer summary should be completed to ensure that a smooth transition occurs.

HOME HEALTH TO ANOTHER COMMUNITY PROVIDER

Home health social workers often assess patient and family needs to discover the need for other community resources. Some of these resources include: Social Security Administration, Medicaid, Medicare, Area Council on Aging, Meals on Wheels, support groups, and many others. The agency must provide enough information to the community provider while insuring that all HIPAA laws and confidentiality are maintained. A summary is not sent to these providers. At times the agency staff may provide information for the family and caregiver to follow up on or may make a direct referral.

INTERNAL TRANSITIONS

Home health agencies provide service through a variety of professionals and para-professionals. These include home health aides, social workers, registered nurses (RNs), licensed practical nurses (LPNs), Physical Therapists (PTs), therapy assistants, occupational therapists, speech therapists, and others. It is important that all disciplines communicate as the patient needs and care plan change. For example, the nurse is in the home providing skilled care and notices that the patient's gait is unsteady and that he is having a hard time completing his personal grooming. After physician approval is obtained to add a home health aide and a physical therapist to the team, the nurse needs to provide the physical therapist and home health aide with information about the patient so that collaborative care can provide maximum outcomes for this patient. As patient needs change, case conferences and one-on-one communication provide other avenues for the transition of care.

PHYSICIAN COMMUNICATION

The Medicare Conditions of Participation (COPs) clearly define the physician's role in ordering and overseeing the home health plan of care. The home health agency staff is required to notify the physician of any changes in the patient's condition or plan of care. Some providers will provide a written or electronic summary to the physician before a scheduled medical visit. This keeps the doctor informed of the most recent activity and allows him/her to have a more complete picture to provide appropriate care management and oversight.

The most common form of communication involves a phone call to the physician's office. This allows the nurse or therapist to provide the physician with real time information. Many agencies and physicians develop parameters of care so the physician can define when he would like to be notified. An example of this may be a diabetic patient whose blood sugar is always between 150 and 250. The physician may give an order to call him only if the blood sugar is greater than 250. This process is also seen with vital signs and congestive heart failure protocols.

HOME CARE SERVICES

Many people think "home care" and "home health" are synonymous. While home health refers to an agency that provides specific clinical visits, home care is the full gamut of health services provided in the home setting. These include:

Home Health

- Skilled nursing services
- Rehabilitation services including physical therapy, occupational therapy, and speech therapy
- ADL support with home health aides
- Medical social services
- Other health care support such as a dietician or respiratory therapist

Home Medical Equipment

- Oxygen and other respiratory services
- Medical equipment including beds, wheelchairs, walkers, etc.
- Medical supplies such as diabetic and wound care supplies
- Specialized items including power mobility items and seat lift chairs

Home Monitoring

- Emergency response systems are available to provide quick response at the push of a button. Lifeline and other providers offer peace of mind and independence in the home setting as the patient and family know that someone is always available.
- Telehealth services are provided in many agencies across the United States. These services vary based on equipment and electronic capability but may include, vital sign assessment, weight monitoring, video observation, and question and answer feedback, and blood sugar tracking.

Medication Management

- While home health provides education and assistance for patients and their families, the ultimate goal is to ensure that medications are taken safely, as prescribed. Since home health is only in the home for a short period of time, other avenues of medication management may be sought.
- Pharmacies are providing an increasingly involved role as many now provide a medication management service which allows regular counseling and followup with patients, especially those dealing with polypharmacy. Several insurance providers now pay for this service as they see the many benefits of pharmacy oversight.

Infusion Services

- A safe, cost savings alternative to a lengthy hospital stay, home infusion services are able to provide a variety of intravenous (IV) services in the home setting. Patients are taught how to care for IV lines as well as how to administer IV therapy.
- Enteral services are often provided by infusion companies, including the provision of pumps, bags, nutritional products, and the needed education.

Other

- The health care coach is one of the newer services being offered in limited amounts. The Center for Medicare and Medicaid (CMS) has provided funding in the development of a care transitions model that includes health care coaches. These non-clinical team members are able to provide basic education, support, as well as medication management via telephone of home visits. While the duties and activities vary, an early project in Louisiana was able to reduce 30-day readmissions in the coached population to a surprising 7% compared to the national readmission rate of 17.6% [10].

HOME HEALTH ROLES DURING TRANSITIONS OF CARE

The home health agency will receive either a written or oral referral with transfer report from the referring agent. This will includes current status as well as orders for home health care. The nurse taking this referral will obtain as much information as possible related to current diagnosis, medications, treatments, as well as any infection control issues. The nurse then will provide a comprehensive assessment, as well as a medication review and reconciliation. The nurse then notifies the physician of any additional needs and services.

The admission nurse will then complete a care plan and provide a report to other home health staff, including the therapist, home health aides, and other nurses. Additionally, she will work with a medial social worker to obtain community resources as needed and available.

When the patient is transferring out of the agency to another pro-vider of care the nurse will educate the patient and family prior to the transfer/discharge about all aspects of care including ongoing needs, resources available, coverage requirements (as applicable), as well as final goal status. A transfer/discharge summary will be completed and the clinician will offer a written summary or a verbal report to the next provider of care. This process is in line with the American Nurses Association's *Scope and Standards of Home Health Nursing*. The nurse is responsible for the coordination of system and community resources that enhance delivery of care across the health care continuum [1].

The physical, occupational, or speech therapist receives an initial report from the home health nurse or, if only therapy services are ordered, receives information from the referring agent. A therapy evaluation/assessment is completed and a plan of care is developed with approval from the physician. The therapist will provide reports to other home health staff to promote consistency and collaboration in the plan of care. Each will work with the medical social worker (MSW) to obtain community resources as needed and available. Ongoing reports of changes in care plan and progress should be reported during case conference and as needed. When the patient has completed therapy services, the therapist will complete a discharge/transfer summary.

The MSW will receive an initial report from the home health nurse or therapist and then will complete a social work evaluation/assessment. It is important to note that the social worker should be involved only if psychosocial issues are interfering with the plan of care. Examples include when a patient cannot afford their medication or their depression interferes with the home exercise program. The MSW will facilitate the acquisition of community resources as needed and available and provide ongoing reports of changes in the care plan as well as progress to the home health team. Upon discharge, the MSW will complete a discharge/transfer summary.

The role of the home care coordinator is unique at each agency; however, it has evolved over the years. As previously noted, the HCC is responsible for making the transition from the hospital to home care as seamless as possible. In today's busy acute care environment, it is often the coordinator who provides home health nurses with the most up-to-date progress and orders from the acute care setting.

All providers will need to be sure that guidelines are followed when using home care coordinators in the acute care setting. Medicare has very specific guidelines on the requirements for hospital discharge planning services. Home care providers cannot provide this service in place of the hospital; however, once the referral is made, the HCC may participate in all aspects of the hospital to home care transition process.

Home care coordinators may also assist the agency and the home health nurses in the start of the care (admission) process. The Home Health COP 484.10 states that the agency must provide the patient with a written notice of their rights before the beginning of care or treatment. This allows the HCC to begin consent, education, and documentation processes while the patient is still in the hospital. Frequently this better informs the patient of what to expect from home care while reducing the time of the initial visit.

Telehealth, though slow to catch on in the home care community, has taken off in recent years and now is seen as a pivotal part of home care today. The benefits, cost savings, and improvement in quality of life have been documented in the literature. Today's high tech environment will impact the transition and communication processes in many ways. More doctors are using smart phones, electronic medical records, web cams, and other devices to keep in touch with their patients and other health care providers.

Managed care organizations are using the Internet as a tool to educate their patients. They offer classes on nutrition, weight loss, exercise, disease management, etc., in an effort to keep the patient knowledgeable and in charge of his condition while reducing overall health care costs.

A variety of monitors are used by physicians, HMOs, home health, while others are bringing wireless care into the home. Some of these services include: sensors for patient location or for falls, peak flow meter readings for asthma sufferers, medication compliance devices that alarms caregivers of medication errors or mismanagement, wireless scales, BP monitors, thermometers, oximetry, and others.

Home care has always been about taking care of people where they preferred to be cared for—at home. While cost savings and outcomes are validated, the time has come to recognize home care as a pivotal part of the transition process and health care continuum. As acute care dollars continue to shrink, home care will be viewed and appreciated as the better alternative. As this outpatient service grows, providers must ensure that the transition process continues to improve so that all patients and providers can work together to get the best outcomes possible.

REFERENCES & RESOURCES

[1] American Nurses Association, *Home Health Nursing: Scope and Standards of Practice*, Nursesbooks, 2008.

[2] P. Anderson and D. Mignor, *Home Care Nursing: Using an Accreditation Approach*, Thomson Delmar Learning Corporation, 2008.

[3] Center for Medicare Advocacy, Inc., "Discharge Planning," Retrieved from: http://www.medicareadvocacy.org/Print/FAQ_DischargePlanning.htm, 2010.

[4] Department of Health and Human Services, "Home Health Conditions of Participation," Retrieved from: http://edocket.access.gpo.gov/cfr_2005/octqtr/42cfr484.1.htm, 2005.

[5] A. Kinsella, "Telehealth and remote monitoring focus on target health management," *Remington Report*, 4(18):16–18, 2010.

[6] L. Landro, "Keeping Patients from Landing Back in the Hospital," *The Wall Street Journal*, 2007, December 12. Retrieved from http://www.inqri.org/AbouSubL-1399.html

[7] T.M. Marrelli, *Handbook of Home Health Standards* (5th ed.), Mosby, 2008.

[8] National Alliance of Caregiving, "A Family Caregiver's Guide to Hospital Discharge Planning," (nd). Retrieved from: http://www.caregiving.org/pubs/brochures/DischargePlanner.pdf

[9] M. Naylor, "Transitional care: A critical dimension of the hone healthcare quality agenda," *Journal for Healthcare Quality*, 1(28):48–54, 2006.

[10] L. Remington, "Emerging technology is re-connecting healthcare," *Remington Report*, 2(18):4–6, 2010.

[11] L. Robinson, "CMS-funded care transitions health care quality improvement project cuts hospital readmission rate in coached population," *Remington Report*, 4(18):10–13, 2010.

[12] M.P. Silver, R.J. Ferry and C. Edmonds, "Causes of unplanned hospital admissions," *Home Healthcare Nurse*, 28(2):71–81, 2010.

[13] E. Surburg, "Home health to hospice: The case for a smooth transition," *Home Healthcare Nurse.*, 26(9):515–520, 2008.

The Home Visit

By Pamela Teenier, RN, BSN, MBA, CHCE, HCS-D, COS-C, and
Lelah R. Marzi, RN, MBA, BSN, COS-C, HCS-D

The home visit is a critical piece of any patient's recovery from or adaptation to a new or exacerbated disease. The home visit is frequently a transition between a hospital stay and independence, a means to identify the support needed to prevent a hospitalization or the help needed for a patient to remain in his home. A home visit can be broken into three sections:

- The **pre-visit**, which includes a review of patient information, determining a plan, and making the initial phone call to the patient
- The **home visit**, which includes all of the activities that will need to be completed while in the patient's home and involves 8 steps
- The **post-visit**, which includes communicating with other members of the home care interdisciplinary team and completing documentation.

By following a logical process for home visits, the clinician can stay focused, stay in control of the interview, gather all the information necessary to complete the assessment, and formulate with the patient reasonable and attainable goals.

THE PRE-VISIT

The preparation for the home visit starts by reviewing available information regarding the patient. Home care begins with a referral. This

Clinical Case Studies in Home Health Care, First Edition. Edited by Leslie Neal-Boylan.
© 2011 John Wiley & Sons, Inc. Published 2011 by John Wiley & Sons, Inc.

may come from a hospital or physician's office. This referral should contain basic information about the patient including diagnosis, address, and date of birth. If the patient is being discharged from a facility, there might also be a history and physical, discharge summary, and medication list. The referral is accompanied by an order from the physician to initiate care. The order will delineate, often very briefly, what the nurse is expected to do for this particular patient. As the nurse prepares for the home visit, she/he should always review orders for the patient. It is critical that orders be followed exactly as written. Each state has a survey process that will verify that each clinician has followed all orders received from the physician.

If the patient is already established in home care and has been receiving care from professionals in other health care disciplines, then the nurse who is coming in on the case should review existing orders and discuss the patient with the other clinicians who have already been seeing the patient. This initial review will give the nurse a picture of the patient and allow a plan for nursing visits to be developed. The plan for this initial visit may be simply to assess and admit the patient to home care. For existing patients, it is important to provide care that is coordinated with that provided by the other clinicians who are already on the case.

Based on this plan, the nurse is able to gather needed supplies and forms for ordered treatments such as wound care, infusion therapy, or catheter changes. The last step in the pre-visit is to contact the patient to schedule the visit; however, this is not the only purpose of the initial contact. This is the first opportunity to gather assessment data from the patient. It tells the nurse whether the patient is able to manage the phone in a case of emergency. What is their cognitive status? Can he provide directions? The nurse might also give them a task. For example, on the initial visit the nurse will want to examine all of the medications the patient is taking. The nurse should ask the patient to have all of their medications (over the counter and prescription) available to review together. This contact allows the nurse to start the patient-nurse relationship with a positive rapport and to improve the patient's overall home care experience.

THE HOME VISIT

The actual time spent in the patient's home can be broken into eight steps. Following this process will make the visit organized and focused. Just as nurses are trained to follow a logical head-to-toe process when performing a physical exam, it is important to follow a logical and consistent process for the home visit. These steps may be adapted as warranted by a particular patient's needs. However, it is highly recommended that a process be followed whenever possible.

Step One: Introduction

The nurse's first visit should begin with introductions. It is very important to remember that home visiting clinicians are guests in the patient's home. Following the introductions, the nurse should sit with the patient (and possibly the caregiver and/or family) to review the referral and history information. This review of information that is already familiar to the nurse will allow the nurse to convey to the patient that the nurse is prepared for the visit.

After this brief review, it is helpful to sit back and get the patient's story. Ask the patient what happened to result in this admission to home care. While listening and observing the patient; assess the home environment; the patient's general appearance; and the status of the patient's speech, hearing, and cognition. Other important information about the patient's history and condition may be revealed during this discussion which can be very useful when developing the Plan of Care (POC). The POC includes and augments the complete orders from the physician. A particular format is used that all home care agencies follow. For instance, a patient may say that he fell in the hospital. This may not be in the records from the hospital, but it is still very important to know so that a POC can be developed that includes reducing the risk of injury from falling. Throughout the visit, the nurse should make observations of the home to assess for safety and for the availability of needed resources. This assessment should continue throughout the visit as the nurse gains more information about the patient and evaluates his living environment.

In home care, one must always consider the safety of the patient's environment as it relates to the condition of the individual patient. Homes are as varied as the people who live in them. These are "non-controlled" environments as compared to the controlled environments of hospitals. Be prepared to politely suggest and instruct the patient to alter their home if it is necessary to maximize their safety. An example of this would be asking a patient to remove loose throw rugs to reduce the risk of falling.

As the introduction comes to a close, ask the patient targeted questions to find out what has happened since the last visit (if there have been any previous visits). For example, one might ask if there have been any doctor visits. Has the patient been taking their medications? Have there been any medication changes? Has he had any falls? This will formulate a background picture of the patient and allow the nurse to outline for the patient what the nurse will be focusing on during this visit.

Step Two: Assessment

With the introductions complete, the nurse moves to the assessment of the patient. Although one should always perform complete assessments during all visits, the initial visit is much more comprehensive than the others typically are as it will be the basis of the POC, which may also include other disciplines. In many cases, it will also determine the agency's reimbursement for services.

Always ask the patient for permission before proceeding with this step. "Do you mind if I check your blood pressure and do a physical exam?" The level of detail for each system will depend on the diagnoses. The clinician's judgment is required to identify and to document issues that must be addressed in the POC. Gather subjective and objective information that include the following:

Subjective: Perform a review of systems by asking the patient if he is currently having any problems with any of the following systems. Consult with a good textbook on history and physical examination regarding targeted questions to ask and appropriate physical examination techniques.

HEENT: Headache, scalp lesions, alopecia, visual changes, hearing loss or tinnitus, epistaxis, rhinorrhea, throat pain, dysphagia

Skin: Lesions, rashes, ulcers

Cardiac: Chest pain, palpitations

Pulmonary: Dyspnea, dyspnea on exertion, coughing, wheezing, pain with breathing

Abdomen: Pain, bowel or bladder difficulties, blood in stool or urine, dysuria, dyspareunia, changes in color or odor of stool or urine, changes in ability to control bowel or bladder

Vascular: Extremity pain or swelling, varicosities, history of blood clots

Musculoskeletal: Pain; fractures; osteoporosis; osteopenia; intake of calcium and vitamin D; difficulty moving, walking, ambulating, performing activities of daily living (ADL) or instrumental activities of daily living (IADL)

Neurological/Psychosocial: Confusion, change in mentation, depression, anxiety, suicidal ideation, change in balance or sensation

General: Ask the patient about his nutritional status and ability to meet transportation, housekeeping, and shopping needs. What support systems are in place?

Objective:

Vital Signs

Weight/Height

Pulse oximetry if available

HEENT:

Head: Palpate scalp and hair. Evaluate cranial nerves and check for temporal artery dilatation.

Eyes: Check eyes for PERRLA and to see if EOMs are intact.

Ears: Examine ears if possible.

Mouth and Throat: Look in mouth at dentition and look for masses under the tongue. Check for ulcers. Check for redness or exudates.

Neck: Check for carotid pulses and bruits. Check for thyroid enlargement and lymphadenopathy.

Skin: Check for tenderness and edema. Check for lesions, bruising, ulcers or rashes. Assess turgor and elasticity of recoil.

Cardiac: Listen to heart and check rate and rhythm. Evaluate whether there are murmurs, clicks, gallops or rubs.

Pulmonary: Listen to lungs and check for adventitious sounds.

Musculoskeletal/Neurological: Evaluate mental status. Assess joint function (mobility, fluidity of movement, range of motion and strength), hand grasp, ability to perform the TUG test. Observe gait if possible. Check to see if wheelchair or other assistive device is properly fit and comfortable for the patient.

Abdomen: Check for bruits, bowel sounds, and organomegaly.

As previously mentioned, the environment and support structure that may influence that patient's ability to become safe and independent in his home must also be assessed in home health care. Considering that the ultimate goal is independence and safe functionality of the patient within his family/caregiver unit, one must take into consideration all aspects of the home. This will include obtaining information from family members or caregivers who may be present and assessing the interpersonal dynamics, availability, ability, and willingness of the caregivers.

Part of the initial assessment process includes a review of the medications that the patient is supposed to be taking. These medications include any orals, injectable, inhalants, drops, ointments, oxygen, vitamins/herbals, transdermals, flushes, enterals, and parenterals.

Verify that the medications match any lists provided by the hospital or by the physician's office. Check the expiration dates. Suggest putting away or separating medications not currently prescribed but kept by the patient. Asking the patient to read the labels of the medication containers is an ideal way to assess his vision. Does he require glasses or a magnifying glass to see print? If so, check to see if he can see how many fingers are raised at an arm's length from his face. This is very important to know, as a patient who has serious visual compromise is certainly at a higher risk for falls and other injuries. This data will be included in the POC, if appropriate.

Risks associated with polypharmacy require assessment as part of an evaluation of the safety of the patient. Assess the patient's knowledge and ability to independently handle his medications. What level of assistance is needed for him to be safe? Does he require another person to safely access and administer any of his medications? Does he require the use of a device to access or open the bottles? Does he know what each medicine is for? Ask if he ever has any negative side effects with any of his medications.

During the initial visit a Medication Profile will be completed. At each follow-up visit, it will be updated based on information communicated by the patient. Medication management is frequently included in the home health POC; thus it is critical to always have an up-to-date list.

Step Three: Hands-On Care

In home care, as with other settings, nursing care is delivered based on physician orders. After the initial visit these orders are developed in communication with the physician. Frequently, the initial referral orders will contain a specific order for treatments and procedures. These procedures might include injections, wound care or catheter changes.

Hands-on care includes any assessment or treatment. Examples are checking vital signs, doing transfer or gait teaching, wound care, catheter care or insertion, administration of injectable medications, performing ostomy care instruction or diabetic foot care instruction. Always ask the patient's permission before proceeding with any hands-on intervention, and remember to always explain beforehand what will be done. During each step of the procedure, it is helpful to inform the patient and caregiver of what is being done and why it is being done, especially if they will be learning how to perform the procedure independently. While one should never coerce a patient or caregiver to perform a skilled procedure, many may feel more comfortable and confident to learn if they know each time what the steps are and how each step is done.

Step Four: Instruction

One service provided by home care nurses is the teaching of patients and their family and other caregivers. Clinicians must be knowledgeable on disease process, medications, diet, pain management, and skilled procedures. As teaching is completed, the clinician must also continue to assess the patient's understanding. Many home care patients are seniors. Some older adults do not learn at the same pace as younger patients. If they have to integrate changes into their day-to-day lives, it may take additional time for them to adjust comfortably to the changes. One needs patience to allow each patient to learn at his own pace with continual assessment of his understanding.

Consider that in home care, as in other environments, patients will have different learning styles. Some may be visual learners, others may be auditory learners, and still others may be primarily kinetic learners. In addition, the "student" may be a family member who is older or impaired in some way. Being flexible with teaching styles is imperative in home care.

Many home care agencies offer a wealth of patient teaching materials, written in layman's terms and with illustrations and diagrams, which are valuable resources during this step. If the agency allows it, make two copies of any teaching material, have the patient "sign off" on the copy, and return the copy to the patient's office record. This will represent and augment documentation of that teaching.

Step Five: Evaluation

Once treatments and teaching are complete, the patient's response to the care provided should be evaluated. Did the dressing change increase the patient's pain? Are they tolerating the infusion well? Are they having any reactions to any of the procedures? This step also includes the patient's response to any teaching that was done, including the teaching format—verbal, written, demonstrative. The family response to teaching is also important to note. Is there progress toward patient goals as predicted, or do we need to alter our teaching methods? Does another caregiver need instruction? Do treatments need to be altered? All of these are possible scenarios at this point in the process.

Step Six: Goal Progression

When documenting this information, reference should be made to the goals that were established at the time of admission. Specific terms and stages should identify the progress and show planning towards discharge. Discharge planning starts at admission and occurs throughout a patient's admission. It does not occur on the visit made just prior to the discharge. Establishing goals in home care is really an exercise in negotiation, for the nurse must be able to understand what the patient's personal goals are, as well as what the physician-driven goals are. An example of this is when the nurse may write that the goal is for the patient's knee to reach 120 degrees of flexion. The patient's goal may be expressed as "I just want to be able to go to my grandson's wedding in two months and walk down the aisle." Patient-centered goals should be documented clearly in the assessment of the patient. If the patient is not a "partner" in this effort, then the outcome will definitely reflect it!

Step Seven: Care Coordination

Throughout the visit, the nurse will need to coordinate care with others. Care coordination is a requirement of many state regulations, as well as several certifying bodies such as the Joint Commission on the Accreditation of Healthcare Organizations (JCAHO) and Medicare. Care coordination, or lack thereof, is frequently cited in state surveys.

This communication regarding the patient may be with internal providers, such as members of the home care team; or it may be with external providers such as Durable Medical Equipment (DME) suppliers or community resource providers. With this communication, the nurse may identify and relate changes in the patient's condition, relate supervision of team members such as Licensed Practical Nurses (LPNs), or relate identified educational needs of the patient that may be better addressed by another team member. The nurse may also be communicating discharge planning information to other members.

Step Eight: Concluding the Visit

At this point the nurse will want to discuss the plans for the next visit. The patient and/or caregivers should be involved in all aspects of his care, and concluding the visit is no exception.

At this point in the visit, the nurse may wish to review with the patient and family what was accomplished during today's visit, remembering to emphasize his progress toward patient-centered and physician-ordered goals. This should be specific to what the nurse is teaching the patient or what the patient is demonstrating. Make sure the patient has understood any instructions; and provide homework assignments, things for the patient to complete between visits, such as reading food labels, weighing himself or testing blood glucose. Ensure that there is no unfinished business, and agree on a date and goals for the next visit. Many agencies may require that the patient sign a document as evidence of the visit. This is a requirement of many payers, including Medicare, and may be accomplished during this step.

POST-VISIT

After each visit is complete, there frequently are still several tasks to be completed. During the visit, care coordination was performed, and it will continue after leaving the patient's home. Depending on staffing patterns, there may be more than one nurse to see the patient. However, only one nurse can visit per day unless multiple visits are ordered by the physician. Communication between nurses is a must. Additionally, in home care today, frequently more than one discipline is providing care to a patient. When there is a change in the patient, either an improvement or a decline, this information must be shared with all of the clinicians providing care. For example, if the nurse notices something in the assessment that might have an impact on the physical therapist's (PT's) ability to complete the exercise program with the patient, it must be communicated. Any change in the patient's condition also must be reported to the physician. Changes may need to be made to the POC. Only a physician can give verbal orders and sign orders, although legislation is imminent to allow NPs to give orders.

Documentation in home care is different from documentation in a hospital. The hospital will bill based on days present, tests performed, and medications administered. Home care is reimbursed based on the documentation of the clinicians. Each time one visits a patient; documentation must include the details of the encounter, the progress and any coordination needs that reflect the services provided to the patient. This documentation will occur during the visit and might need to be completed after the coordination is complete. See Chapter 2 for more information regarding reimbursement practices, home care scope and standards, and care coordination.

 ## REFERENCES & RESOURCES

[1] M.D. Harris, *Handbook of Home Health Care Administration* (5th ed.), Jones & Bartlett, 2009.
[2] I.M. Martinson, A.G. Widmer and C.J. Portillo, *Home Health Care Nursing* (2nd ed.), Saunders, 2002.
[3] K.J. Morgan and S.L. McClain, *Core Curriculum for Home Health Care Nursing*, Aspen, 1993.
[4] R. Rice, *Home Care Nursing Practice: Concepts and Application* (4th ed.), Mosby, 2006.

Section 2

Cardiac

Case 2.1 Congestive Heart Failure

By Jeanie Stoker, MPA, RN, BC

This case study illustrates how the home health nurse and several other disciplines works with a younger patient (pre-Medicare) to improve her quality of life and develop mutually agreeable goals. Ms. M is considered a "frequent flyer" at the local community hospital as she is admitted every 2–3 months for an exacerbation of congestive heart failure (CHF) or chronic obstructive pulmonary disease (COPD), including complete respiratory failure requiring intubation 2 years ago. At only 48 years of age she deals with chronic health conditions as well as a multi-generational home environment. There are numerous relatives in the home, along with several dogs and cats. While the individual relationships are unclear, her daughter-in-law states that she is Mrs. M's caregiver. Ms. M is friendly and appears eager to learn and participate in her plan of care. She would like to improve her overall quality of life and wants to be out and about more.

Reimbursement Considerations

The patient is too young to be eligible for Medicare but currently has Medicaid. Her prescriptions are covered by Medicaid, but the state only allows 5 prescriptions per month. The MSW will work with the pharmacist and Free Clinic to seek means to cover more of her prescriptions.

Clinical Case Studies in Home Health Care, First Edition. Edited by Leslie Neal-Boylan.
© 2011 John Wiley & Sons, Inc. Published 2011 by John Wiley & Sons, Inc.

ORDERS FOR HOME CARE

Patient: 48-year-old white female
Diagnoses: Congestive heart failure, respiratory failure, COPD, hypertension, atrial fibrillation, osteoarthritis, sleep apnea, obesity
Current medications:
- Acetaminophen 500 mg 1–2 tabs every 4–6 hours as needed for pain, fever
- Advair Diskus 250 mcg—1 inhalation twice a day
- Cimetidine 200 mg once a day
- Digoxin 250 mcg once a day
- Enalapril Maleate 10 mg once a day
- Furosemide 40 mg once a day
- Oxygen 2 L continuously
- Spironolactone 25 mg twice a day
- Warfarin Sodium 5 mg once a day
- Oxygen @ 2 L per nasal cannula continuously

Relevant past medical history:
- Hypertension controlled with medication
- COPD requiring medication and oxygen
- Sleep apnea: Had a BiPAP but the dog broke it

RN: Skilled observation and assessment
PT: While not originally ordered, after assessment, order was given to "evaluate and determine plan of care (POC)."
MSW: Assess social factors that adversely impact the POC.

THE HOME VISIT

After scheduling the visit to meet the caregiver's time frame, the nurse enters the home, which is a small, two- story house. The home is clean, cluttered, but with clear pathways; and numerous dogs and cats run freely throughout. The daughter-in-law (DIL) greets the nurse and

---

Cultural Competence

Ms. M is a middle-aged, white female who is dependent on others to help with her needs as well as her daughter's. Her cultural challenge will be obesity and the stigma attached to it in America. The team will assist her in focusing on her weight-loss goals and seek outside support for this initiative. They will also need to provide encouragement and reinforcement at every opportunity.

shows her to a living room where the patient is sitting in a large recliner. A bedside commode is in the corner. The nurse notes that Ms. M appears older than her noted age of 48 and is very slow to stand and greet her. Numerous family members are around and are quick to greet the nurse and offer her a place to sit. The family appears very supportive and eager to help Ms. M. They listen very attentively to the nurse's questions and directions.

The nurse works with Ms. M to establish the following goals:

- Ms. M becomes short of breath (SOB) with minimal exertion. She would like to be able to climb her stairs and not to be so SOB at the top.
- "To stay out of the hospital"
  - Patient will be compliant with daily weights.
  - Patient will verbalize 3 signs and symptoms of cardiac distress.
  - Patient will verbalize 3 signs and symptoms of respiratory distress.
  - Patient will verbalize ways to reduce edema.
  - Patient will recall at least 3 foods high in sodium.
  - Patient will verbalize the relationship between sodium intake and edema.
- Ms. M will be able to take all her medications as ordered, including being able to afford them.
- Patient will verbalize purpose, action, and dose of each medication.
- Ms. M will lose weight so she can do more with her family.

Neal Theory Implications

Stage 3: The nurse completes the assessment of the patient and home and sees the need for multidisciplinary intervention. She knows that a physical therapist referral has been made, but she quickly sees the benefit of requesting occupational therapy and respiratory therapy services. While PT and OT are routine services provided in home health, this experienced nurse recognizes that an RT will provide additional support for sleep and oxygen issues. She has the knowledge to realize that the BiPAP is critical to overall improvement of CHF and needs the RT to support her teaching and thus improve compliance. The RT will also focus on O^2 safety in the home. She develops a plan of care that will focus on medication understanding as well as on early exacerbation recognition. She will ask the physician for "as needed" orders for increased edema and weight gain. Although not initially ordered, she will ask for the CHF protocol, too.

(Continued)

Stage 2: The nurse completes the assessment but will leave feeling overwhelmed by the many caregivers and issues. She will work with the PT as the referral has been made but may not see the benefit of the OT. While she has a basic understanding of regulations, she may not be aware that other disciplines can and should work collaboratively on the plan of care. She will call the Durable Medical Equipment company and report the problems but may not ask for an RT visit to coincide with the nurse's visit. As the case progresses and other services are recommended to her, she will call the physician to ask for those orders.

Stage 1: The clinician in this stage will assess the patient and recognize the need for assistance with the case. The age of the patient may surprise her as many new home health nurses are not much younger than this very sick patient. She may feel overwhelmed and unsure of what needs to be done first. Many nurses are not aware of how to develop a care plan for sleep apnea or the impact on the patient's health. She will need much assistance in developing this plan of care as well as education on sleep apnea. While she may be able to complete the CHF POC, additional issues and resources will also need to be addressed. The preceptor or supervisor will need to guide this nurse in the appropriate care and safety issues related to the care of Ms. M.

Based on the history and physical examination, the nurse discovers the following data:

- Ms. M states that her legs hurt every day but not all the time. She describes the pain as "fire" that is relieved with medications and rest.
- She has 2+ pitting edema in both lower extremities.
- A pedal pulse could not be palpated in either foot.
- Ms. M has diminished breaths sounds bilaterally, but no rales, rhonchi, or wheezing.
- Ms. M is currently on oxygen 2 L per nasal cannula.
- Ms. M becomes dyspneic with minimal exertion and states that the nurse has tired her out with this visit.
- She complains of occasional urinary stress incontinence. She uses a bedside commode in the living room as the bathroom is upstairs and she does not feel she can make it that far every time she has to urinate. She goes upstairs to have a bowel movement and is able to do this without difficulty, but she is very tired when she is done.

- Ms. M can perform her activities of daily living (ADL) with minimal assistance but is unable to get in a bath or shower. She bathes herself in the chair or on the toilet.
- While Ms. M denies any depression, she shares that she is anxious about her current health. "I am too young to be this fat and sick."

Relevant Community Resources

Free prescription programs
Free clinic
Home medical equipment (HME) (Durable Medical Equipment)
Pharmacy
Weight Watchers or similar program

? **CRITICAL THINKING**

1. What is the priority for care for Ms. M?
Answer: The priority for care for this patient is disease management, as well as weight control. She is very eager to improve her overall health status but will need a great deal of instruction, oversight, and support to balance her physical symptoms with the need to lose weight. The nurse sees a need for physical therapy for strength training and possibly the development of a home exercise program. While the nurse has already received an order for the MSW, she plans to request a dietician to provide additional nutritional education.

2. What safety issues need to be considered?
Answer: Ms. M is on oxygen, which has obvious fire hazards. The nurse noted when looking around the room that there were ashtrays with extinguished cigarettes in them. She immediately educates the patient and family of the fire hazard and the urgent need to have all smoking taken outside. She also quizzes Ms. M about her back-up oxygen cylinders and discovers that they are in a small cramped closet. She educates everyone about the proper storage of oxygen cylinders; they should be flat and in an area that is well ventilated. They agree to put them under a bed for now. The nurse encourages the family to obtain smoke detectors and a fire extinguisher.

3. What needs should to be addressed by the MSW?
Answer: Social services should become involved when real or potential social issues interfere with the plan of care. The nurse identified several factors. There is a concern that community resources are needed to

assist with medications and that another BiPAP is needed. While Ms. M denies depression, the nurse is concerned about her coping abilities. The MSW can assess and intervene as poor coping skills could have a great effect on Ms. M's ability to reach her goals. The social worker may also be able to assist with weight loss support programs.

4. What will the physical therapist (PT) do to support the goals for Ms. M?
Answer: The PT will do an assessment to determine Ms. M's needs and goals for therapy. The PT will also assess the home environment and develop a plan to improve ambulation and strength. As disease management and weight loss goals go hand in hand, the therapist will also establish a home exercise program that the patient can do on her own. This will need to be monitored and progress charted to ensure that there is a balance between dyspnea and exercising. Due to Ms. M respiratory status, the PT will also need to complete an O^2 saturation level prior to and at the end of each exercise program. Any abnormalities will need to be reported to the doctor and care may be altered for that visit.

5. Is there anyone else who should be called into this case?
Answer: Yes. The nurse should call the physician for orders for an occupational therapist (OT), a dietician, and respiratory therapist (RT).

6. What will each of these disciplines do?
Answer: The OT will reinforce the teaching and interventions of the nurse and the PT as they all collaborate to meet the patient's goals. Additionally, the OT will teach Ms M. energy conserving methods to improve her ability to complete ADL and improve her overall independence.

A dietician is not always part of the home care team as it is usually not recognized as a required or reimbursable visit. As agencies continue to strive for better outcomes, other disciplines such as a dietician will be able to strengthen the knowledge and skills in the interdisciplinary team. A dietician would serve well on this case as the patient needs to learn the details of a 2 gram sodium diet while focusing on weight reduction. Multiple medication interactions and side effects will also be considered by the dietician as she develops the optimal dietary plan. This plan then can be reinforced by other members of the team.

A respiratory therapist (RT) would also be a valued team member to work with Ms. M. The nurse has already noted issues with oxygen safety and BiPAP noncompliance. The RT will assess the cardiac and respiratory status and oxygen utilization and report findings to the physician and other health care providers. The RT may be able to seek other solutions to help the patient meet her oxygen requirements as well as sleep apnea needs.

Rehabilitation Needs

Physical therapy
Occupational therapy
Respiratory therapy

 BACK TO THE CASE

The nurse reviews the finalized goals and recommendations for other disciplines. The patient is hopeful and demonstrates a deep desire to follow the plan of care. Others in the home are eager to help, and two family members offer to learn the exercise program so that they can all "get healthier together." Everyone agrees that all smoking will now occur outside. The physician is called and provided a report as well as a request for an RD and RT. She agrees to the plan and orders the additional disciplines. The pulmonary specialist is called to request a new BiPAP. The physician says he will provide the new prescription only after seeing the patient as it has been a while since she has been to his office. The patient agrees to set this appointment up soon.

? **CRITICAL THINKING**

1. How will the members of the interdisciplinary team communicate with one another?
Answer: The team has become larger, and some members are outside the home health office walls. The hospital RD and the RT each agree to provide a written report each month and attend case conferences. Any changes in the condition or plan of care will be communicated by the primary nurse.

Interdisciplinary Care Plan

Problem	Plan	Interventions	Evaluation
Knowledge deficit regarding disease process, CHF symptoms	Patient will verbalize understanding of symptoms of CHF and respiratory distress in one week.	Teach patient about specific signs and symptoms including weakness, weight gain SOB, and edema.	Patient will participate in self-care management and be able to recall symptoms.

(Continued)

Problem	Plan	Interventions	Evaluation
Knowledge deficit regarding disease process, CHF symptom management, and interventions	By 3 weeks, the patient will verbalize 3 examples of when to call the home health agency or physician.	Teach patient about specific signs and symptoms, 2+ lbs weight gain, increased SOB, increased swelling in ankles or abdomen.	Patient and/or family will call agency if any symptoms occur.
Fluid volume excess	Within 24 hours, patient will be able to recall correct medication regime if there is a 2 lb wt gain.	Teach patient to weigh each day with same clothes and an empty bladder. Teach medication regime.	Patient will obtain a set of scales, weigh each morning, and record it in the weight log.
Knowledge deficit: Sodium influence in CHF	Within one week, patient and caregiver (CG) will be able to verbalize relationship between sodium intake and edema.	Teach patient and CG about high sodium foods and physiological response.	Patient will be able to recall diet and its impact if edema increases.
Knowledge deficit; low calorie diet	Within 2 weeks, patient and CG will be able to plan and prepare a balanced low calorie meal.	Teach patient and CG about healthy food choices, food pyramid, and healthy low cost food items.	Patient will lose 1–2 lbs per week not related to fluid changes.
Cardiac output decreased	Within 4 weeks, patient will be able to ambulate greater distances and walk up the stairs without SOB. Within 24 hours, patient will use O^2 as ordered	PT will provide strengthening exercises. Nurse will teach about energy conserving activities. RT will educate and assist with O^2 support	Patient will be able to ambulate up the stairs to complete toileting and ADL needs independently.
Altered mobility	Within 4 weeks, patient will be able to ambulate up the stairs.	PT will provide strengthening exercises and a home exercise program.	Patient will be able to ambulate up stairs with minimal exertion.
Knowledge deficit: Sleep apnea	Within 1 week, patient will schedule and see pulmonary physician. Patient will verbalize importance of utilization of BiPAP	Nurse will assess compliance and teach possible outcomes of non-compliance.	Patient will understand the risk associated with non-use of BiPAP and will comply.

REFERENCES & RESOURCES

[1] American Nurses Association, *Home Health Nursing: Scope and Standards of Practice*, Nursebooks, 2008.

[2] P. Anderson and D. Mignor, *Home Care Nursing: Using an Accreditation Approach*, Thomson Delmar Learning Corporation, 2008.

[3] T.M. Marrelli, *Handbook of Home Health Standards* (5th ed.), Mosby, 2009.

[4] Agency for Healthcare Quality and Research, "Taking Care of Myself: A Guide When I Leave the Hospital," Retrieved from http://www.ahrq.gov/qual/goinghomeguide.htm, 2010.

Case 2.2 Atrial Fibrillation

By Jeanie Stoker, MPA, RN, BC

This case study illustrates how the home health nurse works with the patient and spouse to develop goals for chronic care and declining health. While the nurse estimates a life expectancy of less than 6 months, the patient and wife are not ready to discuss end-of-life needs. Mr. G is admitted to home health after recurring admissions to the hospital for congestive heart failure (CHF) and atrial fibrillation requiring a pacemaker during this most recent hospitalization. He is also managing Diabetes Type 2 with oral medication. While Mr. G has required minimal assistance in doing the things that are important to him, he is now dealing with new limitations. He and his wife feel very comfortable in managing his needs and living independently of additional family support.

Reimbursement Considerations

The patient has Medicare and meets all qualifications for Medicare home health. In addition, he has a Blue Cross/Blue Shield supplemental policy. The HomMed monitor is provided at no cost to Medicare or the patient.

Clinical Case Studies in Home Health Care, First Edition. Edited by Leslie Neal-Boylan.
© 2011 John Wiley & Sons, Inc. Published 2011 by John Wiley & Sons, Inc.

ORDERS FOR HOME CARE

Patient: 87-year-old Caucasian male

Diagnoses: Congestive heart failure, atrial fibrillation, hypertension, type 2 diabetes, abnormality of gait

Current medications:
- Omeprazole 20 mg once a day
- Levothroid 100 mcg once a day
- Digoxin 125 mcg, ½ tablet once a day
- Spironolactone 25 mg twice a day
- Crestor 10 mg once a day
- Cozaar 50 mg, ½ tablet twice a day
- Ferrous Sulfate 325 mg once a day
- Combivent 2 puffs every 4–6 hours as needed for SOB or wheezing

Relevant past medical history:
- Hypertension controlled with medication
- Iron deficiency anemia
- Esophageal reflux

RN: Skilled observation and assessment

PT: While not originally ordered, after assessment an order was given to "evaluate and determine plan of care (POC)."

 THE HOME VISIT

The nurse initiates home care services and visits Mr. and Mrs. G in their single level home. The home is clean, uncluttered, and well organized as Mrs. G assumes the role of head of house and primary nurse for her husband. Mr. G is sitting in a recliner with his legs elevated but slowly gets up to greet the nurse warmly. He states he is very happy to be home and appreciates the nurse being able to help keep him there.

As the primary provider, his wife takes his health care needs very seriously. She shows the nurse a diabetic cookbook and demonstrates her knowledge of a low sodium diet by pointing out in the refrigerator the foods she has bought for him.

When the nurse reviews routine home safety instructions, including fall prevention and infection control, the patient and wife seem very aware of measures to keep the home safe. Hand hygiene and clear pathways are observed by the nurse.

Mr. G is concerned about his condition; and he verbalizes to the nurse that, though fluid was drained from his abdomen, his stomach remains large. He is tired of going in and out of the hospital and is eager to work with the home health staff to prevent or reduce the frequencies of admission.

Cultural Competence

Ms. G is an elderly Caucasian male who is newly dependent on his wife for personal and medical needs. His cultural challenge will be giving up the head-of-household role and allowing his wife to direct him with medications, MD orders, and basic needs. The team will assist him to focus on what he can do and the success he obtains when the agreed upon goals are met. There will also need to be a focus on the couple as a team, successfully working together to achieve goals!

Along with his wife, he reviews with the nurse his expectations; and they all agree on the following goals:

Goals

- Patient and caregiver verbalize understanding of 2 GM NA, low carbohydrate diet.
- Patient and caregiver verbalize purpose, action, and dose of each medication instructed on.
- Patient and caregiver verbalize and provide a return demonstration on the HomMed monitor.
- Patient and caregiver will be compliant with daily monitoring and daily weights.
- Patient and caregiver verbalize an understanding of safety and emergency plan.
- Patient and caregiver verbalize an understanding of actions to prevent falls.
- Patient and caregiver verbalize 3 signs and symptoms of cardiac distress.
- Patient and caregiver verbalize 3 symptoms of Digoxin toxicity.
- Patient and caregiver verbalize 3 signs and symptoms of respiratory distress.
- Patient and caregiver verbalize ways to reduce edema.
- Patient and caregiver recall at least 3 foods high in sodium.
- Patient and caregiver verbalize the relationship between sodium intake and edema.
- Patient and caregiver verbalize understanding of signs and symptoms of hyponatremia and hypernatremia.
- Patient and caregiver will monitor blood glucose levels daily.
- Patient and caregiver verbalize 3 signs and symptoms of hyperglycemia and hypoglycemia.

Neal Theory Implications

Stage 3: The nurse at this stage will be able to provide education and support for the chronic condition of CHF. She will need to focus on medication teaching and compliance while addressing symptom monitoring and management. She has attended the H2H conferences that her agency is involved in, and this has provided her with additional education on long term CHF management. She has learned that the 3 areas which lead to rehospitalization are (1) medication compliance, (2) symptom management, and (3) physician follow-up. She realizes that this is her focus of care and will spend most her time educating in these areas. She will also be proactive in assuring that follow-up appointments have been scheduled. She will collaborate with physical therapy to ensure that both are focused on the same outcomes. This nurse will follow up with the telehealth nurse to look for trends when regular visits are not scheduled. She will call the physician if she sees an indication to initiate the CHF protocol. As time progresses, she will also be able to bring up hospice care or palliative care as the opportunity presents itself.

Stage 2: The professional nurse at this level is able to complete the OASIS assessment independently and can identify needs and gaps. She will review the CHF plan of care and begin disease management and medication teaching. The telehealth nurse will inform her of any activities out of the prescribed range, but the stage 2 nurse may not be proactive enough to ask for this information. She will notify the physician of any symptoms and will follow orders as prescribed.

Stage 1: The novice will presume that this is an easy case and may develop some confidence in her home health skills. However, while basic assessment skills are needed, she will need to be proficient in the early signs of CHF exacerbation. If she is advised to follow the protocol, she will need specific direction and a mentor or supervisor to be with her during the first few events. At this time she may not understand the value of telehealth services and will need direction on this as well. She will not be as comfortable discussing end-of-life care and may ask the MSW to help with this. Support of a preceptor or supervisor will be needed in case managing Mr. G.

Based on the history and physical examination, the nurse discovers the following data:

- Mr. G has 3+ pitting edema in both ankles.
- Mr. G has SOB upon moderate exertion, walking less than 20 feet.

- Mr. G has lower extremity weakness and an unsteady gait.
- Mr. G has generalized weakness.
- Mr. G uses a cane to ambulate.
- Rales and wheezes are heard bilaterally, but there is no SOB at this time.
- Mr. G has intermittent reflux and heartburn.
- Mr. G has a healing wound on his right chest wall from the pacemaker insertion.
- Mr. G has diarrhea.
- Mr. G is continent of bowel and bladder.
- Mr. G has ascites with an abdominal girth of 40 inches (down 5 inches).
- Mr. G can provide for his toileting needs independently but his wife assists with bathing.
- Mr. G is on a 2 GM low sodium, low carbohydrate diet.
- Mr. G has no difficulties with speech or swallowing.
- Mr. G monitors his blood glucose independently before each meal.
- Mr. G sleeps well at night, getting 7–8 hours of sleep. He also takes a 30–60 minute nap during the day.
- Mr. G is alert and oriented. He does not appear to be anxious or depressed at this visit.

Rehabilitation Needs

Physical therapy

? CRITICAL THINKING

1. What is the priority for care for Mr. G?
Answer: The priority of Mr. G's care is to maximize his cardiac output. This will be done with care and recommendations made by both the nurses and therapist and as ordered by the physician. Medication management, cardiac conservation activities, early symptom recognition, and strengthening exercise will be priorities for him.

2. What will the nurses do to maximize the cardiac output?
Answer:
a. Cardiac and respiratory assessment at each visit
b. Medication assessment and reconciliation at each visit
c. Daily assessment via HomMed monitor, including BP, pulse, weight, O2 saturation, and questions
d. Educate patient on disease process, signs and symptom management including interventions, other conserving activities.

3. What will the physical therapist (PT) do?
Answer:

a. The PT will conduct a PT assessment to determine Mr. G's needs and goals for therapy.

b. A home assessment will include home safety and fall prevention review.

c. Mr. G will complete strengthening exercises.

d. The PT will develop a home exercise program that he and his wife can do when the therapist does not visit.

4. Are any other disciplines needed at this time?
Answer:

• A home health aide is offered but declined at this time.

• The nurse would like to request a social worker to begin discussion of end-of- life needs and planning. At this time neither Mr. nor Mrs. G are ready to discuss this; but both understand that a social worker is available to discuss coping strategies, health care surrogacy, and other similar needs, as well as long term care support.

 BACK TO THE CASE

The nurse completes the initial assessment and plans to follow up with the physical therapy referral. She offers home health aide services but both Mr. and Mrs. G decline at this time, opting for as much independence as possible. Both are hopeful that physical therapy will improve Mr. G's strength and that he will be able to resume full responsibility of all of his ADL.

The nurse also follows up with the primary care physician to request that this patient be placed on the "CHF protocol". The physician agrees and the protocol is established as follows:

• RN to provide "as needed" visits for cardiopulmonary assessment if set monitor parameters are out of range.

• If weight increases by 2 pounds and fluid retention is suspected, the patient and caregiver is to be instructed to double dose the loop diuretic for 48 hours.

• If weight returns to baseline, resume routine dose of loop diuretics.

• If the patient complains of nausea, vomiting, diarrhea, or other symptoms of dehydration and has a 2 pound or more weight loss, instruct him/her to hold the loop diuretic and call the home health nurse for an evaluation.

• If this does not work, use Zaroxolyn Protocol.
  Zaroxolyn Protocol (Patient must have Zaroxolyn in the home and a physician's order.)

○ If doubled dose of loop diuretic is not effective, instruct patient to take Zaroxolyn 2.5 mg by mouth x1 day 30 minutes prior to doubled diuretic dose, then 5 mg by mouth x1 day 30 minutes prior to doubled diuretic dose.

○ If weight continues to rise or fails to improve, instruct patient and caregiver to call the home health nurse.

• If this does not work use Lasix Protocol (after consulting with the physician).

IV Lasix Protocol

○ Start peripheral line and heparin lock as needed.

○ Draw basic metabolic panel before administering IV Lasix.

○ Give IV Lasix (4 mg/min) 40 mg x1. Give 80 mg of IV Lasix if oral dose of Lasix is more than 40 mg. Double IV Lasix dose after 1 hour if first dose of IV Lasix is not effective.

○ Notify physician if second dose of IV Lasix is not effective.

The protocol is discussed with the patient and wife, and both are eager to do whatever is needed to keep him at home. The patient also comments that the daily monitoring will allow him to have more control over his heart problems.

Relevant Community Resources

Future needs may include:

• An emergency response system such as Lifeline
• A social worker referral for long term needs
• Hospice

?   **CRITICAL THINKING**

1. How will daily monitoring be used to assess the patient and how will findings be communicated?

Answer: The telehealth nurse will download daily monitoring results. She will monitor trends and report any findings out of prescribed ranges to the primary nurse. She will also call the patient to complete a telephone assessment. If indicated, she will arrange for a prn visit to address advancing symptoms. The physician will be notified of any change in the patient's condition and the need for additional intervention.

2. How will the physical therapy team be aware of the patient's cardiac status prior to physical activity?

Answer: The therapist will complete a vital sign assessment as well as O2 Sat before beginning a therapy program at each visit. If the patient has any exacerbated symptoms or abnormal vitals signs, the physician and primary nurse will be notified for further intervention as indicated.

3. How will the members of the interdisciplinary team communicate with one another?
Answer: Team members will communicate by phone and arrange to hold a monthly case conference that includes the patient by phone or in person.

4. Should the nurse consider a hospice referral?
Answer: The nurse should be aware of an opportunity if it presents itself to discuss end-of-life care. If the patient and wife show an interest, the nurse can provide more information, request a social work referral, or ask hospice to visit the patient. Hospice can provide additional resources that may be needed by the patient and family in this environment.

Interdisciplinary Care Plan

Problem	Plan	Interventions	Evaluation
Knowledge deficit regarding disease process, CHF symptoms	Within 1 week, patient and wife will verbalize understanding of symptoms that led to recent hospitalization.	Teach patient and wife about specific signs and symptoms including pain, weight gain, SOB, and edema.	Patient and spouse will participate in self-care management.
Knowledge deficit regarding disease process, CHF symptom management, and interventions	In 3 weeks, patient and wife will verbalize 3 examples of when to call the home health agency or physician.	Teach patient and wife about specific signs and symptoms, 2+ lbs weight gain, increased SOB, increased swelling in ankles or abdomen.	Patient and spouse will call agency if any symptoms occur.
Fluid volume excess	Within 24 hours, patient and wife will be able to recall correct medication regime if there is a 2 lb weight gain.	Teach patient to weigh each day with same clothes and an empty bladder. Teach medication regime.	Patient will be weighed each morning and will increase Lasix if there is a 2+ lb weight gain in 1 day.

Problem	Plan	Interventions	Evaluation
Knowledge deficit: Medication management	By week 9, patient and wife will verbalize purpose, action, and dose of each medication.	Teach patient and spouse about all medications, purpose, action, dose, and side effects.	Patient will safely and correctly take all medications as prescribed and report any adverse reactions.
Knowledge deficit: Sodium influence in CHF	Within 3 days, patient and wife will be able to verbalize relationship between sodium intake and edema.	Teach patient and wife about high sodium foods and physiological response.	Patient will be able to recall diet and its impact if edema increases.
Knowledge deficit; use of the HomMed monitor	In one visit, patient and wife will be able to complete assessment process as directed by verbal cues of the monitor.	Teach patient and wife how to use the monitor and complete a return demonstration.	Daily reports verify utilization and intervention as indicated.
Cardiac output decreased	Within 2 weeks, patient will be able to ambulate greater distances and complete more ADL without his wife's assistance.	PT will provide strengthening exercises. Nurse will teach about energy conserving activities.	Patient will be able to ambulate at least 50 feet with minimal exertion and complete most ADL independently.
Altered mobility	Within 2 weeks, patient will be able to ambulate greater distances.	PT will provide strengthening and balancing exercises.	Patient will be able to ambulate at least 50 feet with minimal exertion.
Knowledge deficit: Type 2 diabetes	Within 3 weeks, patient and wife will verbalize disease management of patient's type 2 diabetes.	Nurse will assess current knowledge and teach on all aspects of care	Patient will be able to identify signs/ symptoms of hyperglycemia, hypoglycemia, blood glucose monitoring, and medication management.

REFERENCES & RESOURCES

[1] American Nurses Association, *Home Health Nursing: Scope and Standards of Practice*, Nursebooks, 2008.

[2] *"Hospital to Home,"* Retrieved from http://www.hospital2home.org, 2009.

[3] T.M. Marrelli, *Handbook of Home Health Standards* (5th ed.), Mosby, 2009.

[4] *"Taking Care of Myself: A Guide When I Leave the Hospital,"* Retrieved from http://www.ahrq.gov/qual/goinghomeguide.htm, 2010.

[5] D. Wetherill, D. Keriakes and L. Seeley, *The Little Book about Congestive Heart Failure*, Robertson and Fisher Publishing Company, 1999.

Case 2.3 Wound following a Coronary Artery Bypass Graft (CABG)

By Jeanie Stoker, MPA, RN, BC

This case study provides an opportunity to look at a complex cardiac and wound case, and to see how cultural diversity and understanding play key roles in outcome obtainment and success. Ms. L previously received home health care because of a recent CABG. At 5 weeks postoperative, she was sent to the hospital by the home health nurse due to drainage from the chest wall site. She has now returned home after an incision and drainage and has a wound vac in place as well as intravenous (IV) antibiotics.

Ms. L is very conscious and protective of the PICC line (right sided) as both she and the nurse observe Mr. L (the caregiver) care for it.

While Ms. L acknowledges the nurse's questions and directions, she and her spouse frequently converse in Spanish. Ms. L has requested that her husband serve as her interpreter.

> **Cultural Competence**
>
> Ms. L is a 56-year-old Hispanic female with serious and chronic health care issues. She has limited resources but does receive 60 hours of CLTC support each week. The home care staff will have to address culturally sensitive issues that may include: language, religion, elder care, family support, and lifestyle patterns. The use of an interpreter and other Hispanic team members will promote a good report with the best possible outcomes.

Clinical Case Studies in Home Health Care, First Edition. Edited by Leslie Neal-Boylan.
© 2011 John Wiley & Sons, Inc. Published 2011 by John Wiley & Sons, Inc.

ORDERS FOR HOME CARE

Patient: 56-year-old Hispanic female

Diagnoses: Coronary atherosclerosis of artery bypass graft, coronary artery disease (CAD), Infected CABG, diabetes mellitus type 2

Current medications:
- 1 g Ceftazidime IV every 12 hours
- Normal saline flush 10 mL flush before and after each IV
- Aspirin 81 mg, 1 three times a day
- Carvedilol 3.125 mg 1 twice a day
- Gabapentin 600 mg ½ tablet three times a day
- Hydrocodone-acetaminophen 7.5 mg–500 mg, 1 every 4–6 hours for pain
- Lasix 20 mg once a day
- Lipitor 20 mg once a day
- Metformin NCL 1000 once a day at bedtime
- Lantus 100 U/ML Vial, 30 units once a day at bedtime sq

Relevant Past Medical History
- Hypertension controlled by medications
- Hyperlipidemia

RN: Skilled observation and assessment, wound care, IV infusion and education

PT: Assess for strengthening program

Reimbursement Considerations

The patient is currently receiving Medicare and Medicaid benefits. These will cover the cost of home health visits, medical supplies, and DME. Her medications are covered by Medicaid in her state, including the infusion drugs and supplies.

THE HOME VISIT

After scheduling the visit to meet the caregiver's time frame, the nurse enters the home, which is a small apartment. The home is cluttered, but adequate walkways are noted. The husband greets the nurse, and it is noted that he is on oxygen with a slightly unsteady gait. He informs the nurse, "I am the nurse for her IV" with a proud grin. A private duty nursing assistant assists him back to his seat while observing and listening to the nurse and patient.

The patient is on the couch and greets the nurse warmly. Many medical supplies are in a large box on the table beside the patient. The patient explains that the two of them live alone but the nursing assistant (NA) helps them 6 days a week. Ms. L says that the wound care is done only by the nurse but that her husband takes care of the IV. The spouse was trained in the hospital and feels "OK" about caring for the infusion. The NA helps with meals, household duties, shopping and drives them to doctor appointments. They also have a daughter who lives 30 miles away and visits occasionally.

Relevant Community Resources

Community long term care (CLTC is a special Medicaid waiver program in the state.)
Social Services will assess additional community needs.
Assisted living may become an alternative for both Mr. and Ms. L
Home medical equipment (HME)
Home infusion pharmacy
Pharmacy

Ms. L is eager to improve her strength and "not be tied to all this medical stuff." With the assistance of her husband as interpreter, she and the nurse agree upon goals for her care:

- Ms. L complains of being tired and wants to be able to complete her bath and change clothes without being so tired.
  - Patient will improve strength and endurance.
  - Patient will be able to participate in self care.
- Ms. L would like to stay out of the hospital and for her wound to heal.
  - Patient will be compliant with IV medication.
  - Patient and caregiver will manage IV administration and PICC line care.
  - Patient and caregiver will verbalize understanding of the wound vac and when to call the nurse. They will not remove the wound vac.
  - Patient will verbalize 3 signs and symptoms of wound infection.
  - Ms. L's chest wound will have 40% tissue regeneration in 30 days.
- Ms. L states that she wants to keep her blood sugar in control as she feels this has contributed to her infection.
  - Patient will verbalize 3 signs and symptoms of hyper-/hypoglycemia.
  - Patient will verbalize 3 ways she can manage her diabetes.
  - Patient will recall diet and work with nurse to improve food choices.
- Ms. L will be able to take all her medications as ordered.
- Ms. L will verbalize purpose, action, and dose of each medication instructed on.

Neal Theory Implications

Stage 3: The nurse at this stage will be able to coordinate a complex plan of care while providing a high level of assessment and intervention. This multifaceted case will require the RN to provide intensive teaching to ensure that IV site care and administration occur when she is not in the home. She will need to be proficient in wound assessment as well as wound vac procedures. Routine wound knowledge will not address the issues in this case. This case is even more challenging as the language barrier may impede teaching and planning, thus she will call the appropriate team members for this. She will also want to address the multidisciplinary needs of the patient and spouse. This will include oversight of the private aide and collaboration with the therapists. She will be able to plan beyond the current scope to determine an alternative action plan if the husband becomes sick enough to be hospitalized.

Stage 2: The professional nurse at this level is able to complete the OASIS assessment independently and can identify needs and gaps. She will ask for an MSW for additional direction and will seek out and take action on all advice to which the the patient agrees. She will be able to set up interpreter services and therapy visits, but will rely on these disciplines for additional direction. She should have documented competencies in IV therapy and wound vac care but will be uncomfortable managing all of this at each visit. She may struggle with addressing diabetic education with other priorities in place.

Stage 1: The novice is often still overwhelmed with all of the regulatory and documentation requirements. She will have the skills to complete a nursing assessment but will need guidance on the best way to answer the OASIS questions as well as proper coding. Upon completion of the initial visit, this nurse will meet with a preceptor or supervisor to be directed regarding additional services and referrals that need to be made. This case could not be adequately managed with a nurse at this level; but with the assistance of a strong preceptor, a novice nurse could assist in jointly managing this case.

Based on the history and physical examination, the nurse discovers the following data:

- There is a midsternal chest wound that is covered by a wound vac. The wound vac is intact and the area around the vac is clean, tan, and dry.

- There is a PICC line in the right forearm. The dressing is dry, intact, and is scheduled to be changed at the next visit. The line extends 0.7 cm from the site. There is no redness, swelling, or pain around the area.
- The patient reports that her blood sugar was 116 this morning before breakfast. She states that it runs between 120 and 140, so she was pleased with this reading. The nurse assesses the blood sugar and finds it to be at 136 two hours after a meal.
- VS: 132/70, 98.8, 84, 18
- Ms. L is 5′5″ and weighs 199 pounds
- Ms. L complains of chest wound pain, level 5 on a scale of 1–10. She states that the pain is relieved with warmth, rest, and medication.
- Pedal and popliteal pulses are weak bilaterally, with 1+ pitting edema
- Ms. L ambulates slowly with a walker. Her gait is unsteady and she becomes tired after walking 10 feet.
- She is able to bathe herself on the toilet with assistance only. She is unable to get into the tub or shower.

Rehabilitation Needs

Physical therapy
Occupational therapy

? CRITICAL THINKING

1. What is the priority for care for Ms. L?
Answer: The priority for this patient is wound healing. This will require multifaceted focus areas to include: wound management, IV therapy management, and diabetic management. The patient is on a wound vac and was seen by the wound care specialist RN in the hospital. If wound healing does not progress as planned, it may be reasonable to request a home consult with this specialist.

2. What safety issues need to be considered?
Answer: Since Ms. L is on IV therapy she will need to be educated on how to safely discard all sharps. The nurse and therapist will also need to focus on fall prevention as Ms. L is considered at high risk for falls. Infection control is also a safety risk. Both the patient and care-giver will need to be taught proper hand hygiene as well as aseptic IV

administration. Mr. L is on oxygen so the nurse will also need to teach everyone about O^2 safety.

3. What will the physical therapist (PT) do to support the goals for Ms. L?
Answer: The PT will do an assessment to determine Ms. L's needs and goals for therapy. The PT will also assess the home environment and develop a plan to improve ambulation and strength. Ms. L is focused on regaining her strength and independence, so the PT will provide a home exercise program that will allow her to work on this in his absence. Since it has been identified that she is at high risk for falls, the therapist will also educate about how to avoid falls as well as how to "fall safely." He will monitor the vital signs before and after each visit to ensure that the patient's overall health is not compromised by the therapy interventions. Any issues or abnormalities will be reported.

4. Is there anyone else who should be called into this case?
Answer: Yes. The nurse should consider asking the physician for orders for an occupational therapist (OT), a dietician, and possibly a wound care specialist.

5. What will each of these disciplines do?
Answer: The OT will reinforce the teaching and interventions of the nurse and the PT as they all collaborate to meet the patient's goals. Additionally, the OT will teach Ms. M. energy-conserving methods to improve her ability to complete ADL and improve her overall independence.

A dietician, while not a part of the traditional home care team could provide additional support and education to the patient and both caregivers. Ms. L wants to improve her blood sugar, and this is the best time to educate her. She will provide diabetic diet teaching as well as reviewing diet diary feedback. This plan can be reinforced by other members of the team

A wound care specialist would be needed to provide additional assessment and recommendations if the wound does not progress as planned.

6. Are there any confidentiality issues with the nurse discussing the plan of care (POC) with the private nursing assistant?
Answer: The nursing assistant should be considered part of the health care team. The patient has the ultimate control of who may or may not have access to any health and personal information. The nurse asked the patient if there were any limitations and she denied any. To insure complete confidentiality, the nurse also asked the patient in private if she wanted the NA to be included in the POC. Ms. L acknowledged that due to her complex health issues, communication limitations, and

her husband's condition that she did want her second caregiver, the NA, to be involved in the POC.

BACK TO THE CASE

The nurse reviews the finalized goals and recommendations for other disciplines. On the second visit the nurse reviews these goals with the patient and both caregivers. The NA notes that she is overwhelmed with taking care of two patients, trying to remind them to take their medications, cooking, and just keeping everyone clean. The nurse plans to request MSW services to see if any other services may be available.

The wound vac is removed at the visit, and wound care is provided in accordance with the MD orders. While the wound is healing, the patient appears frustrated at the size and the amount of time it will take to heal. She is also concerned that her husband is not feeling well and that she needs him to give her the IV each day.

The nurse will ask for a home health order for the spouse. There is a concern that communication may become an issue if the spouse is hospitalized, so a language interpreter visit will be set up to insure a communication plan that will enable all to move toward goal obtainment.

CRITICAL THINKING

1. How will the team communicate with Ms. L if her husband is hospitalized?
Answer: Health providers are required to provide interpretation services. While this may be done by phone, this agency has an interpreter available through a local hospital. The nurse would like to have this person visit to insure all goals and directions are clearly understood. This will also allow them to develop an alternative plan if the spouse is not available.

2. What if the patient and/or spouse cannot administer the IV antibiotic?
Answer: In today's environment, home health agencies are finding it more challenging to provide daily, much less BID visits. While this may be accomplished in the short term, the nurse will need to look at other alternatives. Some of these alternatives include an outpatient infusion center, private duty nursing, or possible rehospitalization. While this issue may never develop, it is good for the nurse to prepare proactively.

Interdisciplinary Care Plan

Problem	Plan	Interventions	Evaluation
Knowledge deficit regarding disease process, CAD	Within 1 week, patient will verbalize understanding of symptoms of CAD signs and symptoms to report.	Teach patient about specific signs and symptoms including chest pain, SOB, weakness and edema.	Patient will participate in self-care management and be able to recall symptoms.
Knowledge deficit regarding disease process, diabetes mellitus (DM)	Within 3 weeks, patient will verbalize management of DM and blood sugar control.	Teach patient about specific signs and symptoms of hypo-/hyperglycemia. Provide diet teaching and diary feedback.	Patient and/or family will be able to keep blood sugar under 140 without periods of hypo-/hyperglycemia.
IV site/ PICC line management	Patient and caregiver will be able to verbalize care and 3 IV problems for which to call the nurse. Caregiver will be able to administer drug after first visit.	Teach patient and caregiver to call the nurse if the IV does not infuse, comes out, or appears infected. Call 911 if severe SOB, itching, etc. during infusion.	Caregiver completes IV infusion successfully. Both caregiver and patient care for line and call nurse if problems.
Infection of a postoperative wound	Within 1 week, patient and caregiver will be able to verbalize signs/symptoms of infection and preventive measures.	Teach patient and caregiver about proper hand hygiene, proper sharps disposal, and signs/ symptoms of infection.	Patient's wound will heal without any additional infections.
Wound care/ wound vac	Within 2 weeks, patient and caregiver will be taught about the wound vac and its efficacy.	Teach patient and caregiver that process of removing all tissue and allowing new growth will maximize wound healing. Only nurse will change vac.	Patient's wounds will heal.

Problem	Plan	Interventions	Evaluation
Altered Mobility	In 4 weeks, patient will be able to ambulate greater distances.	PT will provide strengthening exercises and a home exercise program.	Patient will be able to ambulate 100 feet with a walker with minimal exertion.
Altered ADL independence	Patient will be able to complete ADL without assistance	OT will provide energy-conserving ADL education and intervention.	Patient will be able to complete ADL and possibly a shower without assistance.

REFERENCES & RESOURCES

[1] American Nurses Association, *Home Health Nursing: Scope and Standards of Practice*, Nursesbooks, 2008.

[2] P. Anderson and D. Mignor, *Home Care Nursing: Using an Accreditation Approach*, Thomson Delmar Learning Corporation, 2008.

[3] M.D. Harris, *Handbook of Home Health Care Administration*, Jones and Bartlett Publishers, 2010.

[4] T.M. Marrelli, *Handbook of Home Health Standards* (5th ed.), Mosby, 2009.

Section 3

Peripheral Vascular Disease

Case 3.1 Peripheral Vascular Disease

By Linda Royer, PhD, RN

This case illustrates the importance of diligent management of lifestyle-driven and genetically influenced chronic peripheral vascular disease and the effective role of the home health nurse (HHN), through teamwork, in reducing the demise of diagnosed patients.

Lower extremity arterial disease (LEAD) affects approximately 9 million individuals in the United States; its presence is often silent until life-threatening symptoms become apparent. Resulting impaired circulation, if left untreated, leads to non-healing wounds with serious tissue damage and possible amputation due to infection and gangrene. If treatment is delayed, quality of life declines and health care costs increase tremendously. LEAD is associated with cardiovascular and cerebrovascular diseases; therefore, impending or asymptomatic potential for LEAD should be anticipated in patients displaying those risk factors (hypercholesterolemia, other lipid disorders, hypertension, smoking, obesity, diabetes, physical inactivity, and a family history), begging a thorough assessment. National guidelines have been published; however, LEAD is not recognized in many patients seen by health care providers. It is of higher prevalence than other vascular, diseases including myocardial infarction and cerebrovascular accident.

Background

The HHN has driven 12 miles into the country from his home health agency office in the county's governing center to admit a new patient for services. Mr. B, 68-year-old Caucasian, was a machinist in a metal fabrication plant for 25 years. He retired 8 months ago after undergoing left femoral-popliteal bypass surgery. He and his wife of 38 years have lived all of their married life in the rural farmhouse the HHN is now

Clinical Case Studies in Home Health Care, First Edition. Edited by Leslie Neal-Boylan.
© 2011 John Wiley & Sons, Inc. Published 2011 by John Wiley & Sons, Inc.

approaching. The house is in good repair from outward appearances, the fields stretch for a mile before another farmhouse is sighted, and the yard is fenced and neat. A dozen chickens roam about. The HHN has been informed that good cell phone and Internet service extends to this rural setting. The HNN is greeted warmly at the door by Mrs. B and is ushered into a neat and airy living room displaying pictures of their three grown children and their families. He learns that they all live in the area and are a close-knit family. One daughter-in-law is a licensed practical nurse. Mrs. B states that she works during the school year as a school bus driver.

The HHN received this referral from discharge planners at the regional medical center where Mr. B was treated for a large stage III tibial ulcer on his right leg. He had stumbled over some equipment in his barn, resulting in a wound that would not heal. While in the hospital, he admitted to his physician that he had been experiencing pain in his right leg similar to that of his earlier admission for a left femoral-popliteal bypass 8 months ago. While hospitalized this time, he was diagnostically tested, his medication was adjusted, wet-to-dry dressings with normal saline were applied to his wound, and he received physical therapy (PT) of active and passive exercises to his lower extremities. The home health supervisor was wise to assign this particular HHN to this case, because he is a new HHN with 10 years experience in a cardiac care unit.

ORDERS FOR HOME CARE

Patient: 68-year-old Caucasian male

Diagnoses: Status post left femoral-popliteal bypass of 8 months, peripheral arterial disease (PAD) right lower extremity with absence of claudication, 6-cm stage III anterior tibial ulcer RLE. (Claudication is defined as exercise-induced lower limb ischemia distal to the site of arterial occlusion that is relieved within 10 minutes of rest.)

Medications:
- Atorvastatin (Lipitor) 40 mg once a day by mouth at bedtime
- Amlodipine (Norvasc) 10 mg once a day by mouth in a.m.
- Lisinopril 40 mg by mouth once a day in a.m.
- Cilostazol 100 mg by mouth twice a day
- Low-dose aspirin (80 mg) once a day
- Vitamin supplements of A, B_6 and B_{12}, C, and D.

Relevant past medical history:
- Cardiovascular disease (atherosclerosis)
- Hypercholesterolemia
- Hyperlipidemia (LDL-C)
- Hypertension
- Overweight

RN: Wound care with Mepilex dressing change weekly; diet and physical activity regimen teaching and reinforcement; reinforce importance of appointment-keeping for blood work to monitor inflammatory factors.

PT: Home assessment and rehabilitative ambulatory exercise regimen [2] (American College of Cardiology/American Heart Association [ACC/AHA] Practice Guidelines, p. 47–49).

Reimbursement Considerations

Mr. B has Medicare coverage, Parts A, B, and D. He is able to pay his out-of-pocket expenses with funds from his Health Savings Account his employer set up for employees 10 years ago. He is also drawing Social Security monthly.

THE HOME VISIT

The HHN begins the visit with an environmental scan about the home interior and friendly conversation about the country setting of the home and the family dynamics. He proceeds to focus on the patient's history and current condition and concerns. Mr. B has been a diligent worker at physically challenging jobs most of his life and has always boasted of his strength and endurance. Besides his full-time job he worked his farm in corn and cattle until age 55. The machinist job required standing for long hours on concrete floors and some heavy lifting. In recent years, Mr B's after-work activities have been limited to chores around the home and sedentary relaxation before the TV due to fatigue. His diet for most of his life had been mainly meat, potatoes, and dairy products, with few vegetables and fruits. Consequently, he gained weight to 290 pounds (height 5'10").

He became hypertensive with a blood pressure of 168/106. There is a family history of cardiovascular disease. His older brother died of a myocardial infarction at age 66, and his father suffered with LEAD in the final years of his life.

Surgical intervention for clot removal and a bypass graft on his left leg were done 8 months ago after extreme ischemic calf pain made walking and working unbearable. His surgeon is pleased with his recovery and the quality of perfusion in that extremity. However, Mr. B is not performing regular walking exercise.

The patient had been a smoker most of his life; he quit successfully 1 year ago. Since surgery, some improvements have been made to his diet so that he now eats a few more vegetables each day, eats low-fat dairy products, and has reduced meat intake to lean red meat and chicken. Developmentally, he is a graduate of vocational school where he learned the machinist trade. Mr. and Mrs. B's interest in local and world affairs is evident by the type of reading matter scattered around the house and a news program on TV. A computer screen glows in the nearby office.

Cultural Competence

There is no ethnic or racial diversity in this case. The HHN is from this region of the Midwest and understands beliefs and practices of this couple. He demonstrates sensitivity to the opinions and preferences of the Bs and is able to anticipate future needs.

The patient and his wife collaborate with the nurse regarding the following goals for home care. Mr. B identifies the following:

1. Avoid another surgery through diet, medication, and activity changes.
2. Lose 50 pounds.
3. Get this sore on my leg cleared up. It has me worried. I would hate to get it infected.
4. Create meaning in my retirement years, such as: assisting my pastor in his work, teaching my grandchildren some vocational skills, painting the exterior of this old house, and putting down new flooring inside the house.
5. Reduce the worrying my wife does over me.

Neal Theory Implications

Stage 3: The professional in this stage is accustomed to the necessities of traveling to make home visits. This nurse is also aware of the latest wound-care products that can be used in the home.

Stage 2: The professional in this stage may not feel comfortable collaborating with the physician regarding orders for other disciplines, case managing, working within the patient's environment to manage care.

Stage 1: The clinician in this stage will assess the patient and recognize the need for assistance with the case but may be unsure as to how to proceed in the home setting. In this case, the HHN is in Stage 1 as a new HHN; however, he is comfortable relating and collaborating with the physician and working with another team member—the PT. He may still be unsure of the culture, procedures, and community resources of the home health setting.

Based on the history and physical examination, the nurse discovers the following data:

- BP 142/90 (both arms are similar)
- Apical pulse 84 regular and strong
- Respirations 20 with clear lungs and deep excursions
- Weight on the home scale today is 270 pounds.
- No bruits in the carotid arteries; the upstroke and amplitude of pulses bilaterally are good.
- The referral record history denotes that Mr. B's EKG showed normal sinus rhythm. Because he demonstrates no cardiovascular limitations, he was not put on anticoagulants (except for low dose ASA) to avoid risk of bleeding.
- Good pulses are noted in both femoral arteries, the left popliteal site, and left pedal site; however, the right popliteal and pedal pulses are diminished. The right foot is slightly cool and pale compared to his normal left foot. No edema is noted in either foot.
- The hygiene and integrity of the skin and tissues of the toes and feet are excellent. The footwear consists of cotton socks and supportive shoes.
- Capillary refill bilaterally is spontaneous on left, delayed on right foot.
- The HHN uses the infrared thermometer from the peripheral arterial disease (PAD) kit over large blood vessels sites to identify any localized "hot spots" (an increase of 20 degrees Celsius) that might indicate inflammation. None are found.
- The Ankle Brachial Index (ABI) (the brachial systolic and dorsalis pedis systolic pressures are compared with a Doppler-assisted sphygmomanometer [1, 4]) score is 1.0 in the left lower extremity (normal) and 0.8 in the right lower extremity (borderline perfusion).
- The HHN also notes that the patient's lab values for homoscysteine, C-reactive protein, and lipoprotein-associated phospholipase A_2 (Lp-PLA$_2$) are elevated (perhaps indicating that he never fully recovered vascular integrity after the previous surgery and treatment medications). Research demonstrates that statin medications and ambulatory exercise lower those inflammatory product levels [4, 5]. Drugs and supplements have been prescribed to improve that.
- There are no abdominal bruits.
- Hydration is adequate and there are no difficulties with bowel or bladder function.
- Cursory neurological exam reveals no obvious abnormalities. Sensation is somewhat diminished in sole of right foot when ambulating.
- The patient is able to ambulate with a cane at this time; he could not 2 months ago.

> **Traditional Risk Factors for Cardiovascular Disease and Stroke from the Framingham Risk Score (FRS) Procedure**
>
> Hypercholesterolemia and other lipid disorders, hypertension, smoking, obesity, diabetes, physical inactivity, and family history. Newer research demonstrates that an inflammatory atherosclerotic condition (initiated by high levels of LDL particles clinging to vessel walls) is the cause which can be evaluated with certain markers in the blood: C-reactive protein (CRP) and lipoprotein-associated phospholipase A_2 (Lp-PLA$_2$). The *Adult Treatment Panel III Cholesterol Guidelines of the National Cholesterol Education Program* has determined a simple screening method for determining how to utilize these markers: count the number of FRS (risk factors). If 2 or more, test the Lp-PLA$_2$. Patients over 65 with one risk factor should be tested [5].

The wound on the mid-anterior lower leg is inspected after removal of the dressing. The edges are clean. There is no eschar, but a moderate amount of yellow drainage oozes from the center where the fascia can be seen. Thus far, there have been no obvious signs of infection, either by visualization, blood work, or culture. The nurse measures the wound as 6 cm across, approximately 2 cm deep. There is tenderness to the touch around it. The nurse has brought a new Mepilex dressing which he applies after cleansing the wound with normal saline and drying it with sterile gauze. He instructs the wife in this aseptic procedure as he does so.

> **Mepilex Dressings**
>
> Mepilex dressings are composed of a soft polyurethane vapor-permeable membrane (wound contact side) bonded to polyurethane foam that collects exudates in nonstick fashion and maintains a moist environment at the wound surface, causing no additional trauma to the wound. It can be sized and shaped by cutting with sterile scissors and held in place with a gauze pad and a retention aid (tape or wrap). It is changed according to the amount of drainage and the need for inspection (http://www.dressings.org/Dressings/mepilex.html).

? CRITICAL THINKING

1. What should be the priority of care for Mr. B?
Answer: The primary priority is restoring circulation integrity to the right lower extremity (RLE), thus avoiding the extreme measure of amputation. It is possible that Mr. B will still need another surgery similar to that done on his left lower extremity (LLE). The secondary priority is to facilitate healing of the wound.

2. What should be some concerns and interventions of the home health nurse as he thinks about the psychosocial support structure of this couple?
Answer: Of concern is the comprehension of necessary lifestyle changes that must be made and Mr. B's level of motivation to do so. The nurse should commend Mr. B's smoking cessation accomplishment and highlight that as one of the most difficult behavior changes there is to make. If he can succeed in that, he can probably make other changes. The nurse should review the physician's orders, the medications, and the supplemental vitamins. The nurse might direct Mr. and Mrs. B to reliable sites on the Internet (such as The PAD Coalition; http://www.padcoalition.org) for reinforcing information.

3. What should the nurse teach the couple about nutrition and diet?
Answer: Encourage them to convert to a vegetarian diet with low-fat dairy products and limited eggs and eventually to convert to a strict vegetarian. Stress the need to lower cholesterol, LDL, and triglyceride levels and explain that the drugs alone might not make the corrections needed. On subsequent visits he will provide educational dietary resources. Address salt intake and encourage reduction. Discuss reading food labels. Give suggestions of using herbs to season.

4. What additional orders/referrals are appropriate?
Answer: Dietician visits to educate them.

5. What else should the nurse teach Mr. and Mrs. B?
Answer: Resume walking about his farm and playing with the dogs. Supervised exercise has thus far demonstrated the most progress in mitigating claudication [6]. Studies have shown that 6–8 months are needed. PT will not be covered that long under Medicare, so a plan must be created for sustaining the regimen set up by the professional. Mr. B assures the HHN that family members can be recruited; an accountability system will be arranged.

BACK TO THE CASE

Mr. Blackwell states that his wife has such a sense of humor and interest in life that she is able to encourage him and keep his spirits positive most of the time. They have a close connection with their church and can call on the members for assistance when needed. The family off-spring are close and attentive. The HHN asks that the daughter-in-law who is an LPN be present at the next visit so that he may teach her how to care for the wound and support the diet changes.

The HHN, Physical Therapist, and PCP will consult together on patient goals, lifestyle change teaching, monitoring of wound healing, assessment of circulation and pain (claudication), changes in laboratory values over time, and overall health status on a weekly basis. The HHN and the PT will develop a smooth transition plan for patient and family to assume the exercise regimen when Medicare reimbursement ends.

Interdisciplinary Care Plan

Problem	Plan	Intervention	Evaluation
Deficit in circulatory perfusion RLE	To effect improved perfusion in RLE adequate enough to avoid surgical intervention over next 3 months.	HHN will closely monitor weekly for 3 months via ABI and infrared thermometer testing. HHN will ensure that patient has blood work done to check inflammatory markers as ordered. HHN will support the instructions PT prescribes for activity regimen. HHN will instruct in diet (see below).	HHN is looking for ABI index to improve to 1.0 and for absence of "hot spots" over vascular structure of RLE. HHN expects to see inflammatory markers reduce with improvements in patient's lifestyle.
Deficit in skin (dermal) integrity d/t injury	Patient's wound will reduce to stage II in 1 month and heal by 3 months.	HHN will instruct patient, wife, and the LPN family member in aseptic wound care to be done "as needed" as exudates build up and after showering. (Wound to be protected from shower water.)	Weekly wound inspection and discussion with patient and family should reveal healing at progressive stages.

Problem	Plan	Intervention	Evaluation
Knowledge deficit in care of wound		HHN will monitor wound weekly (observe, measure, document).	
Knowledge deficit of disease process	Patient and family will verbalize the significance of patient's risk factors and the progression to current state of disease while also acknowledging their familial risks.	HHN will lead them to reputable internet sites for educational videos and text concerning CVD and PAD. HHN and PT will also reinforce the importance of lifestyle with each visit.	HHN will look for demonstration of adoption of healthy lifestyle.
Knowledge deficit of diet	Patient and wife will verbalize and demonstrate the importance of a cardiovascular-healthy diet.	HHN will instruct (through internet resources and written materials) in low-salt, low-fat, high fiber, low sugar diet. Minimal meat and 5 servings per day of fruits and vegetables will be stressed.	Patient and wife are internet savvy enough to learn from popular, evidence-based websites and guidance from HHN to preclude need for dietician.
Physical activity	Patient will adopt a regular exercise regimen to improve skeletal, muscle, and circulatory health.	PT will assess patient and prescribe, demonstrate, and guide in a walking, aerobic, and strength exercise program along with an accountability monitor for patient and family to assure compliance.	Success will be demonstrated in the ABI and thermal thermometer assessments, in vital signs, and wound healing, as well as patient's testimony of well-being.

REFERENCES & RESOURCES

[1] E. Asongwed, S. Chesbro and S. Karavatas, "Peripheral arterial disease and the ankle-brachial index," *Home Healthcare Nurse*, 27(3):161–167, 2009.

[2] Author, "American College of Cardiology/American Heart Association practice guidelines for the management of patients with peripheral arterial disease (lower extremity, renal, mesenteric, and abdominal aortic)," 2005.

[3] P. Bonham, B. Flemister, M. Goldberg, P. Crawford, J. Johnson and M. Varnado, "What's new in lower-extremity arterial disease? WOCN's 2008 clinical practice guideline," *Journal of Wound, Ostomy, and Continence Nursing*, 36(1):37–44, 2009.

[4] P. Bonham and T. Kelechi, "Evaluation of lower extremity arterial circulation and implications for nursing practice," *The Journal of Cardiovascular Nursing*, 23(2):144–152, 2008.

[5] L. Braun, "How inflammatory markers refine CV risk status," *American Nurse Today*, 5(5):30–31, 2010.

[6] R. Oka, "Peripheral arterial disease in older adults: Management of cardiovascular risk factors," *The Journal of Cardiovascular Nursing*, 21(5S):S15–S20, 2006.

Section 4

Pulmonary

Case 4.1 Chronic Obstructive Pulmonary Disease (COPD)

By Lisa A. Gorski, MS, HHCNS, BC, CRNI, FAAN

This case study demonstrates how the home health nurse works with the patient with chronic obstructive pulmonary disease (COPD) and their family to decrease the patient's risk for disease exacerbation and hospitalization and to help the patient remain safely in the community. The patient is a 75-year-old African American female who also has diabetes, arthritis, and heart failure (HF). She lives independently in her home with some assistance from her daughter; but she is weak, has chronic dyspnea, and has fallen in her home in the past, although she has not sustained injuries. She has been referred to home care after 6 hospitalizations over the past 18 months for exacerbation of her COPD symptoms. Attention to medication management issues, management of her dyspnea, and patient education emphasizing early recognition of COPD symptoms are essential in helping this patient stay at an optimal level of wellness in her home.

Cultural Competence

Ms. R is African American. The nurse and therapists will need to help Ms. R to recognize the importance of regular appointments with her physician and the importance of calling at the first indication of signs or symptoms. Studies show that patients with lower incomes and lack of social supports are more likely to use emergency departments as their regular places of care.

Clinical Case Studies in Home Health Care, First Edition. Edited by Leslie Neal-Boylan.
© 2011 John Wiley & Sons, Inc. Published 2011 by John Wiley & Sons, Inc.

ORDERS FOR HOME CARE

Patient: 75-year-old African American female
Diagnosis: COPD
Current medications:
- Furosemide 20 mg once a day
- Advair Diskus 100/50 mcg (fluticasone and salmeterol) 2 puffs once a day
- Lantus insulin 10 units subcutaneous every night
- Metoprolol tartrate 50 mg once a day
- Prednisone 30 mg once a day x1 day, 20 mg once a day x1 day, 10 mg once a day x1 day and then discontinue
- Azithromycin 250 mg once a day x2 days and then discontinue
- Nexium 40 mg twice a day (esomeprazole)
- Ventolin 100 mcg (albuterol) metered dose inhaler 2 puffs every 6 hours as needed
- Acetaminophen 350 mg every 4–6 hours as needed for pain

Relevant past medical history:
- Type 2 diabetes mellitus
- Heart failure and blood pressure controlled with medication
- Arthritis. History of falls at home.

RN: Assess and evaluate. Medication management. Teach patient and family disease management.

Reimbursement Considerations

This patient qualifies for Medicare. Based upon Medicare criteria, the patient must be homebound and require skilled care. Skilled care includes assessment, medication management interventions, and other patient education. Due to her functional limitations, especially her shortness of breath, Ms. R is currently homebound. As she recovers from her recent COPD exacerbation and increases her activity with PT and OT intervention, she will likely no longer be homebound. Discharge and transition to an outpatient pulmonary rehabilitation program may be considered depending upon her progress.

THE HOME VISIT

The patient lives in her own small home that is relatively clean. The patient's daughter answers the door and lets the nurse in but promptly goes to her room. The patient walks in using a cane. She moves slowly into the kitchen asking the nurse to follow her. After introducing herself, the nurse begins to perform the initial assessment, first explaining agency services and expectations. Ms. R is cooperative during the home visit. While in the kitchen, the nurse asks Ms. R about meals and how she adheres to her diabetic and low sodium diet, noting on the referral information that her most recent HgA1C level was 6.8%, reflective of good diabetic management. Ms. R receives two delivered meals per day. She prepares breakfast by herself—usually milk, cereal, and coffee.

To assess her living situation and her ability to safely ambulate and transfer, the nurse asks the patient to give her a tour of her single level home. Laundry facilities are in the basement and Ms. R explains that her daughter does her laundry as she does not feel safe going down the stairs. The bathroom is small; there is a raised toilet seat, a shower grab bar, a hand-held shower, and a tub bench present. Ms. R explains that her daughter helps her get into the tub; but, once in, she is able to bathe herself. The bedroom is small and somewhat cluttered. Medicine bottles are noted on a bedside table, and some inhalers are visible on a shelf above the bed. The nurse asks permission to obtain all of the medications and bring them into the kitchen. Ms. R is agreeable and mentions that there is another plastic bag of medications in the corner. As Ms. R and the nurse walk around the home, the nurse notes Ms. R's increased breathlessness with the activity. They return to the kitchen where the nurse completes the rest of the physical assessment. She focuses on the respiratory assessment, asking the patient to rate the level of breathlessness during their tour and after sitting down for a few minutes. She uses a 0–10 scale, showing the patient a copy of the scale. She asks the patient about the usual activities that produce shortness of breath. The patient explains that she is most short of breath during bathing and activities of daily living such as getting dressed. The nurse further asks the patient about the circumstances surrounding her hospitalizations, what happens just before she goes into the hospital. Ms. R explains that she starts becoming more short of breath; and when it gets worse, she goes to the emergency room. The nurse notes that most of the hospitalizations occurred during the winter months in the cold climate where she lives. She asks Ms. R about flu and pneumonia vaccines. Ms. R states that she always gets her flu vaccine, and she *thinks* she had a pneumonia vaccine.

The nurse then completes a thorough respiratory assessment. She auscultates Ms. R's lungs, listening for any adventitious sounds and notes that her lungs are clear. She notes no evidence of accessory muscle use. She asks Ms. R if she has a cough, which currently she does not, and then asks about coughing prior to her hospitalization. Ms R. remembers then, that in addition to "bad" shortness of breath, she was coughing more. The nurse assesses for any evidence of edema in her extremities, also noting the rapidity of capillary refill in her finger and toenail beds. She proceeds to check Ms. R's vital signs and also checks her oxygen saturation using a pulse oximeter. Her saturation level is 93%.

The patient is due for a "puff" of her inhaler during the visit, so the nurse asks Ms. R to show her how she uses her inhaler. As Ms. R and the nurse go through her medications, the nurse notes that there are several duplicates, that 3 different pharmacies have been used, and that there are numerous expired and old prescription bottles.

Relevant Community Resources

Home meal services
Outpatient pulmonary rehabilitation programs

As she completes the assessment, the nurse asks Ms. R about her goals and what she expects from home care. Ms. R simply states she wants to live in her home and not "end up in a nursing home." As they discuss her care, they both agree that a major goal is to try and stay well at home and stay out of the hospital.

Based upon the history and physical assessment, the nurse identifies the following:

- Ms. R has difficulty managing her oral medications.
- Ms. R does not use her inhaler correctly.
- Ms. R has no difficulty consistently administering her single dose of daily insulin in the evening/ Her diabetic management is adequate at this time, as reflected by her HgA1C.
- Ms. R does not recognize early signs of COPD exacerbation that could be managed at home.
- Ms. R is a frequent emergency department (ED) user, believing that if you feel sick, you go to the ED.
- Ms. R has significant dyspnea when performing activities of daily living (ADL) and with ambulating distances in the home over 20 feet.
- Ms. R has some assistance with instrumental ADL (e.g., laundry) and ADL from her daughter.
- Ms. R uses her cane safely within the home, and her bathroom is adapted to allow her to safely use the toilet and the bath.
- Ms. R has some mild pain associated with her arthritis but it is managed to her satisfaction with over-the-counter analgesics.

? CRITICAL THINKING

1. Why did the nurse ask questions about the circumstances surrounding her previous hospital admissions?
Answer: An important overarching goal of home care is to keep patients out of the hospital and at an optimum level of wellness in their com-

munity. So the question must be asked: why is she in the hospital so often? The nurse should investigate and address potential contributory factors. Such information is helpful in providing relevant patient education. While it is not *always* possible to identify a specific cause with exacerbations of COPD, known factors include environmental causes such as extreme weather, exposure to irritants in the home such as visitors who smoke, or exposure to infections such as colds. Clues might include the times of the year when hospitalizations happen. It is also important to understand the symptoms associated with worsening of Ms. R's condition because the nurse will want to focus education on early recognition of those symptoms that would allow intervention and possibly avoid hospitalization. Ascertaining vaccination status is critical for patients with COPD. Ms. R obtains her annual flu vaccine but is uncertain whether she has ever received the pneumococcal vaccine. Pneumococcal disease occurs year-round and COPD patients should receive the vaccine at least once in their lives; in high risk patients, it may be given every 5–10 years.

2. Why did the nurse ask the patient to rate her shortness of breath?
Answer: Dyspnea has been referred to as the "sixth vital sign" for patients with COPD, just as pain is commonly called the fifth vital sign. Dyspnea is a disabling symptom associated with great distress and suffering for patients with COPD, which is a progressive disease. Exacerbations occur with increasing frequency over time. Increasing dyspnea is the major symptom associated with COPD exacerbation. Tools such as numerical rating scales are recommended and are useful in assessing the patient's current state and effectiveness of interventions such as medications. Like pain, dyspnea is a subjective symptom, and it is important for the nurse to accept the patient's self-report. Early recognition of exacerbation is essential to allow early treatment and reduce the risk of hospitalization.

3. How should the nurse address the patient's belief in use of the ED whenever she feels sick?
Answer: Because the patient's dyspnea is the symptom that causes the patient to seek care, patient education addressing early identification of worsening breathlessness is critical to early intervention. Use of a "stoplight" tool is helpful to many patients as it ties in symptoms to "green" (feeling good), "yellow" (caution, potential worsening of condition and need to take action), and "red" (emergent care). Helping Ms. R identify her yellow zone symptoms, which might also include a cough and increased fatigue, is critical. Then the nurse can work with the patient in developing an "action plan" of steps to take, such as calling her home care nurse or doctor right away and using an as-needed inhaler. The goal is to improve the patient's self-care management of her disease, and to try to avoid, whenever possible,

the ED. In fact, in many instances, early symptoms can be managed at home.

4. Why did the nurse ask the patient to demonstrate her inhaler use?
Answer: This could be another possible factor in Ms. R's COPD exacerbations. It is well-documented that most patients do not use their inhalers correctly. An important aspect of COPD medication management is inhaler use. If the patient does not use the inhaler correctly, dyspnea associated with the disease is not going to be well managed.

5. What is another priority of care for Ms. R?
Answer: A major priority of care for Ms. R is safe management of her medications. Poor medication management is a factor in chronic disease exacerbations and a documented cause for potentially preventable hospitalizations. The nurse will help Ms. R simplify her medication management. This will include discarding or setting aside any medications the patient is not currently taking, helping the patient identify a system that will help her remember to take her medications and stay on track with refills. It will also be important to assess if there are financial issues, making it difficult for Ms. R to order and pay for her refilled medications on time.

6. Is there anyone else who should be called into this case?
Answer: Yes. The nurse should discuss the need for occupational and physical therapy (OT and PT) services with the patient and the physician, obtaining orders for the services.

7. What would an OT and PT do?
Answer: The OT will further assess the patient's performance of ADL and IADL, both in terms of safety and in relation to her dyspnea. The OT will work with Ms. R to identify ways to conserve her energy while performing her ADL. This might include storing household items in ways to limit reaching and bending, pacing activities by breaking them into smaller steps, and helping Ms. R to be realistic about how much she can do. The PT and the OT will work with the patient in developing a home exercise program, as part of a pulmonary rehabilitation program. Pulmonary rehabilitation for patients with COPD is a well-recognized, evidence-based intervention. Major components of pulmonary rehabilitation include lower and upper extremity exercises and patient education addressing self-management, as well as prevention and treatment of exacerbations. Pulmonary rehabilitation is associated with improvement in level of dyspnea and in overall quality of life. Some home care agencies provide formal pulmonary rehabilitation programs and some may initiate an exercise program and refer the patient to a formal outpatient program following home care. Both the OT and PT will teach Ms. R breathing techniques to use during ambulation and

other activities, as well as exercises including pursed lip breathing, and will monitor response to activity using a pulse oximeter.

Rehabilitation Needs

Occupational therapy
Physical therapy

BACK TO THE CASE

The nurse helps Ms. R with her medications, giving her a pillbox to help with organization and monitoring her adherence. Her daughter, although a somewhat reluctant and shy caregiver, agrees to help and will place the pills in the box every week. Due to the patient's insurance coverage, it turns out that there are not significant financial problems related to medications. The patient is just overwhelmed with keeping track of prescriptions and refills. The patient likes the pillbox because it is easier than opening all the bottles and her daughter will let her know when refills are needed. The nurse contacted Ms. R's physician and found out that she did have a pneumococcal vaccine 2 years earlier. She talked to the physician, discussing the need and rationale for getting a PT and OT involved in Ms. R's care, and obtained the order for those services. During a visit about 3 weeks into home care services, Ms. R rates her shortness of breath as worse and states she has had a dry cough over the weekend. The nurse points out that these are symptoms in her yellow zone of her action plan. Ms. R has orders for use of her as-needed bronchodilator inhaler. The nurse instructs her to use a dose during the home visit, which she does with good technique. The nurse completes a respiratory assessment and notes no evidence of accessory muscle use and that Ms. R's other vital signs are stable other than a slight decrease in her oxygen saturation to 91%. The physician is notified because this represents a change in her condition; there are no further orders at this time other than activating the as-needed inhaler use. The nurse collaborates with the physician, stating she will follow up with a home visit the next day to reassess Ms. R's respiratory status and response to the medication intervention, obtaining the order for the extra home visit. The next day, symptoms are improved. The nurse uses this opportunity for patient education, helping the patient recognize the importance of early intervention in averting symptoms and also helps the patient recognize that while the outcome was good, she should not have waited 2 days before letting the nurse know about her worsening dyspnea and cough.

Neal Theory Implications

Stage 3: The professional in this stage is comfortable in collaborating with other disciplines and recognizes the benefits to interdisciplinary care for COPD management. The nurse recognizes that patient education alone is inadequate in helping the patient to self-manage and that the PT and OT will provide the patient with additional tools and strategies to manage COPD. The nurse becomes confident in identifying early signs of disease exacerbation and uses this patient's situation to help the patient make the connection among early recognition, early treatment, and a positive outcome of *not* going into the hospital.

Stage 2: The nurse in this stage recognizes a lack of knowledge in chronic illness management and will seek out and use care guidelines to guide practice. She may still feel uncomfortable asking a physician for orders for additional disciplines or extra home visits but will find care guidelines helpful in providing rationale for such decisions.

Stage 1: The nurse at this stage may be comfortable performing a thorough respiratory assessment but may be less clinically competent and confident in assessing and investigating causes of disease exacerbation. She may lack specific knowledge, for example, may assume that a long-term patient with respiratory disease would know how to use her inhalers and wouldn't feel comfortable asking the patient to demonstrate her skill.

? CRITICAL THINKING

1. Why did the nurse obtain an order to assess the patient the next day?
Answer: When treating a potential COPD disease exacerbation, it is important to assess Ms. R's response to the as-needed inhaler treatment. A thorough reassessment of her respiratory status is warranted. If there is no improvement or if the symptoms significantly worsen, the physician should be notified and emergent care may be needed.

2. How will the nurse, the PT, and the OT work together to ensure the best patient outcome?
Answer: Communication and discussion about progress toward goals is essential. An interdisciplinary care plan will outline the specific areas

of intervention by the nurse, the PT, and OT. All of the clinicians should be consistent in assessing the level of dyspnea with activities during their visits and should reinforce patient education about identifying and responding to early signs of exacerbation. Ongoing communication between each discipline, via the telephone and through documentation, is essential.

Interdisciplinary Care Plan

Problem	Goal/Plan	Intervention	Evaluation
Knowledge deficit regarding disease process	Patient will verbalize the importance of minimizing COPD exacerbation triggers. Patient will identify early signs of COPD exacerbation.	Teach patient about causes of COPD exacerbation and how to minimize them. Contact physician about whether patient had pneumococcal vaccine. Teach patient about early signs, using the Stoplight tool and teach the importance of reporting.	Patient will participate in self-monitoring of disease signs/ symptoms. Patient will utilize strategies to reduce risk of disease exacerbation.
Ineffective medication management	Patient will utilize a method to improve adherence with taking medications.	Teach patient about importance of medications in optimizing disease management. Work with patient and daughter to use a pillbox and medication list to improve adherence. Teach patient about importance of sharing current and updated medication list at every doctor visit and if going into the hospital.	Patient will take medications as ordered.
Self-care deficit regarding proper use of inhaler	Patient will demonstrate correct technique for inhaler use.	Teach patient how to use inhaler properly. Obtain spacer for use with inhaler.	Patient will have less dyspnea.

(Continued)

Problem	Goal/Plan	Intervention	Evaluation
Dyspnea with ADL performance	Patient will use energy conservation strategies.	Contact physician for order for OT. Teach patient to use energy conservation measures.	Patient dyspnea is interfering less with ability to perform ADL.
Dyspnea with ambulation	Patient will demonstrate improvement in distance walked and with less dyspnea.	Contact physician for order for PT. Develop home exercise program to improve endurance.	Patient's dyspnea is interfering less with ability to ambulate and exercise.

REFERENCES & RESOURCES

[1] V.L. Carrieri-Kohlman and D. Donesky-Cuenco, "Dyspnea management," *Evidence-Based Nursing Care Guidelines: Medical-Surgical Interventions*, B.J. Ackley, B.A. Swan, G.B. Ladwig and S.J. Tucker (eds.), pp. 263–273, Mosby Elsevier, 2008.

[2] H. Mead, L. Cartwright-Smith and K. Jones et al., "Racial and ethnic disparities in U.S. healthcare: A chart book," Retrieved from the Web August 30, 2010. http://www.commonwealthfund.org/usr_doc/Mead_racialethnicdisparities_chartbook_1111.pdf 2008.

[3] National Heart, Lung, and Blood Institute (NHLBI) World Health Organization (WHO) Workshop, "Global strategy for the diagnosis, management, and prevention of chronic obstructive pulmonary disease: Executive summary," Retrieved from the Web August 30, 2010. http://www.goldcopd.org/Guidelineitem.asp?l1=2&l2=1&intId=2180 2009.

[4] Registered Nurse Association of Ontario, *Nursing Care of Dyspnea: The 6th Vital Sign in Individuals with Chronic Obstructive Pulmonary Disease (COPD)*, Registered Nurse Association of Ontario, Retrieved from the Web August 30, 2010. http://www.rnao.org/Storage/67/6135_REVISED_BPG_COPD.pdf 2010.

[5] A.L. Ries, G.S. Bauldoff and B.W. Carlin et al., "Pulmonary rehabilitation: Joint ACCP/AACVPR evidence-based clinical practice guidelines," *Chest*, 131:4S–42S, 2007.

Case 4.2 Pneumonia

By Leigh Ann Howard, RN, MSN

This case study examines the complexities of home care for a woman with multiple needs and how family dynamics play a role. Mrs. Z, a 78-year-old woman, has just been discharged from the hospital after being admitted for high fever, cough with green sputum, and decreased appetite. She fell at home and called 911. She was found to have pneumonia and broken ribs. She is the primary caregiver of her husband, who has dementia. Mrs. Z was driving and doing most activities independently before being admitted to the hospital.

 ORDERS FOR HOME CARE

Patient: 78-year-old woman
Diagnosis: Community acquired pneumonia with new oxygen (O^2)
Current Medications:
- Metoprolol 25 mg twice a day
- Azithromycin 250 mg once a day for 10 days
- Furosemide 40 mg twice a day
- multiple vitamin once a day
- Metformin 500 mg twice a day
- Prednisone Taper 20 mg for 2 days, 10 mg for 2 days, 5 mg for 2 days, 2.5 mg for 2 days
- Codeine 15 mg every 4–6 hours as needed for pain

Clinical Case Studies in Home Health Care, First Edition. Edited by Leslie Neal-Boylan.
© 2011 John Wiley & Sons, Inc. Published 2011 by John Wiley & Sons, Inc.

Relevant past medical history:
- Heart failure
- Diabetes
- Occasional falls

RN: Assess and evaluate

Reimbursement Considerations

The patient is old enough for Medicare. Medicare does have home-bound requirements. The patient is in an acute state and will qualify for Medicare home health care services.

THE HOME VISIT

The nurse arrives at the home to assess and evaluate the patient. A "frazzled" middle-aged woman answers the door. She ushers the nurse into the bedroom where the person whom the nurse assumes is the patient is resting in bed. The three exchange greetings, and the nurse starts the admission process. After verifying the patient's name and date of birth, the nurse begins the assessment.

Mrs. Z is pleasant throughout the visit but is visibly fatigued and is slow to answer questions. She is alert and oriented to time, place, self, and situation and introduces the younger woman as her daughter. Mrs. Z states that her daughter flew home to care for her father while Mrs. Z was in the hospital. Her daughter is anxious to get back home as she has teenaged children and a full-time job. Mrs. Z tells the nurse that she thinks she was so worn down by caring for her husband that she was not caring for herself. She was getting progressively sicker until she fell in the home and awoke in the hospital.

Mrs. Z's daughter interrupts at this point and asks what time they can expect the nurse every day "so I can get back home. I have a very important job." The nurse explains to the daughter what home health nursing is and believes that there is confusion between what the daughter believes is home health care and reality.

Cultural Competence

Mrs. Z is Caucasian. She has been the primary caregiver and finds herself in a new role needing to receive care. Her daughter has been overwhelmed caring for her parents and having her family so far away. It is important that they support each other with the help of any community resources as available.

The nurse notes that the couple lives in a one floor condo unit. The bathroom is handicapped accessible and the area is not cluttered. The husband is sitting in a recliner in the living room reading a magazine. He says "Hi" to the nurse and goes back to reading his magazine.

The nurse continues her assessment of the patient and the home. The patient is friendly during the process and says she "enjoys the company". The nurse notes that the patient's daughter is very anxious and impatient during the home visit.

The nurse works with Mrs. Z to establish the following goals:

- To be able to care for her husband again
- To be independent with activities of daily living (ADL)
- To not rely on her daughter as much for her total care
- To identify caretaker support systems in place to help her care for her husband

---

Neal Theory Implications

Stage 3: The nurse in this stage understands how and why the caregiver role of the patient for her husband with dementia must be considered in the plan of care. The daughter is anxious to return home. The nurse in this stage understands that the family is the patient entity and that the family must be considered when planning any care for the patient.

Stage 2: The nurse in this stage understands that arrangements must be made to provide care of the patient and her husband during this time but may not be aware of the resources that are available or how to access them.

Stage 1: The nurse in this stage is most likely to focus care on the patient and may be less aware of the implications the loss of the caregiver role by the patient has on the family dynamics and on the patient's self-image. This nurse may be less likely than nurses in other stages to include the family in the plan of care.

The history and physical exam uncovers the following data:

- Mrs. Z is having difficulty with pain on deep breathing and is only taking shallow breaths.
- Mrs. Z has very diminished lung sounds.
- Mrs. Z is new to oxygen, and it is set at 2 liters.
- Mrs. Z has lower and upper extremity weakness.
- Mrs. Z has only been standing at the bedside for bathing and using the bedside commode.

- Mrs. Z is still raising slightly yellow tinged sputum.
- Mrs. Z is unable to state her medications, what they are for and when to take them.
- Mrs. Z has +2 edema to her lower extremities.
- Mrs. Z has been continent of bowel and bladder.
- Mrs. Z has diabetes and has been having elevated blood sugars.
- Mrs. Z reveals that she has not been careful to change positions frequently.
- Mrs. Z has slight redness to her coccyx.
- Mrs. Z denies any pain or frequency with urination.
- Mrs. Z denies any problems with swallowing or speech.

? CRITICAL THINKING

1. What are some priorities for Mrs. Z's care?

Answer: Mrs. Z must be taught to splint her ribs with a pillow when coughing to help raise secretions and decrease her pain. She can be taught to do this with a pillow to splint her ribs. She and her daughter must be taught to change positions frequently, even though it may be painful in order to help prevent development of pressure sores. The nurse will speak with Mrs. Z's daughter about staying longer as Mrs. Z cannot care for herself and her husband at this time. It is also extremely important to teach and document oxygen safety.

2. What other disciplines should be involved?

Answer: Home health aides (HHA) will help in bathing the patient and with basic care needs. Occupational therapy (OT) will assist in helping the patient with ADL. Physical therapy (PT) is needed for strength and balance training and to develop and implement an exercise plan. A medical social worker (MSW) will assist with setting up community and family resources and support for the daughter. The patient may be able to receive in-home support for housekeeping, meal preparation, and errands. Long-term planning and possible assisted living placement can also be discussed. Enrolling Mrs. Z in the agency's telehealth program would also be beneficial.

Rehabilitation Needs

Physical therapy
Occupational therapy
Social worker
Home health aide

3. What would telehealth do for the patient?
Answer: Telehealth is proven to help decrease re-hospitalizations. It will allow for vital signs to be assessed every day without a nurse making a home visit every day. The telehealth nurses would be able to see any changes in patient status, blood pressure, oxygen, heart rate, and weight. Also, with Mrs. Z's history of heart failure it is very important that she get in the habit of checking her weight every day.

4. What would be some important teachable topics?
Answer: Educate on heart failure to include heart failure medications, daily weight checks, and diet. The importance of changing positions frequently needs to be taught and reinforced to help with the prevention of pressure ulcers. Medication management is also important. Mrs. Z may benefit from using a pill box to help organize her medications. Also, education is needed to be sure she knows what medications she is taking, why she takes them, and any special considerations. Fall prevention is also important as Mrs. Z is at risk for another fall. She should be reminded to call for help and use a cane or walker as appropriate.

Relevant Community Resources

Housekeeping services
Alzheimer's support groups when the patient is able to attend
Friends and family in the area who can help provide care

BACK TO THE CASE

The patient's daughter pulls the nurse aside and is tearful about leaving her parents. She says that she knows they are not ready to be alone, but she is not sure what else to do. The nurse asks the daughter if it is possible to take a leave from work in order to get things in order for her parents. They discuss having a social worker visit to help discuss community resources and possible assisted living. The daughter is in agreement with this.

The nurse discusses enrolling the patient in the agency's telehealth program. She explains that this will allow Mrs. Z to check her blood pressure, weight, pulse oximetry, and heart rate. These will be checked every day by the nurse in the agency office who can alert the doctor as necessary. The nurse reviews the medications with the patient and her daughter. The daughter states that she will pick up a pillbox to help keep all of the medications in order. She and the patient appear more at ease than they appeared on the nurse's arrival. The nurse reviews the pain medication and the patient states that she will use the pain medication before she gets to the point where the pain is intolerable. The nurse reviews the patient's blood sugars and discusses the diabetic diet with the patient and her daughter. Her daughter states that they have been eating take out foods as that is what has been easier. The nurse discusses with the daughter and the patient the importance of following a diabetic diet and quick meals that would be appropriate for the patient to eat. They will continue to keep a log of blood sugars for the nurse to review at the next visit. The patient states that she will try and get up twice a day to sit in the bedside chair. They agree that the patient will try and do deep breathing exercises frequently throughout the day to prevent further pulmonary issues. The nurse notes that the patient's daughter has relaxed quite a bit throughout the visit. She tells the nurse she feels more competent to care for her mom and will start calling family and community resources to prepare for her return home. The nurse also discusses assisted living, and the patient states that she is open to that as long as she and her husband can stay together.

Interdisciplinary Care Plan

Problem	Plan	Interventions	Evaluation
Gas exchange, impaired	Patient will continue with O2 use, deep breathing and splinting when coughing. She will use her pain medication more appropriately to help keep her pain level down and help her take deep breaths with less pain within 1 week.	Teach patient about the importance of deep breathing and coughing. Reinforce the use of splinting her cough and appropriate use of pain medication.	Patient will discuss methods to decrease her pain when coughing and deep breathing. She will continue to have clear lung sounds.
Pain, acute	Patient will use pain medication appropriately to prevent her pain from becoming intolerable within 1 week.	The nurse will educate the patient regarding pain and proper use of pain medications.	The patient will state decreased pain levels verbally and by pain scale.
Weakness generalized	Patient will have increased strength within 2 month.	Physical and occupational therapies will work with the patient to increase strength and teach exercises to maintain strength.	Patient will have more endurance to sit up in her chair or ambulate to her kitchen.

Problem	Plan	Interventions	Evaluation
High risk for impaired skin integrity	Patient and daughter will state the importance of the patient changing position by 1 week.	Nurse will educate the family on the importance of frequently changing position to prevent skin breakdown. PT/OT will work with the patient to gain strength making it easier for the patient to change position.	Patient will be free of skin breakdown issues and will increasingly become more independent with position changes.
Injury, high risk for	Patient will have increased awareness of risk for falls within 2 weeks.	The nurse will educate the patient and daughter about the importance of using a cane or walker for ambulation. PT/OT will work with the patient to increase strength.	The patient will be free from falls and demonstrates use of walker or cane for ambulation.
Potential for ineffective family coping	The patient and family will be able to cope with the increased needs of aging parents and the possibility they will continue to need increasing care within 3 months.	The nurse will continue to provide help and support. MSW will also be set up to assist the patient and family in setting up community resources in addition to supporting the family in making the necessary decisions and long term care planning.	The patient and the family will have increased resources for help and emotional support. They will demonstrate use of these resources.

REFERENCE & RESOURCE

[1] S. Schmitt, "Community-acquired pneumonia," *Current Clinical Medicine*, W.D. Carey's (ed.), pp. 717–724, Saunders, 2009.

Case 4.3 Tuberculosis

By Leigh Ann Howard, RN, MSN

This case study illustrates how the home health nurse works with a tuberculosis (TB) patient. This patient, Mr. Y, is a 32-year-old man who is a cafeteria worker at a local inner city school. His family immigrated here when we was a young man. He has limited English speaking skills, but he can read some in his own language. A few months ago he took a trip to visit family in his home country. He has always been active until the past few weeks when he started feeling ill. He has had a severe cough for the past few weeks, as well as loss of appetite, fever, and weight loss. He has been out of work for the past week and a half due to his symptoms. The patient has a young child at home, and he and his wife are expecting another child. He presented to the emergency room (ER) after developing chest pain. A sputum culture was positive for TB, and the chest x-ray was abnormal. He admits to coughing up blood. The patient says that he was afraid to tell his family this and was in denial that there was a problem. Patient education and strict adherence to TB medications is a must. Before making the home visit, the nurse reviews the agency's TB policy and ensures that the N95 mask fits properly and has a seal. The patient has requested that a male nurse be sent to visit him.

Clinical Case Studies in Home Health Care, First Edition. Edited by Leslie Neal-Boylan.
© 2011 John Wiley & Sons, Inc. Published 2011 by John Wiley & Sons, Inc.

Cultural Competence

Mr. Y is the primary caregiver for his family and comes from a very patriarchal background. He feels strongly that he is to provide for their needs and that all decisions must go through him. Health care information is not to be shared with the entire family and is to be kept private. The home care team will respect this way of life while including his family in his care. Health assessments can be done privately and out of earshot of family members if so desired. The home health agency respects the patient's request to send only male nurses. The nurse discusses with Mr. Y that there may be situations when that is not possible. Mr. Y appreciates that the agency is doing everything they can to accommodate this request as part of his cultural considerations.

 ORDERS FOR HOME CARE

Patient: 32-year-old male
Height: 5'7"
Weight: 130 pounds
Diagnosis: Tuberculosis
Current Medications:
- Isoniazid (INH) 900 mg
- Rifampin (RIF) 600 mg
- Pyrazinamide (PZA) 600 mg once a day
- Ethambutol (EMB) 750 mg once a day

Relevant past medical history: None noted.
RN: Assess, evaluate, direct observation therapy (DOT), monitor adherence to medication regime.

 THE HOME VISIT

The nurse arranges a visit time through an interpreter service, and the interpreter will meet the nurse at the patient's home. The nurse meets the patient for the first time. The patient is friendly but obviously anxious about his diagnosis. He states that he is relieved to see the nurse arrive. The home is clean, but slightly cluttered with children's toys. The nurse is greeted by a friendly dog and a toddling 18-month-old. A young woman obviously in the later stages of pregnancy, whom the nurse assumes is the patient's wife, comes out from the kitchen. She greets the nurse through the interpreter, apologizes for the house being a mess and thanks the nurse for coming. The nurse introduces himself to the patient, spouse, and child.

The nurse asks where would be a good place to talk and fill out the paperwork. The patient's spouse guides the toddler with her down the hall to another room, and the nurse and patient sit at the kitchen table. The patient is friendly and hospitable to the nurse. The nurse obtains a health history and asks how things have been going for the patient.

The patient expresses stress and fear around his health and need to work in order to continue to care for his wife and child. He is concerned about them. The patient is also concerned about being out of work for some time and is worried about finances.

Reimbursement Considerations

The patient's insurance needs fall under the local department of health as he is a patient with TB. He and his family may be eligible for Medicaid or other health services through the state.

The nurse examines the patient, and works with Mr. Y to establish the following goals:

- To remember to take his medications as prescribed
- To be able to state medication side effects and to know when to alert the physician
- To be able to cope effectively with this diagnosis
- To return to work as soon as medically possible

Neal Theory Implications

Stage 3: The nurse is aware of community resources and how they can help the patient. The nurse understands the implications of this public health problem and makes a concerted effort to alert all those who need to know about the patient and his disease in order to care for him without exposing themselves to the disease.

Stage 2: The nurse may not be fully aware of the implications of tuberculosis as a public health problem but should know about the personal protective equipment required by the agency. The nurse may not be fully aware of community resources that are available to help this patient and the family.

Stage 1: The professional in this stage may be able to recognize a need for other disciplines and resources but may not know how to incorporate them into the situation.

The nurse discovers the following data during assessment:

- Mr. Y denies having any cough.
- Mr. Y is having some difficulty sleeping due to anxiety.
- Mr. Y is anxious about the possibility of forgetting to take his medications.
- Mr. Y reports a 15-pound weight loss since last month.
- Mr. Y continues to have a decreased appetite and nausea.
- Mr. Y denies coughing up blood tinged sputum at this time.
- Mr. Y does continue to have slight chest pain.
- Mr. Y still has fatigue.
- Mr. Y has a history of depression.
- Mr. Y has periods of lose bowel movements

? CRITICAL THINKING

1. What other referrals may the nurse want to make?
Answer: The nurse may want to obtain a physician's order and make a referral for a social work visit. The social worker may know where the patient can go for help to meet both his emotional and financial needs. This may help the patient feel more in control and better able to cope with the situation.

Rehabilitation Needs

Social worker

2. What strategy may the nurse use to help the patient remember his medications?
Answer: The nurse may have access to pillboxes that can be used to help the patient organize his medications, or the patient can have a family member purchase one. The nurse can assist and observe the patient fill the box for the week. The nurse would review the importance of keeping the pillbox in a safe place where his child could not reach them. This would also help the patient to feel more empowered and a part of his care.

3. How might the nurse educate this patient on his medications?
Answer: The nurse can obtain written medication information in the patient's native language. Another idea would be to make a chart for the patient with drawn or photographed pictures of the medication and pictures of the side effects.

> **Relevant Community Resources**
>
> Community supports within cultural group
> Financial resources/food pantry

BACK TO THE CASE

The nurse begins to question the patient about his medications and discovers that the patient is not very knowledgeable about them. The patient is able to properly state when to take the medications, but he is not informed about the side effects and special considerations. He states that he just cannot remember much as he is in such fear about the diagnosis and worried about his family. He states that he is afraid he will forget to take his medications. The nurse presents him with a free agency medication box. The patient is happy about this, feels that this will help him keep everything organized, and feels that he has a little more control over his situation.

Mr. Y and the nurse also review the medication information sheets that the nurse prepared in the patient's own language. Mr. Y states that he is having trouble understanding the information on the sheets. The nurse asks him if pictures and drawings would help. He agrees that he thinks that would be the most helpful. The nurse plans a visit time to see Mr. Y the next day and plans to bring pictures or drawings of the medications.

The nurse calls the patient's physician and relays how the visit went. The nurse requests an order for the social worker to help Mr. Y cope with his situation and identify community and financial resources. The physician is agreeable to this and thanks the nurse for the information.

Interdisciplinary Care Plan

Problem	Plan	Interventions	Evaluation
Knowledge deficit surrounding disease process	Patient will acknowledge verbal understanding of tuberculosis within 3 days.	Teaching will include culturally relevant and appropriate materials and the use of interpreters as needed.	Patient will participate in educational activities. He will verbalize knowledge with the nurse.

(Continued)

Problem	Plan	Interventions	Evaluation
Impaired gas exchange	By the next visit, the patient will alert the nurse and physician with any changes in respiratory, issues including cough.	Discuss and teach signs and symptoms to be alert for. Alert physician's office that patient will alert them immediately should there be changes.	Patient is able to list to the nurse symptoms that would need to be made known to the physician. Patient also verbalizes the reasons why it is important to do this.
Nutrition altered: Less than body requirements	Patient will be able to discuss appropriate nutritious foods within 3 weeks.	Nurse and patient will discuss nutritious foods with consideration to the patient's culture.	The patient will gain 1 pound a week by eating nutritious foods until he reaches the appropriate weight for his height and age.
Fear	Patient will verbalize fears regarding taking care of his family and his diagnosis within the first week.	Nurse will discuss feelings of fear and validate those feelings. Nurse will contact physician to see if treatment for depression should be initiated and collaborate with community resources for counseling.	Nurse will evaluate and document the patient's moods in addition to questioning the patient about feelings of fear.
Knowledge deficit regarding medications	Within 3 weeks, the patient will be able to discuss medications and when to take them.	Nurse will teach the patient with appropriate materials regarding the medications. This may mean pictures, charts, and graphs.	Patient will be able to tell/show the nurse his medications, when he takes them, and when to notify the doctor. This may include using pictures, charts, and graphs.

REFERENCE & RESOURCE

[1] O.C. Ioachimescu and J.W. Tomford, "Tuberculosis," *Current Clinical Medicine*, W.D. Carey's (ed.), pp. 789–795, Saunders, 2009.

Section 5

Gastrointestinal

Case 5.1 Stomach Cancer

By Sharron E. Guillett, PhD, RN

This case study illustrates how the home health nurse works with the family of a non-English speaking patient to provide end-of-life care in a culturally appropriate manner for a patient with a gastrointestinal cancer. The patient is a 94-year-old Vietnamese female, diagnosed with end-stage pyloric cancer and dementia. She lives with her daughter and son-in-law who report that she has recently begun to wander at night and has fallen attempting to get to the bathroom. The family is determined to care for her at home. Integrating supportive therapies with cultural practices is essential to providing quality care for the patient and her family.

 ORDERS FOR HOME CARE

Patient: 94-year-old Vietnamese female
Diagnoses: Dementia, pyloric cancer, hemorrhoids
RN: Assess and evaluate.
Current medications:
- Reglan 10 mg once a day 6 hours as needed
- Bextra 10 mg once a day
- Docusate 100 mg once a day
- Nexium 40 mg once a day at bedtime
- Zantac 150 mg twice a day
- Prevacid 5 mg once a day

Clinical Case Studies in Home Health Care, First Edition. Edited by Leslie Neal-Boylan.
© 2011 John Wiley & Sons, Inc. Published 2011 by John Wiley & Sons, Inc.

- Xanax 0.5 mg at bedtime
- Skelaxin 200 mg three times a day
- KU-Zyme 1 cap four times a day

Relevant past medical history: Arthritis

THE HOME VISIT

The nurse arrives at the patient's home, which is a small, two-story condominium. The home and yard are well kept. There is one short flight of steps to a covered porch where many pairs of shoes are arranged outside the door. A woman dressed in white pants and a uniform smock greets the nurse at the door. The woman smiles but apparently does not understand or speak English. She bows slightly and motions for the nurse to come in. The nurse returns the bow, shows the woman her stethoscope, takes off her shoes in the entry hall, and waits to be taken to the patient. A woman who does speak English comes down from the second floor and introduces herself as the patient's daughter. The daughter takes the nurse to the kitchen where the patient is lying on a daybed against the back wall of the room. This is where the patient stays during the day and sleeps at night. It is near the bathroom.

The woman who answered the door is introduced as the "cook". It appears that the cook provides meals and supervision for the patient while the daughter is at work. The daughter works at a nearby accounting firm that serves Vietnamese clients. A rather disheveled looking gentleman then comes downstairs and is introduced as the son-in-law. He works nights and sleeps most of the day, but he is home in case there is a problem with the patient. He speaks English but not as well as his wife. After making introductions, he returns upstairs to sleep.

The nurse turns her attention to the patient, who is wearing a long-sleeved garment over a short-sleeved top, a knit hat, long pants, socks, and slippers. She is covered with a blanket. It is warm in the kitchen, so the patient appears overdressed. Her skin is pale, but her face is flushed. The nurse bows slightly and introduces herself to the patient. The daughter translates, explaining to Ms. W why the nurse has come. Ms. W smiles (she is edentulous) and motions for the nurse to sit next to her. Once the nurse is seated, Ms. W points to her abdomen, her back, her knees, and her head. The daughter explains that Ms. W has chronic constipation and pain in her knees because of arthritis. The head and back pain are the result of a recent fall. It is the falls that have prompted the request for home care services.

Further questioning reveals that Ms. W has begun to get up in the night to use the bathroom and has fallen several times. The daughter now sleeps in the kitchen on a cot that she places next her mother's bed. The nurse notes that there is a walker and portable commode folded up and not in use. The daughter explains that Ms. W will not use either one. The nurse notes that there are a number of medication containers on a bedside table along with a number of containers written in a foreign language. The daughter explains that they also have a traditional physician who provides them with herbal medicines. She does not know what they are made of but says that their purpose is to improve appetite and strength. The nurse begins the assessment by examining Ms. L's head and back for signs of injury. Finding no redness, bruising, or tenderness, the nurse continues with the standard admission assessment.

Cultural Competence

Ms. W is Vietnamese and still follows traditional therapies. Like the Chinese, many Vietnamese people believe in the concept of yin and yang. This concept is based on the belief that health requires balancing the positive and negative forces of the universe and that illness results if there is an imbalance between these forces. Food is commonly used as treatment [2], but in Ms. W's case food use is limited due to her pyloric mass.

Older Vietnamese people commonly consult an herbalist and mix Western medicine with traditional therapies. The daughter needs to be taught the potential dangers of mixing herbs and Western medications.

Many Vietnamese believe pain and illness are experiences to be endured and therefore do not take medications prescribed for pain relief. This may explain in part why Ms. W has 2 pain relievers ordered and 4 medications related to stomach acidity. It may be that the physician believes the medication is not working when in fact it is not being taken.

Her daughter and son-in-law feel strongly about keeping Ms. W at home and allowing her to die there. The family needs to know that they can change their mind at any time and that hospice care is available for them at home as well as in a health care setting.

Ms. W is pleasant and cooperative, smiling often. The daughter provides the history and reports the following: Ms. W denies stomach pain, nausea, or vomiting but feels bloated most of the time and does complain of "gas" and "heartburn". She feels the need to defecate frequently but is unable to pass stool. Currently she has "small BM" only every "couple of days," intake is minimal and consists primarily of soups and Ensure. There has been a 5-pound weight loss over the last few weeks, which is making the patient weak. The daughter believes that Ms. W is more confused lately and that this plus the weakness are causing her to "fall a lot".

The nurse examines Ms. W and finds her vital signs within normal limits; lungs are clear; skin is dry and intact with turgor consistent with her age. Nail beds are blue tinged, and conjunctivae are pale. The abdomen is slightly distended but soft and nontender, and bowel sounds are present. Ms. W is able to stand without assistance and takes a few steps. She is weak but steady.

Reimbursement Considerations

The patient is eligible for residential care, but the family has requested a Medicaid waiver for the elderly and disabled in order to have home care. Ms. W's level of care score is 6, which allows her to have only 25 hours of care per week. This not enough to provide an overnight caregiver Monday through Friday. The nurse, as case manager on this case, will need to negotiate with the home care agency to utilize respite hours beyond those originally allowed.

When the exam is completed, the nurse explains that Ms. W qualifies for residential care and asks the daughter what her goals are. The daughter explains that they are aware that Ms. W is terminal and that if she continues to refuse food she will likely die. The family has decided to keep Ms. W at home and to let her die at home. She reveals that they do occasionally have her "transfused" at the doctor's office when she is "very weak".

The nurse establishes the following goals for Ms. W:

- Prevent further weight loss
- Prevent injury
- Manage therapeutic regimen
- Provide palliative care
- Minimize disruption of family members' health and cohesion

Neal Theory Implications

Stage 3: The professional in this stage is confident and collaborates with other disciplines both within and outside of home care. She contacts the herbalist to determine what traditional "medicines" are being given to the patient and makes sure the medical provider is aware of the complementary therapy being utilized. The nurse is respectful of cultural ways but firmly and gently advocates for the patient.

Stage 2: The professional in this stage may not feel comfortable contacting the herbalist or questioning the family's methods. She may accept the family's refusal for outside help without exploring the reasons for the refusal, overlooking significant resources that would be of benefit.

Stage 1: The clinician in this stage will assess the patient and recognize the need for assistance with the case, but the language barrier and cultural health habits may create uncertainty as to how to proceed in the home setting.

Based on the history and physical examination, the nurse discovers the following data:

- Ms. W has profound weakness but is able to take a few steps unassisted.
- Ms. W has reflux and occasional epigastric pain.
- Ms. W has arthritic pain in the knees.
- Ms. W consistently consumes 2 or 3 cans of Ensure per day.
- Ms. W is confused at night and at risk for injury.
- Ms. W is taking many meds for the same diagnosis and combining them with unknown herbal therapies.
- The daughter and son-in-law are sleep deprived and experiencing increased stress due to caregiver responsibilities.

? CRITICAL THINKING

1. What is the priority of care for Ms. W?
Answer: The priority of care must always be safety. The factor that places patients at the highest risk for falls is a history of falls. The nurse and Ms. W's daughter need to explore possible solutions for minimizing the likelihood of injury. Since Ms. W tends to fall at night, a health aid who will assist Ms. W to the bathroom at night is essential. Other strategies include leaving a dim light on during the night, removing all scatter rugs, providing bathroom rails and grab bars, and using side rails on the daybed.

2. What is the priority for Ms. W's family?
Answer: The priority for the family is respite care. Ms. W's daughter is overwhelmed with the responsibility of caring for her mother, managing her job, and keeping her marriage stable. She is not sleeping at night, which is affecting her work; and she is reluctant to have "outsiders" in the home while her husband is sleeping for fear his rest will be

disrupted and his job will be jeopardized. It is essential that the family develop a trusting relationship with the nurse as case manager, and it is important for the health care team to show respect for the family's living patterns and to keep disruptions to a minimum.

Relevant Community Resources

Housekeeping services
Respite care
Hospice or palliative care services

---

3. Is there anyone else who should be called into this case?
Answer: Yes. The nurse should call the physician for orders for a home health aide (HHA), dietician (D), and a medical social worker (MSW). Considerations should be given to starting hospice care in the home. This option should be discussed in the home and with the physician.

4. What will each of these disciplines do?
Answer: The HHA will visit Ms. W biweekly to help her bathe and dress, put the dirty laundry in the washing machine, and tidy the bathroom and Ms. W's living space.

The dietician will assess Ms. W's nutritional intake and caloric needs and develop a diet plan that incorporates her cultural preferences, promotes elimination, and retards gastric reflux. The MSW will assist the family in finding respite care at night so the daughter can get sufficient sleep and so that Ms. W will remain safe at night. The MSW will also work with Ms. W's family to find culturally relevant hospice/palliative care resources to provide quality end-of-life care for both Ms. W and her family.

BACK TO THE CASE

The nurse explains to Ms. W's daughter that her mother can be kept comfortable while the daughter is at work and safe while the daughter sleeps, with a minimum of outside help. The nurse assures her that the team will respect their cultural practices and beliefs and that the goal is to support the family in providing care, not to take their place The nurse calls the primary care provider (PCP) to discuss the multiple medications addressing reflux, acidity and pain and requests that duplicates be discontinued. The physician agrees to discontinue Zantac, Prevacid, and Skelaxin.

| ? | **CRITICAL THINKING** |

1. How will the members of the interdisciplinary team communicate with Ms. W, the daughter, and the "cook?"
Answer: Ms. W's daughter will write out some key phrases for salutation and courtesies and some key terms such as "pain," "bathroom," "hunger." A picture board will be used. Ms. W's daughter is also available by phone at her workplace.

2. What will happen after each discipline makes its initial visit?
Answer: Team members will communicate by phone and arrange to hold a monthly case conference that includes the patient's daughter by phone or in person. Each team member will reinforce what the other members are doing with the patient and family. Each team member will be alert to changes that indicate a decline in the patient's condition warranting a shift from promoting health to providing a peaceful dignified passing.

Interdisciplinary Care Plan

Problem	Goal/Plan	Intervention	Evaluation
Risk for injury due to falls	Patient will be free of injury.	Provide nighttime caregiver. Keep dim light on in patient's room. Get side rail for daybed. Install safety bars in bathroom. Remove scatter rugs and clutter.	Patient will navigate environment without injury.
Pain in knees	Patient will have reduced pain in lower extremities within 2 weeks.	Encourage patient to take pain meds as ordered. Get prescription for liquid analgesics. Teach alternative pain management strategies.	Patient states pain in knees is a 2–3/10.
Altered elimination: constipation	Patient will maintain bowel pattern.	Promote high fiber liquids. Teach family members to assess and document character and quantity of stool. Assess bowel sounds at each visit.	Patient has small formed bowel movement every 1 to 3 days. Abdomen remains soft. No impaction evident.

(Continued)

Problem	Goal/Plan	Intervention	Evaluation
Altered nutrition: Less than body requirements	Patient will increase calorie intake.	Contact dietitian to plan diet that is consistent with patient's diagnosis and food preferences. Provide small, frequent liquid meals.	Patient's weight will remain stable.
Caregiver stress	Daughter will identify resources that decrease burden of caregiving. Daughter will report getting adequate rest.	Provide daughter with list of community resources as well as MSW contact numbers. Provide information related to home and agency hospice care. Encourage daughter to express feelings about caregiving (personal and use of resources).	Daughter is sleeping in her own room. Daughter and her husband are able to maintain employment. Daughter verbalizes satisfaction with caregiving arrangements.

REFERENCES & RESOURCES

[1] American Association of Colleges of Nursing. http://www.aacn.nche.edu/elnec

[2] V. Edmonds and P. Brady, "Health care for vietnamese immigrants," *Journal of Multicultural Nursing & Health*, 9:52–58, 2003.

[3] National Cancer Institute. http://www.cancer.gov

[4] Vietnam-Culture.com. http://www.vietnam-culture.com.

Case 5.2 Malnutrition/Anemia

By Linda Royer, PhD, RN

This case illustrates the complexities that a chronic disease generates and the ingenuity required of an intuitive home health nurse. Mrs. B, a 72-year-old Caucasian female, was served by a nonprofit home health Agency 8 years ago when she needed physical therapy after a knee replacement brought on by rheumatoid arthritis (RA). At that time she and her spouse were educated about self-care management including diet, medications, and activity. She was discharged satisfactorily after 2 months. In the interim, her husband died, her daughter and family moved 1,200 miles away, and her son was convicted of a felony and is serving 15 years in prison. Her son's wife takes no interest in Mrs. B's well-being, even though she lives in the same neighborhood.

Cultural Competence

Mrs. B may feel like an outsider because her son is incarcerated, and she may need support.

The experienced nurse from that agency visits in the morning, knowing that the visit will take about 1½ hours and that some referrals will have to be initiated. She drives alone to a low socio-economic neighborhood that she is familiar with in a middle-sized city. Driving down Mrs. B's street she takes note of single and multiple dwellings in a mixed state of order and repair or disrepair. At the corner Quick

---

Clinical Case Studies in Home Health Care, First Edition. Edited by Leslie Neal-Boylan.
© 2011 John Wiley & Sons, Inc. Published 2011 by John Wiley & Sons, Inc.

Mart, about a dozen Hispanic would-be laborers linger in the parking lot looking for an invitation to work. The homes on Mrs. B's block have uncluttered yards and a new coat of paint, the result of a cooperative neighborhood improvement campaign in the Spring. The patient's two-story bungalow is half painted; her trash is overflowing the receptacle; the dog run at the side yard has odorous excrement piles. Mrs. B has been living alone with her cocker spaniel, Fritz, as her companion and "protector."

Previous trips to this neighborhood for other patient referrals have revealed that a national chain grocery store is 3 blocks away. A bus line runs through the neighborhood. An ambulatory postman delivers mail, and police regularly patrol so that the crime rate has declined in the past 3 years.

Mrs. B has been referred to home health for professional case management by the hospitalist physician who managed her overnight inpatient hospital stay for abdominal pain and tarry stools, the third in as many months. She was discharged yesterday.

Reimbursement Considerations

The patient is enrolled in Parts A, B, and D of Medicare. She has no private insurance, but she receives a small pension from her career as an employee of the telephone company. She also receives Social Security payments (from which her Medicare A and B premiums are deducted). While she was hospitalized, Medicare Part A covered her expenses (provided the institution "accepts assignment" or charges no more than Medicare). She was strongly advised by the patient representative there to apply for Medigap insurance (Medicare Supplement Insurance). Part A also covers home health services as long as they are medically necessary, particularly as she is homebound (cannot leave the home without assistance). Part B covers her primary care—both medical and preventive. Unfortunately, Medicare does not cover routine dental care or dentures. Because she has Parts A and B, she applied for Part D of Medicare, which covers her medication costs. At the beginning of each year she must meet the deductible before the coverage resumes. And there is a small out-of-pocket co-pay required when prescriptions are filled. Because of her limited array of medications, she probably will not run the risk of dealing with the "donut hole"—the coverage gap when expenses for her drugs have reached $2,830 and further purchases are out of pocket until they reach $4,550 when Part D resumes for the rest of the year. In fact, Mrs. B has wondered if the monthly premiums for Part D are really necessary, particularly if they total more than the actual cost her medications would be without it.

ORDERS FOR HOME CARE

Patient: 72-year-old African American female

Diagnoses: Gastritis, gastric bleeding, tarry stools, iron-deficiency anemia (Hgb = 9.5; normal minimum = 12), secondary to mismanagement of rheumatoid arthritis

Medications:
- Iron 325 mg once a day
- Celebrex 100 mg twice a day

Relevant past medical history:
- 3 recent hospitalizations for gastrointestinal bleeding
- Uncontrolled pain due to RA of hands, right shoulder, knees, and back
- Overuse of analgesics
- Weight loss; malnutrition

RN: Assess and evaluate home setting; case manage; monthly phlebotomy for reticulocyte count and hemoglobin and hematocrit.

THE HOME VISIT

Mrs. B welcomes the nurse cordially. She is frail and thin and appears weak. She can ambulate only a few steps before she becomes dyspneic. A quick environmental scan of the home inside reveals unswept floors and bedclothes on the couch where she has been sleeping for sometime because of her inability to negotiate the stairs to her bedroom and bathroom on the second floor. Dirty dishes are in the sink and on the counter, some with moldy food in them. Only a few food items—mostly soup cans—are seen beyond the open cupboards. There is dry food in the dog's dish. The kitchen screen door is unlatched so that the dog may go outside as needed.

The nurse accepts the chair Mrs. B offers her and attends actively to the immediate past history related to her about her illness. As she talks, it becomes evident that she is of average intelligence and developmentally consistent with her age. She examines her affect for signs of depression and counts her respiratory rate and depth for adequate oxygen support while she places an oximeter clamp on her finger. She notes the paleness of her conjunctivae and skin turgor quality for hydration and looks for edema of the lower extremities, all this while building rapport and listening to Mrs. B's discourse. She then gains permission to assess her blood pressure and auscultate her heart and lungs. The nurse continues with her assessment by asking about her urinary habits, color of urine and characteristics of any bowel movements she may have had since arriving home. She is eager to gain a diet recall from Mrs. B because of apparent lack of food supplies and household management. Mrs. B offhandedly brushes her off with the statement, "I eat mostly cream soups and milk to soothe my stomach; I get along all right." The nurse opens the refrigerator to see only some dairy products, eggs, white bread, and sodas. "I don't like vegetables, and fruit is too acidy," she says. "How are you sleeping at night?" the nurse asks. "I don't sleep too good; my jumpy legs keep me awake a lot."

The OASIS assessment is conducted and, supplemental to that, the Patient Health Questionnaire–2 is used to screen for depression. Once the assessment is complete, the nurse begins to formulate her nursing diagnoses and her plan of care. The nurse notes the following data:

- The patient's facial affect is somewhat flat; she smiles very little and wears a worn, pinched expression as she rubs her knees and knuckles. She obviously is in pain and struggles to look unconcerned about it. On inquiry, the patient does have her prescriptions and has taken her analgesic this morning with a small glass of milk.
- The O^2 saturation by oximeter is 89. Because of her pain the patient breathes shallowly and strains. Her nail beds are pale and venous return is slow. Breath sounds are clear, but respirations are shallow. Her heart rate is 90, BP is 96/66. There is 1+ edema of her ankles and feet; her feet are bright pink.
- The patient's skin is dry and turgor reveals slight tenting. The nurse hands her a fresh glass of water to drink during the visit. Mrs. B reports that her urine is very dark yellow and of low volume. Further questioning revealed she drinks water by the sips— approximately 2 glasses per day. She has seen no tarry stools today.

The nurse asks Mrs. B: "What most concerns you now?" The answer is surprisingly, "The care of my dear Fritz. I can't take him for walks like I used to. We would walk through the neighborhood and visit with the neighbors. Now, he just lies around watching me. I can't even go out with him in the yard as often as he needs, so the yard is looking and smelling pretty bad."

Relevant Community Resources

Housekeeping services from a contractual provider. Mrs. B will have to pay for those services.
Area Agency on Aging: To provide transportation to the Senior Center for socialization and oversight.
Support groups for individuals with RA and for families of the incarcerated

When asked to continue, she mentions the following:

- "My jumpy legs . . . they bother me so at night that I can't sleep. I remember my father had this problem." (Restless leg syndrome is common with arthritis and anemia and may diminish with successful treatment. The cause is uncertain and a cure is unsure. [NINDS; Reuters])
- "My pain and the threat of more bleeding in my stomach."
- "My teeth are bad; they say I need to have them all out and get dentures. I dread that . . . and it costs so much."
- "I miss my son and my daughter and the grandchildren. She had to move with her husband because his company sent him. He got a raise by doing that. She hated to go and leave me. She calls every week, but she is busy, works, too. My son is in prison, you know. I haven't been able to see him in 4 months; he is only about 30 miles away. My daughter took me before they moved away."

The nurse asks the patient to identify some immediate goals the team can work on together and notes the following:

- To feel stronger and as pain free as possible
- To clean up her house and get the outside paint job completed; to find someone to clean up her yard
- To be able to go upstairs to her room again

Neal Theory Implications

Stage 3: The nurse in this case is comfortable synthesizing her observations of the patient and her environment with the services she can provide through the home health agency, and she is knowledgeable of community resources. She is also confident in the capabilities of other disciplines on the team and can plan interventions incorporating them. The nurse began to plan her approach to care as she drove through the neighborhood and walked to the front door of Mrs. B's home.

Stage 2: The professional in this stage may not feel comfortable collaborating with the physician regarding orders for other disciplines, case management, and working within the patient's environment to manage care.

Stage 1: A newly-hired nurse may have had orientation and education about home care but is still hesitant in garnering professional and community services, since she is not yet familiar with them and has not formed relationships with contacts. She has much to

(Continued)

learn about the roles and functions of the other team members. Having never worked with an occupational therapist before, she is unaware that improvements can be made in mobility and coping with RA by this discipline. Medicare regulations are a confusing maze to her thus far, and how to interpret changes in health care reform will pose difficulty for some time. She has worked with certified nursing assistants before, but she is still unsure of the reimbursement boundaries on the functions of the home health aide.

There are many concerns in this home, and the nurse realizes from experience with chronically diseased elderly people that changes toward improved quality of life often take time with incremental steps of acceptance of new lifestyle practices. However, she realizes that facilitating a safe and relatively symptom-free lifestyle will create emotional and mental health, physical strength, greater interest in social relationships and, ultimately, less expense to the health care system that serves her.

? CRITICAL THINKING

1. What are the priorities for this case?
Answer: While many critical observations have been made concerning the patient, her lifestyle, and her environment, the foremost problem is facilitating the healing of her stomach and restoring her gastrointestinal system to normal function. Each time she experiences a bout of gastric bleeding, her body stores weaken more than before, eliciting a recurrence of anemia. In fact, elderly patients with chronic RA are typically anemic, not necessarily due to depleted iron stores. Other priorities from the patient' point of view are to put the house in order, meal preparation, and food shopping until the patient has strength enough to accompany a home health aide to the store where they can select foods the patient will accept. Housekeeping services will clean the home and do the laundry on a weekly visit.

2. Are there referrals that are appropriate at this time?
Answer: Yes—a dietician to assess, teach, and develop a nutritious meal plan. The dietician should include the aide on a joint visit to plan the shopping and menu planning; An Occupational Therapist (OT) to teach joint-saving, safe, and strengthening activities and to assess the home for safer, conservational adjustments; a medical social worker (MSW) to determine economic assets and needs and to address the

bitter relationship with her daughter-in-law and possible community support for home management, supervision of the dog's health and care, future independent shopping, and social relationships, such as the Senior Center. Also, the MSW can address the need for better contact with the patient's son.

Rehabilitation Needs

Occupational therapy

BACK TO THE CASE

There is a difference between anemia of chronic disease (which Mrs. B may naturally have due to the RA) and iron-deficiency anemia. Scientists note that chronic anemia in the elderly is due to the inability of the body to utilize the iron that is stored in the reticuloendothelial system. In fact, the iron stores may be increased, but unavailable [10]. The HHN, the dietician, and the aide will work together with her in developing a healthful eating lifestyle with foods high in vitamins and minerals in the texture and frequency that aids healing. The nurse has attended a conference on health care needs of the elderly in which anemia was addressed as a public health crisis—3 million+ elderly (65+) in the U.S. are anemic. Even in mild cases the risk for functional impairment and increased mortality is of concern [5]. Common physical performances of standing, rising from a chair, and walking decline; and more co-morbidities are brought on through weakness.

Secondary to that problem is the administration of analgesics. Providers have tried several analgesics with Mrs. B with varying degrees of success. Celebrex is a new one for her. It is important that she take it as prescribed along with proper nutritional intake and adequate fluids to avoid gastric side effects. The nurse will need to monitor the effectiveness of this new medication and observe for any side effects. Common side effects with Celebrex are: constipation, diarrhea, dizziness, gas, headache, heartburn, nausea, sore throat, stomach upset, and stuffy nose. Gastrointestinal (GI) side effects have included nausea (3.5% to 9.09%), upper abdominal pain (7.32% to 10.4%), dyspepsia (2.8% to 8.8%), abdominal pain (1.3% to 8.5%), vomiting (less than or equal to 7.3%), diarrhea (4.9% to 10.5%), gastroesophageal reflux (4.7%), and flatulence (2.2%). Constipation, diverticulitis, dry mouth, dysphagia, eructation, esophagitis, gastritis, gastroenteritis, hemorrhoids, hiatal hernia, melena, stomatitis, tenesmus, tooth disorder, intestinal obstruction, intestinal perforation, GI bleeding, colitis with bleeding, esophageal perforation, pancreatitis, cholelithiasis, and ileus have been reported in less than 2% of the patients (http://www.Drugs.com).

The nurse will instruct Mrs. B to take Celebrex whole with meals to reduce side effects, to avoid adding other nonsteroidal anti-inflammatories to her regimen, to avoid drinking alcoholic beverages, and to report any of the above symptoms to her physician or the nurse. To augment the pain-relieving properties of Celebrex, Mrs. B might use a topical agent such as Bengay or Voltaren Gel on her painful joints, which will then bypass the stomach and bring local relief.

Rest is important to building strength, and the patient's restless leg syndrome is disturbing her rest and sleep in the evening and night. To avoid resorting to prescription drugs, the team will work with natural interventions, such as warm baths, increased exercise during the day, and her improved diet. Once her anemia is corrected, the problem may retreat.

The team will monitor the patient's state of emotional health as improvements are made in her care management. Should the need for intervention become apparent, a referral to psychological services will be sought from the physician.

Education and assistance in activities of daily living (ADL) until strength is gained and she gives evidence of managing herself satisfactorily are important to Mrs. B's independence and self-determination. It is prudent to empower her toward restoration of health rather than to provide minimal services and see her move to a nursing home.

? CRITICAL THINKING QUESTIONS

1. What will the other team members do?
Answer: The dietician will visit 2 or 3 times to assess and teach restorative dietary practices and will guide the aide in collaborative meal planning and cooking. She will also consult with the nurse. The OT will assess flexion, movement, and capability of Mrs. B's hands and arms and will teach conservation movements and strengthening activities that will safely maintain use of her extremities. The OT will also give suggestions for assistive devices if necessary and for adjustments in the features of the home to facilitate movement and necessary activities.

The MSW will examine Mrs. B's economic assets to test for eligibility for any further or long-term services under state or federal programs, and she will assist her in choosing and applying for supplemental insurance. She will introduce her to senior services through the Area Agency on Aging and to support groups for both individuals with RA and for families of incarcerated individuals. She will look for supportive dynamics of the neighborhood to obtain help for yard cleanup and exterior painting. Mrs. B indicated that she used to attend the Baptist church; the pastor will be contacted with her permission so that their outreach services might be extended to her. Finally, she will attempt to meet with the daughter-in-law to facilitate reconciliation with Mrs. B and work toward a helping relationship between them. The aide will assist with bathing and other aspects of hygiene and prepare one balanced meal for her daily times 2 weeks and then reduce her visits to 3 per week. A housekeeper will clean the home and do the laundry in Mrs. B's washer and dryer.

2. How will the team communicate?
Answer: Since the hospitalist physician ordered case management, the nurse is confident that she can make referrals to the rest of the team. Once all have made their first visits and assessed from their perspectives, they will meet in the office to discuss their management plan and create collaborative goals that the nurse will share with Mrs. B at her next visit. The team will meet again for a case conference in a month to determine progress.

Interdisciplinary Care Plan

Problem	Goal/Plan	Intervention	Evaluation
Knowledge deficit regarding management of arthritis, medications, and nutrition, as evidenced by (AEB): weakness, blood loss, weight loss, pain, inadequate diet recall	Patient will describe the relationships among adequate therapeutic nutrition, fluid balance, restorative mobility techniques and regular exercise, and responsible medication regimen in 1 week and will demonstrate changing behaviors compliant with the above in 3 weeks.	The nurse will establish a restorative care plan among a multidisciplinary team and continue to teach patient about her chronic condition, reinforcing education of other members. The nurse will monitor vital signs, weight, draw labs as ordered and interpret to patient. The dietician will teach and demonstrate proper diet with support of the aide.	With a goal of self-care management aided by family and community support, the nurse will measure knowledge and behavior change weekly, collaborating with the physician toward discharge from home health in 3 months.

(Continued)

Problem	Goal/Plan	Intervention	Evaluation
Potential risk for mental/ emotional disruption— depression, sleep loss, AEB: flat affect, expressed anxieties, poor coping strategies with chronic disease	Patient will experience hope, peace, and confidence in self-care management once condition is improved, a support system is in place, and strategies are learned for coping with discomforts of chronic disease.	Team will monitor for decline in depressive symptoms and anxieties; and nurse, aide, and OT will introduce acceptable treatments for RLS and insomnia.	Once anemia has been corrected, diet has been improved, and strength has been gained, expect to see decline in RLS and to see improved sleep, leading to improved mental health.
Hygiene and environmental deficits	Patient will assume self-care once strength is gained and pain diminished. The clean home environment will elicit motivation and pride.	Provide home health aide, intensely at first, to assist with hygiene of self, facilitate adequate nutrition. Shop for, cook, and serve one meal per day M-F for 2 weeks, and then 3 times per week. Housekeeper will restore cleanliness and order to home environment. MSW will recruit individuals to clean up the yard.	Expect patient to manage hygiene independently in 2 weeks and to assume easy household tasks in 3 weeks.
Financial concerns	Potential for decline into need for institutional housing if medical and nursing needs are not met. Potential for decline to poverty status if unable to assume self-care and homestead management. Uncertainty about financial supports and future health care costs.	MSW will assess financial needs, concerns, and desires of patient and will advise and refer to community sources as needed.	Patient will demonstrate responsibility toward financial obligations and homestead management.

Problem	Goal/Plan	Intervention	Evaluation
Lack of social support—familial and community	Potential for risk of further depression without meaningful contact with family and neighbors. Cannot continue in home without support of custodial services of the community.	MSW will establish contact and a plan of regular communication with the daughter and her family. She will attempt to improve relationship with nearby daughter-in-law for regular support. She will collaborate with prison authorities and community sources to establish a visiting schedule with her son.	Family and community supports will be put in place to effect stability of patient in her home by discharge time (3 months).

REFERENCES & RESOURCES

[1] "Celebrex," Retrieved June 9, 2010, from http://www.drugs.com/celebrex.html

[2] L. Goodnough and A. Nissenson, "Anemia and its clinical consequences in patients with chronic diseases," *The American Journal of Medicine*, 116(7a): 18–19, 2004.

[3] C. Jacelon, "Managing the balance: Older adults with chronic health problems manage life in the community," *Rehabilitation Nursing*, 35(1):15–24, 2010.

[4] "Modified Pyramid for Elderly." http://nutrition.tufts.edu/1197972031385/Nutrition-Page-nl2w_1198058402614.html

[5] V. Picozzi, "Anemia in the elderly: a Public Health crisis in hematology. ASH Special Symposium: Anemia in the Elderly," *Hematology*, 2005:528–532, 2005.

[6] T. Sheeron, C. Reilly, M. Weinberger, M. Bruce, J. Pomerantz, "THE PHQ-2 on OASIS-C: Identifying geriatric depression among home health patients," *Home Healthcare Nurse*, 28(2):92–102, 2010.

[7] A. Harding, "Restless leg syndrome runs in families, study confirms," *Reuters News Service*. Retrieved June 9, 2010, from http://www.reuters.com/article/idUSTRE64A4CV20100511

[8] "Restless leg syndrome, National Institute Neurological Disorders and Stroke (NINDS)," Retrieved June 9, 2010, from http://www.ninds.nih.gov/disorders/restless_legs/detail_restless_legs.htm.

[9] W. Shiel, "Restless leg syndrome, MedicineNet," Retrieved June 9, 2010, from http://www.medicinenet.com/restless_leg_syndrome/article.htm

[10] D. Smith and W. Sheckler, "Anemia in the elderly," *American Family Physician*, 62(7):1565–1572, 2010.

Section 6

Genitourinary

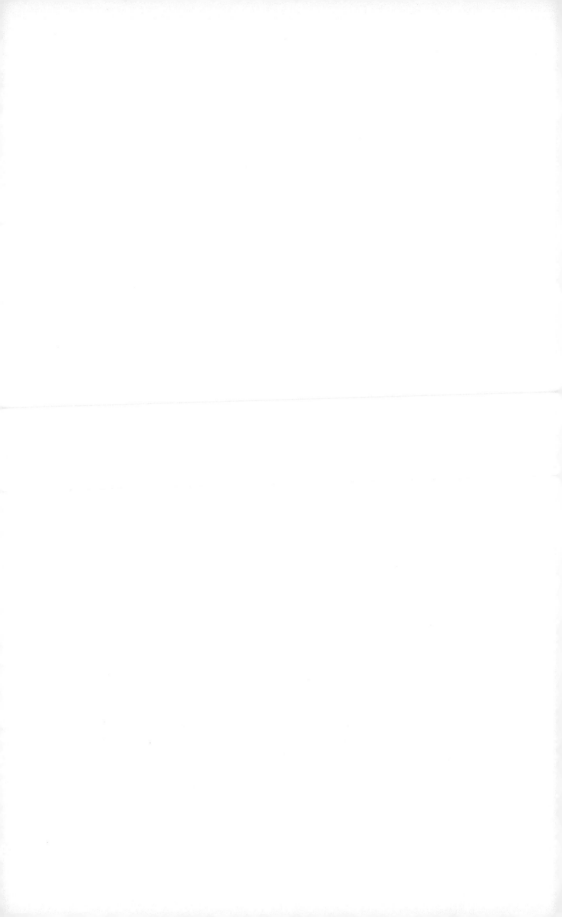

Case 6.1 Neurogenic Bladder

By Kathleen Francis, RN, MSN, CWOCN

This case illustrates how the nurse works with the patient and her significant others to achieve positive outcomes by individualizing the plan of care to meet the goals and expectations of the patient. By assisting the patient and her family in adapting to her illness, the nurse can increase the patient's independence and improve the patient's ability to maintain her health.

Mrs. J is a 51-year-old female with a past medical history of multiple sclerosis (MS), hypertension, and hypothyroidism, who is admitted to the home health agency for skilled nursing services management of her Foley catheter. The patient was recently hospitalized for sepsis secondary to urinary tract infection (UTI). Mrs. Jones is known to the agency and has received multiple services in the past related to her disease progression, such as skilled nursing, physical therapy (PT), occupational therapy (OT), and medical social work (MSW). Prior to hospital admission, the patient was able to manage her neurogenic bladder with

Cultural Competence
Mrs. J is a white American female. Her family is very supportive and available to assist her in any way necessary. The patient would like to be as independent as possible. The team will need to provide positive feedback to the patient and family members and encourage their ongoing support as the patient works toward maximizing her functional status to improve her quality of life.

Clinical Case Studies in Home Health Care, First Edition. Edited by Leslie Neal-Boylan.
© 2011 John Wiley & Sons, Inc. Published 2011 by John Wiley & Sons, Inc.

clean intermittent catheterization (CIC), but she has had increased difficulty performing CIC secondary to reduced manual dexterity as her disease has progressed. She reports that she has had some recent difficulty with constipation. The patient also receives weekly self-administered intramuscular injections.

 ## ORDERS FOR HOME CARE

Patient: 51-year-old female
Diagnoses: MS, neurogenic bladder, indwelling Foley catheter
Current medications:
- Baclofen 20 mg tablet by mouth three times a day
- Diovan 80 mg tablet by mouth once a day
- Avonex 30 mcg by intramuscular injection once weekly
- Levofloxacin 250 mg by mouth once a day for 10 days
- Synthroid 100 mcg by mouth once a day

Relevant past medical history:
- Hypertension
- Hypothyroidism

RN: Assess and evaluate. Manage Foley catheter. Change Foley catheter monthly. Instruct patient and caregiver about catheter care. Assess patient's ability to self-administer Avonex (interferon beta 1a). Instruct the spouse as needed to ensure continued independence with this treatment regimen.
PT: Assess and evaluate.

Reimbursement Considerations

The patient is too young to be eligible for Medicare and has too much income and too many assets to qualify for Medicaid. If she was employed and became disabled for 24 months, she may be eligible for Medicare; however, she has not been employed since her daughter was born. She may be eligible for Medicaid in the future. At present her health care is covered under her husband's policy, which is managed care insurance. Their insurance policy does not limit the number of home care visits. However, insurance company approval is required for all services, and the services must be deemed necessary.

The nurse, as the case manager, will need to negotiate with the insurance company for any needed approvals. In addition, the nurse (as well as the PT, OT, and MSW) will need to thoroughly document all services. Upon discharge, the insurance company will likely ask for a copy of the record to verify and review the episode of care. If the insurance company identifies that the visit documentation is incomplete, they will request reimbursement for those visits.

THE HOME VISIT

On admission, the visiting nurse identifies that the patient lives with her spouse and two teenage children in a single-family home. The house and grounds are well kept, clean and non-cluttered, with a ramp access located next to her driveway. The home is a three-bedroom, two-story structure with a bedroom and bathroom located on the first floor. The patient's husband and teenage daughter are present and assisting her during the admission. Both have verbalized that they are able and willing to learn, as needed, all aspects of her care. The nurse conducts the initial assessment interview with the patient's husband and daughter present. However, the physical assessment is performed in the patient's bedroom to maintain her privacy.

The patient is alert and oriented and able to respond appropriately. The patient denies any food or medication allergies. The skilled nursing assessment indicates that the patient is afebrile with a temperature of 98.7 degrees Fahrenheit; her blood pressure is 130/80 mmHg; her apical/radial pulse is 88/88 with a regular rhythm. Her respiratory rate is 20/minute, with no adventitious sounds on auscultation. Her abdomen is soft, non-tender when palpated, with bowel sounds auscultated in all four quadrants of her abdomen. There are no abdominal bruits on auscultation. The patient denies any bowel problems and reports that she has regular bowel movements (BMs) every other day. Her last BM was one day ago, per patient report. Her skin is soft, dry, of normal color, and intact with no skin lesions or pressure ulcers. She appears well nourished.

The patient is able to ambulate with a rolling walker and close supervision. The patient utilizes the following durable medical equipment (DME) to perform her activities of daily living: a wheelchair with a high-end pressure redistribution cushion, a wheeled walker, and a wheelchair lift.

The Foley catheter is a 14-French silicone type catheter connected to a bedside urinary drainage bag. The catheter is intact and patent, draining clear amber urine in good amounts. The patient has expressed difficulty ambulating with the bag in tow and is fearful that she may dislodge the tube or fall over it.

Relevant Community Resources

MS support group
Community agency for independent living

Mrs. J denies any feelings of depression or sadness. However, she verbalizes frustration regarding the need for the urinary catheter and drainage bag and wishes she could return to her previous level of functioning. She expresses anxiety and embarrassment related to her altered body image. She mentions that she is fearful of having intercourse with the catheter in place and would prefer to return to her prior level of functioning.

The patient does not appear to have a hearing deficit. She is wearing eyeglasses and informs the nurse that they are progressive-type lenses that she wears all of the time for both distance and near vision. She is able to read the medication labels with her corrective lenses in place. She denies the presence of pain that may interfere with her ability to perform activities of daily living, and she appears to be free of pain when she moves about.

Rehabilitation Needs

Physical Therapy
Occupational therapy

When the nurse has completed gathering data and her assessment, the nurse and patient identify the following goals:

- The patient will be free of infection.
- The patient will have increased endurance and improved manual dexterity.
- The patient will return to her previous level of functioning.
- The patient will be able to manage her neurogenic bladder utilizing CIC.
- The patient will be able to self-administer her injection.

Based on the history and physical examination, the nurse discovers the following data:

- The patient has a good support system available.
- The patient has increased fatigue, requiring assistance with some of her activities of daily living (ADL).
- The patient has poor endurance.

Neal Theory Implications

Stage 3: The professional in this stage collaborates with other disciplines both within and outside of home care and is autonomous with the clinical aspects of the case and the logistical aspects of working with the agency. This nurse understands and appreciates the limitations of the patient's environment but also how the environment and the patient's lifestyle can be utilized to optimize self-care management and quality of life.

Stage 2: The professional in this stage may not feel comfortable collaborating with the physician regarding orders for other disciplines, case managing, working within the patient's environment to manage care. This nurse may not be confident enough to request the orders needed from the PCP or to make recommendations that might have to be defended in a discussion with the PCP.

Stage 1: The clinician in this stage will assess the patient and recognize the need for assistance with the case but may be unsure as to how to proceed in the home setting. This nurse may not understand how to translate hospital practices regarding catherization and the use of indwelling catheters to the home setting in which CIC and clean technique is used and the patient manages her own catheterization.

- The patient has anxiety related to her altered body image.
- The patient is continent of bowel.
- The patient has neurogenic bladder dysfunction.
- The patient is at high risk for a urinary tract infection that will have an impact on her neurogenic bladder management.
- The patient does not have difficulty with speech or swallowing.
- The patient has normal visual acuity.
- The patient is sexually active and has increased anxiety secondary to the presence of the indwelling catheter.

? CRITICAL THINKING

1. What is the priority for care for Mrs. J?
Answer: Since Mrs. J is not exhibiting difficulty ambulating with assistive devices and her home is equipped with the necessary DME, safety is established. However, she has verbalized difficulty ambulating with

the urinary drainage bag, and this may create a fall risk. The nurse can provide and instruct the patient on the safe way to utilize a leg bag apparatus in place of the urinary drainage bag while she is out of bed and ambulating. This would require the nurse to instruct the patient on the proper way to change the bags without contaminating the tubing so that the patient is not at an increased risk for infection.

2. What is the next priority for her care?
Answer: The next priority for care is to keep the Mrs. J free from infection. She has an indwelling catheter to manage her neurogenic bladder dysfunction. She will require instructions on catheter care and management. In addition, she has verbalized dissatisfaction with this method of urinary incontinence management. PT and OT services can help Mrs. J return to her optimal level of functioning.

3. What goals do you think the PT can help Mrs. J to achieve?
Answer: The PT will determine the patient's needs and goals for therapy. The PT can teach the patient exercises to increase endurance and to strengthen her upper and lower extremities. Once her endurance is improved, she may be able to self-administer her injection, manage her urinary incontinence (UI) with CIC, and have an increased level of functioning.

4. What goals do you think the OT can help Mrs. J to achieve?
Answer: The OT can assist the patient to become independent in the self-management of UI and injection administration. The OT will evaluate the patient's needs and goals and can instruct the patient about the use of assistive devices to achieve her goals. The OT will also instruct the patient regarding exercises that she can do to increase her endurance and manual dexterity.

5. Is there anyone else who should be called to this case?
Answer: Yes. The patient should have an MSW evaluation to assist the patient with long-range planning and community linkage. The patient has verbalized anxiety related to her altered body image and may require additional counseling for sexual dysfunction (real or perceived) due to the presence of the indwelling catheter.

Neurogenic Bladder

Urinary continence is generally defined as the ability to store urine in the bladder until the bladder can be evacuated at a socially acceptable time [1, 5, 6]. Continence is a result of the complex interrelationship of psychosocial, physiologic, and mechanical factors [5, 6]. Urinary bladder elimination involves relaxing the pelvic floor muscles, contracting the detrusor muscle, and simultaneously opening the urethral sphincter to achieve complete emptying of the bladder [4–6]. An intact neurological system is essential for these activities to occur [3, 5, 6].

Multiple sclerosis (MS) is a chronic, demyelinating, autoimmune condition that affects the central nervous system. Although the clinical course of MS is unpredictable, it generally presents with a pattern of relapsing and remitting symptoms that may result in increased functional loss [11]. Patients with MS commonly have bladder storage problems and incontinence, such as urinary retention, bladder spasticity, overactivity, and incomplete emptying of the bladder [7, 11].

When the neurologic lesion affects the spinal segments C2 to S1, the associated bladder symptoms are termed reflex UI or neurogenic bladder and can result in damage to the upper urinary system due to the occurrence of detrusor sphincter dyssynergia (DSD) [5, 6]. DSD is described as the loss of coordination between the bladder and the urethral sphincter. The detrusor muscle contracts, but the sphincter does not consistently relax, resulting in an obstruction of the bladder outlet [5, 6]. DSD obstructs urine flow, causing large amounts of residual urine to be left in the bladder. This can result in upper urinary tract distress, with damage to the renal parenchyma, by increasing the potential for bacteriuria and urinary tract infections [3, 5–7].

Management of Reflex UI

CIC is a common method utilized to manage reflex UI. CIC involves insertion of a straight catheter into the bladder at specified time intervals, usually every 4 to 6 hours, depending on the individual. CIC can be considered as a management option for patients who have sufficient manual dexterity or a willing caregiver to perform the catheterization and a bladder capacity greater than 200 cc (required to prevent bladder and renal complications) [1–3, 8]. Generally, if the patient has the functional ability to dress and feed him or herself, they have the functional ability to perform CIC[3]. The advantages associated with this method include regular, complete bladder evacuation for the patient and a reduced effect on the patient's body image with an unaltered appearance of the genitalia. Studies indicate that the long-term compliance with this method is substantial [2, 5, 6].

The long-term use of an indwelling catheter for the management of reflex UI has been associated with multiple complications, including infection, bladder spasms with urine leakage, urethral erosion, calculi, bladder cancer, and hematuria [5, 6, 9]. In addition the long-term use of indwelling catheter has the highest rate of patient dissatisfaction [5, 6]. Because of this, indwelling catheter use should be reserved for those patients for whom it is the best option. When an indwelling catheter is selected as the best management option for the patient, serious thought should be given to the creation of a suprapubic cystostomy as this alternative can eliminate the risk for urethral erosion. However, it does require a minor surgical procedure for placement [5, 6].

Catheter Care and Patient Instructions

Indwelling catheter placement is accomplished using strict aseptic technique. Ensuring that the catheter is well lubricated will prevent urethral trauma. Once the catheter is in place and the balloon is filled according to the manufacturer's recommendations, the catheter should be secured. Unsecured catheters can lead to complications, such as urethral erosions, bleeding, and bladder spasms [10]. For the ambulatory patient, a leg bag may be preferred as it is less cumbersome and easier to conceal. The patient can then attach the catheter to a larger drainage bag at night, when they go to bed. The nurse can instruct the patient to attach the nighttime drainage system directly to the leg bag using the bottom spout so they can maintain a closed system and reduce the risk of catheter-associated urinary tract infections [10].

Patients and caregivers should be instructed on routine care of the indwelling catheter intended to prevent complications. Instructions should include the positioning of the drainage bag and tubing, measures to maintain a closed system and prevent contamination, catheter stabilization, and adequate fluid intake [10] (Table 6.1.1).

If CIC is utilized to manage reflex UI, the patient is typically taught to self-catheterize using clean technique. Teaching the caregiver or family members can increase compliance if the patient becomes ill and

TABLE 6.1.1. Points to emphasize when teaching caregivers.

Indwelling Catheter Care

- Keep drainage bag off the floor, and position drainage bag below the level of the bladder at all times to prevent reflux.
- Keep drainage tubing straight and free of kinks, and don't allow the tubing to fall below the level of the drainage bag.
- Empty the drainage bag when one-half to two-thirds full to avoid undue traction on the catheter.
- When emptying the drainage bag, do not allow the spout to come in contact with the collection container or the floor.
- Disinfect the urine collection containers after each use.
- Drainage bags can be cleaned with a vinegar solution of one part vinegar to three parts water (1:3) or a bleach solution of 1 ounce bleach and 10 ounces of water (1:10).
- Adequate fluid intake is important to prevent catheter-associated urinary tract infections by promoting a constant flow of urine.
- Limit caffeinated beverages and avoid bladder irritants such as alcohol, smoking, carbonated beverages, artificial sweeteners, heavily spiced foods, and citrus fruits and juices as these can increase bladder spasms.
- Perineal cleansing is recommended, and the ambulatory patient can shower. The area can be cleansed gently avoiding catheter manipulation as this can increase catheter-associated urinary tract infection (CAUTI).
- The use of petroleum based creams or ointments should be avoided as this can degrade the catheter material.

unable to self-manage. Patient and caregiver instructions should include pharmacologic and non-pharmacologic methods to reduce bladder spasms and urinary leakage between catheterizations. If necessary, the physician can include an anticholinergic, such as oxybutynin, to the patient's medication regimen. Some common side effects include dry mouth and constipation. Frequently, the patient may reduce fluid intake to avoid urine leakage that occurs in between catheterizations. Patients should be instructed to avoid fluid restrictions unless instructed to do so by their doctor, as concentrated urine can irritate the bladder causing increased detrusor spasms. Instead, the nurse should encourage adequate fluid volume intake with fluids evenly distributed throughout the day and avoidance of high volume intake over a short period of time [5, 6] (Table 6.1.2).

TABLE 6.1.2. Points to emphasize when teaching patients and caregivers.

Clean Intermittent Catheterization

- The CIC can be performed using clean technique.
  a) Instruct patient or caregiver to wash their hands prior to performing the CIC.
  b) Instruct the patient to identify the urethral opening (females use a mirror).
  c) Lubricate the tip of the catheter and insert the catheter gently.
  d) Resistance may be felt as the catheter passes the sphincter. Instruct the patient to use steady gentle pressure to advance the catheter until urine starts to flow.
  e) Once the urine is drained, the patient can gradually remove the catheter to ensure complete emptying of the bladder.
  f) Instruct the patient to wash their hands and the catheter when they have completed the catheterization procedure.
- The catheters can be washed in antiseptic soap and water. If needed, they can be flushed with a syringe.
- Once the catheters are cleaned, they can be air dried and placed in a plastic container or storage bag.
- CIC frequency should be every 4–6 hours.
- Normal bladder capacity is approximately 500 cc, limiting fluid intake and ensuring timely CIC will prevent overdistention of the bladder.
- The volume of urine in the bladder should be maintained at or below 450 cc.
- If the patient consistently has urine volumes >450 cc, increased CIC frequency may be required.
- Avoidance of caffeine and bladder irritants (see Table 6.1.1) can reduce the incidence of bladder spasms and urine leakage between CIC.
- Signs and symptoms of urinary tract infection, including new or increased urinary leakage between catheterizations, cloudy or foul-smelling urine, or not feeling well should be communicated to their primary care physician for evaluation.
- Always take a "travel kit" when leaving home. The kit should include all of the necessary supplies for catheterization away from home.

The visiting nurse explains to the patient that she may be able to achieve independence with her UI management and with her injection, pending additional therapy. Since the patient has been able to self-manage in the past using CIC, then she may be agreeable to a plan of care that includes returning to this management option. The nurse may suggest PT and OT evaluations to achieve this goal. PT can have a positive effect on the bladder management program by maximizing the patient's wheelchair mobility and endurance and occupational therapy can be instrumental in developing any needed assistive devices [3, 5, 6].

The patient and her family are agreeable to the plan. The nurse explains that she will need to instruct the patient and family on the care of the indwelling catheter (see Table 6.1.1) as this will not be removed without an alternative plan for UI management and physician approval. The nurse instructs the patient about safety and ensures that the catheter is secured on the patient's anterior thigh with tape to prevent inadvertent removal. Since the patient has expressed anxiety related to the tube and drainage bag, the nurse can use this opportunity to discuss some of the feelings (self-image) that the patient may have regarding the indwelling catheter. The nurse recommends an MSW referral. The patient's initial reaction to this suggestion is negative. However, she reluctantly agrees with the encouragement of her husband.

The nurse calls the primary care provider (PCP) to report her assessment, findings, and recommendations. The nurse asks the PCP for additional orders:

- MSW evaluation for resource and community linkage and for long range planning
- OT: To assist the patient to have increased endurance and improved manual dexterity so that she can self-manage her UI via CIC
- The nurse also asks the physician if the patient can use a leg bag rather than the urinary drainage bag during the day to prevent falls and increase patient acceptance.

The nurse also discusses the patient centered goals for care, which are that the patient would like to return to her previous level of functioning. The PCP approves the plan of care with the additional orders. As for the UI management, the PCP states that the patient will need to be evaluated by urology before any changes in UI management can occur.

Interdisciplinary Care Plan

Problem	Goal/Plan	Intervention	Evaluation
Weakness in upper and lower extremities	Patient will have increased strength in all extremities within two months.	PT will help the patient engage in increasing levels of physical activity and exercise. Teach patient strengthening exercises.	Patient is able to participate in self-care activities related to increased strength.
Fatigue	The patient will have strategies to manage fatigue within 1 month.	Exercise Promotion PT will help the patient engage in increasing levels of physical activity and exercise. Exercise can reduce fatigue and help the patient build endurance for physical activity. The OT can provide the patient with assistive devices and teach the patient energy conservation techniques. Encourage the patient to use assistive devices for ADL and IADL: long-handled sponge for bathing Encourage the patient to identify tasks that can be delegated to others. Delegating tasks and responsibilities to others can help the patient conserve energy.	The patient will report less fatigue and increased ability to self-manage activities of daily living.
Risk for infection related to indwelling catheter	The patient will be free from infection.	Monitor for signs of infection: cloudy urine, sediment in urinary drainage system, abdominal pain, fever, malaise, etc. Teach the patient/family catheter care. Teach hand washing. Encourage adequate fluid intake (>2000 cc/day). Instruct the patient on medication regimen and antibiotic treatment. Ensure medications are taken as directed. Teach patient and caregiver the signs and symptoms of infection and when to report these to the physician or nurse. See Table 6.1.1 for indwelling catheter care instructions.	The patient remains free from urinary tract infection.

(Continued)

Problem	Goal/Plan	Intervention	Evaluation
Neurogenic urinary incontinence	The patient will be able to self-manage her UI using CIC within 2 months.	PT/OT services to increase patient's ability to self manage/increase manual dexterity Followup with urology related to patient's ability to manage UI with CIC. Teach patient CIC procedure using aseptic technique. Ensure adequate fluid intake. Teach/instruct patient on medication regimen (antispasmodic) as ordered. See Table 6.1.2 for CIC instructions.	Patient has increased manual dexterity and is able to self-manage UI with CIC using aseptic technique.
Ineffective coping: individual and family	The patient and family will be able to cope with her disease process and altered body image.	Assist family in setting realistic goals. Encourage family members to seek information and resources that increase coping skills. Refer family to social service or counseling.	The patient will verbalize acceptance of her altered body image. The patient will have resources for emotional support and use them.

REFERENCES & RESOURCES

[1] B.T. Benevento and M.L. Sipski, "Neurogenic bladder, neurogenic bowel, and sexual dysfunction in people with spinal cord injury," *Physical Therapy*, 82(6):601–612, 2002.

[2] Consortium for Spinal Cord Medicine, "Consortium Bladder Management for Adults with Spinal Cord Injury: A Clinical Practice Guideline for Health Care Providers," Retrieved July 25, 2010, from http://www.pva.org/site/DocServer/Consumer_Guide_Bladder_071410.pdf?docID=13861 2010, June.

[3] K.F. Francis, "Management of bowel and bladder continence following spinal cord injury," *Ostomy/Wound Management*, 53(12):1–9, 2007.

[4] M. Gray, "Anatomy and physiology of the urinary system," *Fecal and Urinary Diversions: Management Principles*, J. Colwell, M. Goldberg and J. Carmel (eds.), pp. 163–183, Mosby, 2004.

[5] M. Gray, "Pathology and management of reflex incontinence/neurogenic bladder," *Urinary and Fecal Incontinence: Current Management Concepts* (3rd ed., Rev.), D. Doughty (ed.), pp. 187–221, Mosby, 2006.

[6] M. Gray, "Physiology of voiding," *Urinary and Fecal Incontinence: Current Management Concepts* (3rd ed., Rev.), D.B. Doughty (ed.), pp. 21–50, Mosby, 2006.

[7] J. Litchfield and S. Thomas, "Promoting self-management of multiple sclerosis in primary care," *Primary Health Care*, 20(2):32–39, 2010.

[8] G.C. Pellatt and T. Geddis, "Neurogenic continence. Part 2: Neurogenic bladder management," *British Journal of Nursing*, 17(4):904–913, 2008.

[9] J.M. Smith, "Indwelling catheter management: From habit-based to evidence-based practice," *Ostomy/Wound Management*, 49(12):(June 5, 2010) doi. http://www.o-wm.com/content/indwelling-catheter-management-from-habit-based-evidence-based-practice 2003.

[10] J.M. Smith, "Current concepts in catheter management," *Urinary and Fecal Incontinence: Current Management Concepts* (3rd ed.), D.B. Doughty (ed.), pp. 269–304, Mosby, 2006.

[11] J. Winland-Brown and J. Rhoads, "Neurologic problems," *Primary Care: The Art and Science of Advanced Practice Nursing* (2nd ed., Rev.), J.W.-B. L.Dunphy, B. Porter and D. Thomas (eds.), pp. 78–84, F. A. Davis Company, 2007.

Case 6.2 Urostomy Care

By Kathleen Francis, RN, MSN, CWOCN

This case illustrates that the nurse can assist the patient in verbalization of feelings of anxiety related to his disease process and change in body image and in identification of realistic goals to maximize level of function and independence. In addition, the nurse can offer suggestions that will help the patient adapt his altered personal needs (urostomy care) to his cultural beliefs.

Mr. B is a 62-year-old African American Muslim male with a past medical history of type 2 diabetes mellitus, gastroesophageal reflux disease, hypertension, hyperlipidemia, and bladder cancer, who is status post radical cystectomy and pelvic lymph node dissection with the construction of an ileal conduit for urinary diversion (urostomy). The patient is married with 5 adult children, and has been employed for 33 years as a lawyer for a local law firm. He is the sole breadwinner in the household and is anxious to return to work.

Cultural Competence

Mr. B is an African American Muslim male. Observant Muslims pray 5 times a day.

It is very important to observe strict personal hygiene during prayer, and therefore a ritual cleansing process is required before prayer. It is important that the team ask Mr. B about his religious practices so the team can act appropriately to assist Mr. B in a way that is conducive to his practices. Mr. B may want to change the bag prior to each prayer. Therefore a 2-piece system is most convenient for him; otherwise, the skin may be damaged by frequent removal of the adhesive [2].

ORDERS FOR HOME CARE

Patient: 62-year-old African American, Muslim male

Diagnoses: Bladder cancer, surgical removal of the bladder, and creation of ileal conduit for urinary diversion

Current medications:

- Benazepril 20 mg by mouth once a day
- Simvastatin 40 mg per day by mouth once a day in p.m
- Glucophage 500 mg by mouth twice a day
- Omeprazole/sodium bicarbonate 20 mg by mouth once a day
- Cephalexin 500 mg by mouth twice a day
- Acetaminophen 650 mg by mouth every 4–6 hours as needed for pain

Relevant past medical history: Hypertension

- Diabetes
- Gastroesophageal reflux disease
- Bladder cancer

RN: Assess and evaluate patient for safety and postoperative management of ileal conduit. Teach patient self-management techniques. Assess and evaluate midabdominal incision line; monitor it for signs and symptoms of infection.

Follow-up appointment with urologist in 1 week for evaluation and removal of stents.

Follow-up appointment in 2 weeks with oncology.

Reimbursement Considerations

The patient is 62 years old and may qualify for Medicare. However, he is employed and has managed health care (HMO) coverage through his employer. Most HMO coverage plans limit home health care service visits to no more than 120 per year, and/or they require HMO authorization for continued home health care visits. The nurse will need to ensure that he/she documents and communicates the need for continued home health services to the managed care case coordinator to obtain authorization for all home health service visits. Some agencies have a managed care department that can obtain the written reports from all disciplines and communicate these reports (via electronic records) to the HMO to secure needed approvals. If the HMO does not issue approval for home health care services, the patient will need to be informed so that he can make the decision to accept the services for a predetermined fee. Many home health care agencies have systems in place to obtain needed authorizations for services. In addition, some HMO's do not cover the cost of disposable supplies, such as dressing supplies and gauze. The patient may need to contact his insurance company to find out the details of his coverage regarding ostomy supplies.

THE HOME VISIT

The patient lives with his wife and 3 adult children in a private 2-story home. The home is clean, well kept, and uncluttered; but there is an odor of urine in the air. The patient is found sitting on the living-room sofa. He is dressed in loose fitting gym pants and a t-shirt. His wife is nearby and offers to get his papers from the hospital and the list of medications. She appears happy and relieved to see the nurse, while the patient does not appear happy at all. Upon questioning, the patient admits he is anxious and states, "I don't like being ill, and I have no idea where this is all going. I really do not like the 'not knowing'!"

Once the preliminary questions are answered, the visiting nurse asks the patient if he would prefer to complete the physical assessment in the privacy of his bedroom. He agrees, but would like his wife to look on so she too can learn how to pouch his stoma. Mrs. B follows them into the bedroom, reluctantly. During the removal of the pouch and examination, her facial expression is one of disgust. The nurse notices that the patient appears embarrassed, and the wife tries to busy herself doing other tasks rather than looking at the patient's abdomen.

The patient is alert, oriented, and able to verbalize. His skin color is normal, with normal temperature and texture. He appears well nourished with a height and weight of 6'2" and 200 pounds. However, the patient reports that he has, "lost about 25 pounds over the last 3 or 4 months." His vital signs are as follows: blood pressure is 140/88, heart rate (apical/radial) 72/72, regular with no ectopic beats noted; respiratory rate 24, lungs clear with no adventitious sounds noted. No edema noted in his extremities. Capillary refill is less than 3 seconds. Strong bilateral pedal pulses are palpable, his toes are warm and mobile, and his feet are free from injury. His abdomen is soft, with bowel sounds audible in all four quadrants; the midline incision is well approximated with staples; the healing ridge is palpable; periwound is intact, with no erythema noted. The right lower quadrant stoma is pink, well budded, with urinary stents visible in the os and draining amber urine. The stoma is pouched with a two-piece pouching system connected to a gravity drainage bag. The nurse notes that the wafer is taped at the corners. Upon questioning, the patient reports that there was some urine leakage, so he taped it to secure the bag. He admits that he does not know how to change the wafer and was afraid to try it alone.

The patient reports that he does not have pain and has not had to take his pain medication. He is able to ambulate independently. He has normal vision but requires reading glasses and is able to read the medication labels with his reading lenses.

After obtaining the assessment data, the nurse asks the patient to identify his goals. They are as follows:

- He will be independent with his urostomy care.
- He will be able to resume activities (personal/sexual/religious).
- He will be able to go back to work.
- He will return to his previous level of health and be cancer free.

Neal Theory Implications

Stage 3: The nurse in this stage will be knowledgeable and comfortable managing a urostomy and teaching the patient and family about its care. He will immediately see the value in including the WOCN and the MSW in the patient's care.

Stage 2: The nurse in this stage might be inclined to manage the urostomy the way it would be managed in the hospital setting without taking into account the home environment, the patient's religious/ethnic priorities, and the wife's difficulty accepting the situation.

Stage 1: The nurse in this stage may be uncomfortable managing the patient's care in the home and might need guidance from a more experienced home health nurse to arrange the care and interdisciplinary team.

Based on the history and physical exam, the nurse identifies the following data:

- The patient has a support system available (wife).
- The patient's incision is healing well with no signs of infection.
- The patient's urostomy is draining amber urine in good amounts via patent stents.
- The patient's urostomy pouch is leaking.
- The patient is unable to self-manage the urostomy.
- The patient's wife was not able to assist effectively.
- Mrs. B's reaction to the urostomy may impact negatively on the patient's ability to accept it and return to his previous level of health.

- The patient and his wife are having difficulty coping with the change in his body image.
- The patient and his wife are having difficulty coping with the change in his health status.
- The patient will need to be independent with his urostomy in order to return to work.

? CRITICAL THINKING

1. What is the priority for Mr. B?
Answer: The priority for Mr. B is to prevent infection. He has an abdominal incision that is not yet fully healed; and if his ileal conduit continues to leak, it may impair the wound healing process and cause a wound infection. Pouching the stoma with an appropriate pouching system that does not leak and helping Mr. B to self-manage it will prevent the ileal conduit from leaking and possibly contributing to postoperative wound infection.

If urine leakage is allowed to remain on abdominal skin, the peristomal area will become denuded and prone to fungal infections which will have a negative effect on the pouch seal, as a weeping peristomal area will not allow an adhesive barrier/wafer to adhere to the area and it becomes difficult to obtain an adequate seal.

2. What can skilled nursing services do to help Mr. B reach his goals?
Answer: Skilled nursing services can assess and monitor the patient's wound for progress toward healing and can instruct the patient regarding when to notify the nurse or the physician. The nurse can assist the patient to become independent with his urostomy care and can also help him to become more at ease with his changed status by maintaining a nonjudgmental approach. She can offer suggestions to the patient and his wife related to self-management, troubleshooting, and ADL tips to help the patient return to his previous level of functioning.

3. Is there anyone else who should be called into the case?
Answer: Yes. Since the patient and his wife have demonstrated difficulty in accepting the change in the patient's body image and health status, the patient should have a medical social worker (MSW) evaluation for long-range planning and community resource linkage.

Rehabilitation Needs

Medical social worker
Wound ostomy continence specialist
Patient may require ongoing psychological counseling.

If the nurse is unable to obtain adequate pouch seal, he may suggest that the patient be evaluated by a wound ostomy continence specialist (WOCN) or enterostomal therapy nurse (ETN). Some home health care agencies have WOCN/ETN available for home health care visits. Others may be able to direct the patient to an ostomy clinic in their region or area. These are usually affiliated with the hospital clinics.

4. What will each of these disciplines do?
Answer: Nursing will assess and monitor the patient's physical and emotional status and continue to monitor his abdominal incision wound for healing progress. The nurse will also instruct the patient about ileal conduit/urostomy care and self-management skills. In addition, the nurse will instruct the patient and wife on dietary concerns (related to the stoma), and about how to obtain needed supplies. He can direct the patient and family to resources available in their community (United Ostomy Association, American Cancer Society). The nurse can initiate sexual counseling, based on the PLISSIT model [1] that involves four levels: permission, limited information, specific suggestions, and intensive therapy. If intensive therapy is needed, the nurse will refer the patient to a specialist for further counseling.

The MSW will evaluate the patient and council him and his family regarding acceptance of his changed body image and health status. The MSW will also be able to assist the patient to identify resources in his community and access to his needed supplies as well as initiate sexual counseling. The MSW may suggest ongoing psychotherapy if the patient demonstrates the need for continued therapy and sexual counseling.

5. How will the members of the interdisciplinary team communicate with each other?
Answer: The members of the team will document their initial assessments, evaluations, and recommendations in the electronic medical record, making this information easily accessible to other members of the team. They can communicate via electronic mail, telephone case conferences and hold a monthly case conference that includes the patient either by phone or in person. Case coordination and communication are essential components of the home health care plan.

BACK TO THE CASE

The nurse removes the leaking urostomy appliance (Figure 6.2.1.) and discovers that the peristomal area is denuded, with weeping satellite lesions noted in the periphery. The stoma is pink, budded; and the mucocutaneous junction is intact with sutures visible. There are 2 stents protruding through the os. These are patent and draining amber urine.

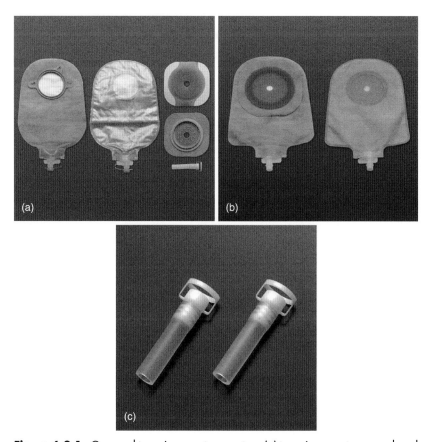

Figure 6.2.1. One- and two-piece urostomy system: (a) two-piece urostomy pouch and barrier; (b) one-piece urostomy pouch, and (c) urinary drainage bag connector. (Photos from Hollister online brochure.)

The patient has some additional pouches and barriers that the WOCN gave him in the hospital. The nurse determines that a WOCN evaluation may be needed and plans to schedule a joint home visit (RN and WOCN) within the week. In the meantime, he demonstrates the process for changing the urostomy appliance to the patient and his wife. The nurse teaches them about peristomal care and cleaning and then dusts the denuded area with stomahesive powder. He measures the stoma, cuts the barrier to the identified dimension, and applies the barrier and pouch. Once the barrier and pouch are applied, the nurse demonstrates how to empty the pouch and how to change the pouch so that the patient can self-manage before prayer.

The RN also demonstrates how to connect the nighttime drainage system so that the pouch does not get overfilled and pull off the abdomen, which would cause leakage under the barrier. The RN also suggests that the patient utilize an ostomy belt to help secure the wafer, especially if the patient will be bending during prayers. The RN instructs the patient to empty the pouch when it is one-third full and that doing this in conjunction with the usage of the nighttime drainage system will prevent urine and moisture from being in contact with the area around the stoma which can contribute to increased bacterial growth [1]. He explains that the barrier and pouch will need to be changed if a leak is detected. This will prevent the skin from becoming irritated and damaged. If that occurs, the wafer may not adhere properly, compounding the problem that may result in additional leakage.

By the end of the initial visit, the patient is able to verbalize the steps in the pouch changing process and he is able to demonstrate emptying the pouch as well as how to connect it to the nighttime drainage bag. He verbalizes his satisfaction with the visit and is looking forward to the WOCN/RN joint visit. He has the telephone numbers for emergency contact, if needed.

The nurse plans the next visit in 48 hours as the pouch will need to be changed at least every 2 days and as needed for leakage due to the current condition of the surrounding skin.

Relevant Community Resources

United Ostomy Association: http://www.ostomy.org/
Friends of Ostomates Worldwide: http://www.fowusa.org/ newsite/page.php?page=home
American Cancer Society: http://www.cancer.org/
Wound. Ostomy Continence Nurses Society: http://www.wocn. org/

After the visit, the RN telephones the physician to discuss the initial assessment and the plan of care. He asks for additional orders: MSW evaluation for counseling and long range planning needs and antifungal powder for dusting the peristomal area. The physician agrees to the proposed plan of care and will call the patient's pharmacy for the order of nystatin powder. This can be dusted around the stoma with the stomahesive powder with each pouch change.

The ileal conduit is the most frequently performed urinary diversion for the treatment and management of invasive bladder cancer [4, 5]. A segment of the ileum is used to form the ileal conduit stoma, and the ureters are then anastomosed to the ileal segment so that the urine can drain through the stoma into an external collection pouch [6] (see Figure 6.2.2.). Because the area of the small bowel is used to form

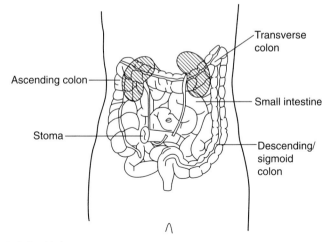

Figure 6.2.2. Abdomen.

Equipment: Skin barrier/wafer, drainable urostomy pouch, scissors, measuring guide, washcloth or soft paper towels, and plastic bag for disposing of old pouch.

1. Empty pouch into toilet.
2. Gently remove current pouch using care not to injure the underlying skin.
3. Gently cleanse around the stoma with water; then pat dry.
4. Measure stoma with measuring guide (up to six to eight weeks after surgery).
5. Transfer the measurement to the cut to fit barrier and cut the barrier opening to the required size.
6. Remove the paper backing and apply the barrier to the abdomen. Hold in place for 30-60 seconds so the pressure and warmth can activate the adhesive.
7. Apply urostomy pouch to skin barrier and test for secure seal; ensure the pouch spout is closed.
8. You can shower with the pouch in place.
9. Use a night drainage bag or get up regularly to empty the pouch during the night.
10. If the skin becomes red, sore, or you have difficulty getting the barrier to stay on, please contact the WOC nurse or your doctor for evaluation.

Figure 6.2.3. Urostomy care procedures.

---

the stoma and the bowel continues to create mucus, the urine that drains into the pouch will have mucus; this should not be mistaken for a sign of clinical infection [5]. In addition, patients with urinary diversions are at increased risk for urinary infection due to their shortened urinary tract system. Teaching the patient hand-washing and stoma care techniques will help the patient to avoid urinary tract infections [1, 5].

Breaking down the steps of stoma care may help to lessen the patient's anxiety when teaching (see Figure 6.2.3.).

Interdisciplinary Care Plan

Problem	Goal/Plan	Intervention	Evaluation
Potential for infection	The patient will be free from infection within 8 weeks.	Monitor the wound for signs and symptoms of infection. Report any unusual findings to the physician for followup. Instruct patient on ostomy self-management to prevent effluent leakage on incision site. Encourage fluid intake of 2000 mL to 3000 mL of water per day to flush the renal system and prevent urinary complications. Instruct the patient on meticulous hand-washing technique prior to pouch change.	The patient's incision will be healed. The patient will be free from urinary tract infection.
Inability for self-care (urostomy) management	The patient is able to demonstrate urostomy care self-management within 8 weeks.	Instruct patient on self-management of his urostomy. Break procedure for urostomy pouch change down to separate steps and instruct on each one (see Figure 6.2.3). Allow patient some time to adjust/accept his stoma while teaching aspects of stoma care.	The patient verbalizes confidence in his ability to independently care for his urostomy.
Anxiety related to current health status	The patient will be able to verbalize feelings of anxiety within 2 weeks. The patient will be able to identify coping strategies to alleviate his anxiety within 8 weeks.	Maintain a calm manner while interacting with patient. Use simple language and brief statements when instructing patient about self-care measures. Encourage patient to seek assistance from an understanding significant other or from the health care provider when anxious feelings become difficult.	The patient will have reduced anxiety levels related to his health status.

Problem	Goal/Plan	Intervention	Evaluation
Ineffective coping for the patient and family	The patient and family will be able to cope with his disease process and altered body image.	Assist family in setting realistic goals. Encourage family members to seek information and resources that increase coping skills Refer family to social service or counseling.	The patient will verbalize acceptance of his altered body image. The patient will have resources for emotional support and use them.

REFERENCES & RESOURCES

[1] J.E. Carmel and M.T. Goldberg, "Preoperative and postoperative management," *Fecal and Urinary Diversions: Management Principles* (1st ed.), J. Colwell, M. Goldberg and J. Carmel (eds.), pp. 207–239, Mosby, 2004.

[2] Coloplast Corp, "Urostomy Background and Consequences," Retrieved September 7, 2010, from http://www.coloplast.com/OstomyCare/Topics/EducationTools/HowUrostomyIsCreated/Pages/UrostomyBackgroundAndConsequences.aspx 2008, 01.

[3] Hollister, Hollister new image online product catalog. Retrieved September 7, 2010, from http://www.hollister.com/us/products/product_series.asp?id=1&family=1&series=14 2010.

[4] D.S. Kaufman, W.U. Shipley and A.S. Feldman, "Bladder cancer," *The Lancet*, 374(9685):239–250, 2009.

[5] L. Nazarko, "Caring for a patient with a urostomy in a community setting," *British Journal of Community Nursing*, 13(8):354–358, 2008.

[6] N. Tomaselli and D. McGinnis, "Urinary diversions: Surgical interventions," *Fecal and Urinary Diversions: Management Principles* (1st ed.), J. Colwell, M. Goldberg and J. Carmel (eds.), pp. 184–204, Mosby, 2004.

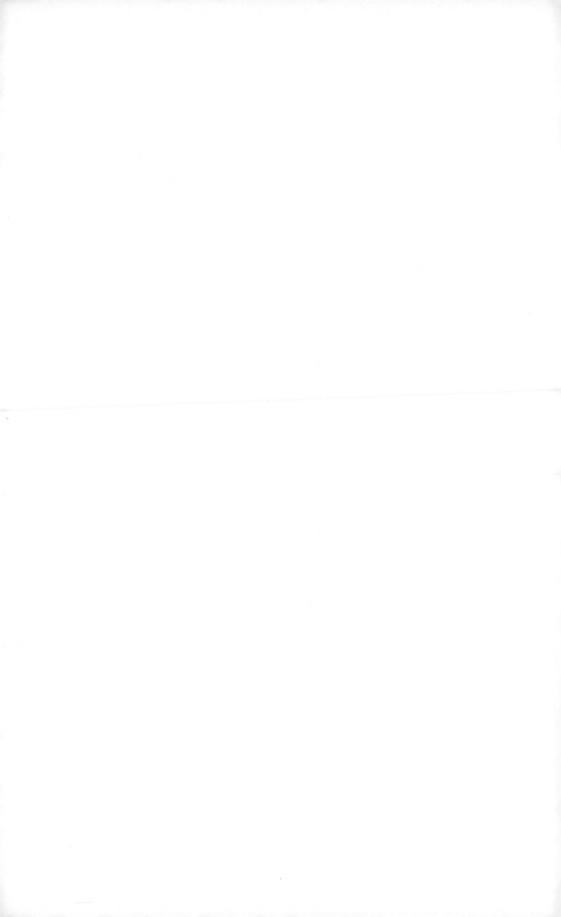

Case 6.3 Urinary Tract Infection and Functional Incontinence

By Kathleen Francis, RN, MSN, CWOCN

This case illustrates how the home health care nurse can work with the multidisciplinary team and the patient to identify mutually agreeable goals that will return the patient to her optimal level of functioning. Mrs. S is a 75-year-old female who is admitted to the home health agency following a right hip total joint arthroplasty. The patient has a history of hypertension, hypothyroidism, osteoarthritis, and coronary artery disease. She had coronary artery stenting 2 years ago. On admission, the patient admits that she fell on her way to the bathroom and fractured her right hip, requiring the recent surgical repair. The patient explains that she takes frequent trips to the bathroom to avoid "accidents," such as urinary leakage.

 ORDERS FOR HOME CARE

Patient: 75-year-old female
Diagnoses: Joint replacement of right hip; gait abnormality; osteoarthritis
Current medications:
- Enalapril 10 mg by mouth once a day
- Hydrochlorothiazide/triamterene 25 mg/37.5 mg by mouth once a day
- Simvastatin 20 mg by mouth once a day
- Warfarin 2 mg by mouth once a day

- Acetaminophen 650 mg by mouth every 4–6 hours as needed
- Ibuprofen 400 mg by mouth three times a day

Relevant past medical history:

- Hypertension
- Coronary artery disease
- Coronary artery stent placement (2 years ago)
- Osteoarthritis.

RN: Assessment and evaluation for home healthcare services. Teach medications, pain management, and disease self-management; assess and evaluate for safety.

PT: Assessment and evaluation.

Labs:

- CBC weekly
- PT/INR weekly

Reimbursement Considerations

The patient is eligible for Medicare. In order for the services to be covered under the Medicare home care benefit, the patient must be homebound. The homecare services must be skilled, necessary, and ordered by the physician who oversees the plan of care. In addition, the services are intermittent and short term, meaning the services do not exceed 40 hours per week or 8 hours per day and the services will be tapered when the patient improves their level of functioning. When the services are reduced or discontinued, the patient will be advised of the changes in the plan of care and will be asked to sign a home health advanced beneficiary notice (HHABN).

 ## THE HOME VISIT

The patient lives alone in a first-floor apartment with six stairs at the entrance. The home is well kept, clean, and uncluttered. A young woman, who identifies herself as the patient's niece, greets the nurse at the door. The patient is found dressed in her bathrobe, sitting up in a living room chair with her walker close by. The table adjacent to the chair is covered with her medications, food tray, and reading material. It seems to the nurse that the patient has placed these items here so that she does not have to walk or move to get them.

The patient appears happy to see the nurse and is pleasant while the nurse reviews the physician's orders for home care, obtains the patient's history, asks the necessary questions, and reviews the medication regimen with the patient. After the initial interview, the nurse asks the patient's permission to complete the physical assessment in the patient's bedroom, to provide more privacy. The patient slowly rises from the chair and ambulates with the walker to her bedroom. Here the nurse notes that the patient has a standard double bed with a dresser and a scatter rug near the foot of the dresser. The nurse also notes that the bathroom is well equipped with grab bars in the tub and a tub/shower chair and a raised toilet seat. The nurse notes an additional scatter rug in the kitchen and a well stocked refrigerator and cabinets.

Mrs. S's vital signs are as follows: BP 136/82; A/R HR 66/66 and regular; temperature: 98 degrees Fahrenheit; respiratory rate: 22. Lungs are clear with no adventitious sounds noted.

Mrs. S is alert and oriented. The patient appears well nourished. She is easily able to answer the nurse's questions. The patient reports that she wears eyeglasses with progressive type lenses for distance and for reading. She is able to read the labels on her medication bottles with the use of her eyeglasses. Her abdomen is soft, non-tender, with bowel sounds on auscultation in all four quadrants. The patient denies any constipation and reports regular bowel movements. However, she mentions that she had a urinary catheter inserted in the hospital and has had some feelings of urgency and frequency since it was removed. She initially denies urinary incontinence. However, after questioning, she admits that she often goes to the bathroom 3 or 4 times a night and may have an "occasional accident," if she waits too long. The patient reports to the nurse that she uses sanitary napkins as containment for when she has to go out, "just in case." She also admits that she frequently stays home to avoid the embarrassment of an accident. When the nurse asks the patient if she has reported any of this information to the doctor, the patient states, "No. It is embarrassing. Besides, what is the doctor going to do? This is a part of old age, and I guess I have to live with it."

Cultural Competence

The patient is a Caucasian, who appears stoic. The nurse will need to observe for subtle signs of pain, when assessing the patient for pain management. In addition, the patient may have anxiety related to her UI, requiring the nurse to approach this topic with understanding and sensitivity. The nurse should ask the patient for permission before discussing this issue.

The patient has a closed incision on her right hip. The margins are approximated with well-defined healing ridge on palpation, and no erythema is noted. There is no edema noted in her lower extremities, and the patient's skin is intact. The patient reports that her pain has been managed with her medication regimen and that it sometimes interferes with her ability to perform her activities of daily living. The patient is able to ambulate on level surfaces with her walker and with close supervision, but she is unable to negotiate stairs. She requires assistance to get in and out of her tub, using the tub/shower chair. She is unable to bend to wash or dress her lower body and requires assistance to complete these activities. The patient currently requires the assistance of her niece for shopping, cooking, and cleaning. Prior to her accident, she was independent and able to manage all aspects of her activities of daily living. The patient mentions that she is anxious to get back to driving so that she does not need to inconvenience her family.

The patient identifies the following goals:

- To live independently
- To get back to driving her car
- To be free from pain
- To be able to go out without fear of urinary incontinence

The Neal Theory Implications

Stage 3: The nurse in this stage recognizes the value of adding other services and how the team can work together to reinforce one another's plans to help the patient attain her goals.

Stage 2: This nurse may focus only on the possibility of a urinary tract infection and the need to resolve that, but may not recognize how the PT or HHA can significantly contribute to the plan of care.

Stage 1: This nurse may focus on the rehabilitation and medication needs of the patient and may not recognize that the environment plays a significant role in the future function of the patient and that functional incontinence must be resolved to prevent future falls.

Based on the history and physical examination, the nurse identifies the following:

- Mrs. S has gait abnormality.
- Mrs. S is at risk for falls.
- Mrs. S is unable to transfer without assistance.
- Mrs. S has urinary incontinence.
- Mrs. S may have a urinary tract infection.
- Mrs. S has pain with some activities.
- Mrs. S is free from wound infection.
- Mrs. S does not have difficulty with speech, hearing, or vision.
- Mrs. S has no history of depression and does not report any feelings of sadness.
- Mrs. S is motivated to return to her prior level of functioning.

Rehabilitation Needs

Physical therapy

? | **CRITICAL THINKING**

1. What is the priority for care for Mrs. S?
Answer: Safety is always the priority. The nurse and the physical therapist (PT) will assess the patient's environment and make recommendations to ensure safe transfers and ambulation in the home and to decrease the likelihood of falls. In this case, the nurse and PT will advise the patient that scatter rugs should be removed as they create a risk for falls, especially when the patient uses durable medical equipment (DME), such as her walker, to ambulate. Since the patient lives alone and has a history of falls, she is at risk for falls and may benefit from a personal emergency response system (PERS) that can be activated if she has another accident.

2. What can the PT contribute to this case?
Answer: The PT can assess and evaluate the patient's environment for accessibility and safety. The PT can assess the patient's ability to ambulate on level surfaces and then graduate the patient to unlevel (outside the home/sidewalk) surfaces. They can teach the patient transfer techniques and how to navigate stairs. If able, the PT will teach the patient how to ambulate using a cane.

3. Is there any other service that may be ordered for this patient?
Answer: Yes. The patient can use a home health aide (HHA) to assist her with bathing and dressing. Based on the nurse's assessment, the patient would be eligible for approximately 2 hours a day for a maximum of 10 hours a week of HHA service. The HHA can assist the patient to bathe, dress, and provide supervision when she ambulates. Once the patient's level of functioning improves, the HHA services will be reduced.

4. What can each discipline (RN, PT, and HHA) contribute to this case?
Answer: The RN assesses and evaluates the patient for safety and safe use of DME. He also instructs the patient on the medication regimen and ensures that the patient can safely manage their medications. The RN also monitors the incision site and instructs the patient on the signs and symptoms of infection. The RN will also instruct the patient on pain management, on urinary incontinence (UI) management, on dietary changes that may decrease urgency, and on timed voiding to reduce the incidence of UI.

The PT assesses and evaluates the patient's environment for safety as well as the patient's ability to ambulate and transfer. They can instruct the patient on ambulation and transfer techniques, the use of DME, and how to navigate stairs. The PT can also teach the patient how to safely transfer in and out of an automobile when she is no longer homebound. In addition, they can instruct the patient on exercises to increase stability and strength.

The HHA will assist the patient with activities of daily living (ADL), such as bathing, dressing, and making meals. The HHA can/may do light cleaning around the patient's home to keep the floors free from clutter and may clean the patient's dishes after meals. The HHA will also provide supervision when the patient ambulates.

UI is defined as the unintentional loss of urine which is sufficient to be a problem or loss of bladder control [1, 3, 8]. The etiology of UI can be multifaceted and difficult to determine. Regardless of the cause of UI, it should not be accepted as the norm or a normal part of aging. UI can be a distressing problem to many patients as feelings of shame are often associated with it [1, 7]. This shame associated with UI can prevent the patient from addressing the topic with their health care provider. The patient may often be reluctant to discuss UI with the nurse. Because of this, the nurse may need to provide the patient with privacy during the assessement and interview. Offering an empathetic and nonjudgmental attitude while collecting the data can also help the patient feel at ease so that they can verbalize their feelings.

The major types of non-transient UI include: functional UI, stress UI, urge UI, overflow UI, and reflex UI. Functional UI results when the patient is unable to get to the toilet. It results in urinary leakage due to either physical or cognitive impairments that prevent the patient from getting to the toilet [1]. Providing these patients with physical therapy and occupational therapy may help to alleviate their UI. For the patient with cognitive impairment, a timed voiding schedule with toileting every 2 hours can help to decrease the episodes of UI. In this case, the patient may have a functional UI secondary to her reduced mobility.

In stress incontinence, the involuntary leakage of urine occurs with physical effort, such as coughing, sneezing, or other physical efforts that cause increased intra-abdominal pressure. The problem results from an incompetent urethral sphincter or a relaxed urethra [1]. The patient will often report that she experiences a small loss of urine with increased physical efforts that she manages with a sanitary napkin. For these patients, teaching them Kegel exercises may help to increase the sphincter tone and reduce the incidence of stress UI. Offering advice on incontinence pads may help the patient to better contain the UI.

In urge UI, the patient has that "gotta go, gotta go" feeling. They have an overactive bladder. The detrusor muscle (bladder muscle) is constantly irritated and will contract resulting in a loss of a large volume of urine. These patients often report frequent trips to the bathroom, sometimes hourly, due to the compelling urge to void [1]. Here the nurse can help the patient to avoid bladder irritants, such as coffee, spicy foods, alcohol, and citrus, and can encourage adequate fluid intake to keep the urine diluted [5]. Anticholinergic medications also help to reduce urgency, but they have systemic side effects that may make therapeutic dosing and patient compliance difficult [5, 7].

Overflow UI results from acute or chronic retention of urine. Lower urinary tract retention is usually due to some type of urethral outlet obstruction, such as that seen with benign prostate hypertrophy and is most often diagnossed in men. However, women can present with outlet obstruction resulting from uterine prolapse. The patient often reports frequent trips to the bathroom with hesitancy, poor urine flow, and feeling like they are not able to fully empty their bladder [6]. Urinary leakage occurs when the bladder becomes irritated with the residual urine and contracts, forcing a small amount of urine to leak. Management often involves surgical interventions and/or use of alpha adrenergic antagonists (alpha-blockers) for patients whose retention is caused by excessive urethral tone or prostatic hyperplasia. They reduce urethral resistance by blocking sympathetic receptors at the bladder neck [6].

Reflex or neurogenic incontinence results in the loss of urine secondary to neurological dysfunction and is typically associated with neurological disorders, such as spinal cord injury or multiple sclerosis [1]. Management is focused on the preservation of renal function by avoiding urinary tract infections and upper renal damage. Specifically, the patient will need a method to evacuate the bladder at regular intervals. This can be achieved by intermittent catheterization or indwelling catheter placement [2].

Another type of urinary incontinence that should be discussed is transient UI. Transient urinary incontinence is caused by reversible factors, such as delirium, infection, atrophic vaginitis and urethritis, pharmaceuticals, psychological conditions, or other conditions that result in excess urine production, fecal impaction, or temporary immobility [1]. A patient who presents with acute onset incontinence or delirium should be evaluated for a systemic etiology, such as infection (usually urinary tract infection in the elderly). Once the cause of the incontinence is known, the incontinence can be alleviated by treating the cause or removing it if it is pharmaceutical. It is important for the nurse to ask the patient if his/her incontinence is a recent development/symptom or if it is chronic. Urinary incontinence is not the norm for elderly patients; the nursing assessment and plan of care should be focused on improvement of the patient's health status. The nurse can develop a plan of care for the patient to meet their needs and implement it to achieve positive outcomes.

BACK TO THE CASE

The nurse explains to the patient that she can return to her previous level of functioning, with the help of RN, PT, and HHA services. The patient is pleased and satisfied with the plan of care and is highly motivated to work toward her goals.

Relevant Community Resources

The Community Agency for Senior Citizens (CASC) or similar local agency for senior citizens: may help the patient access assistance with housekeeping, shopping, etc. so that she can remain independent in the home.

Personal emergency response system (PERS) so that the patient can remain safe at home and call for assistance when/if she has a fall and is unable to get up or to the phone to call for help.

The nurse discusses the "urinary issue" with the patient, and asks the patient to keep a 3 or 4 day diary that lists the patient's intake (foods and fluids) and voiding times. This is designed to get baseline data so that the nurse can instruct the patient about strategies to prevent urinary incontinence.

The nurse calls the primary care physician (PCP) to discuss her findings. He requests additional orders for the HHA services. He also tells the PCP of the patient's report of urinary incontinence and frequency. The doctor orders the additional services and asks the nurse to obtain a urine sample for culture at the next RN visit.

Interdisciplinary Care Plan

Problem	Plan	Interventions	Evaluation
Pain	The patient will have reduced pain and increased mobility within 8 weeks.	Pain management instructions Pain medication regimen Physical therapy Guided imagery	The patient will report reduction of pain and increased mobility.

Problem	Plan	Interventions	Evaluation
Urinary incontinence	The patient will report no urinary leakage or adequate urinary containment within 8 weeks.	Bladder diary Instructions on Kegel exercises Instructions on dietary changes to reduce urge Instructions on containment options Urine culture and sensitivity Monitor for urinary tract infection	The patient reports that she has not had urinary incontinence and/ or urge/frequency.
Gait abnormality	The patient will be able to ambulate independently with a cane within 8 weeks. The patient will be able to navigate stairs independently within 8 weeks.	Physical therapy for strengthening and gait training HHA services to support and supervise daily exercises	The patient will ambulate independently on all surfaces safely.
Potential for falls	The patient will be safe at home.	Removal of unsafe scatter rugs Instruction on safety and keeping a safe environment Use of PERS in home	The patient will verbalize knowledge of safety instructions and will demonstrate that she values safety, as evidenced by removal of scatter rugs.
Inability to perform ADL independently	The patient will be independent with ADL activities.	HHA services to assist patient with ADL activities	The patient will verbalize satisfaction with the level of assistance and demonstrate independence as her functional ability improves.

REFERENCES & RESOURCES

[1] D. Doughty, "Introductory concepts," *Urinary & Fecal Incontinence: Current Managment Concepts* (3rd ed.), D.D. Doughty and D. Doughty (eds.), pp. 1–20, Mosby, 2006.

[2] K.F. Francis, "Management of bowel and bladder continence following spinal cord injury," *Ostomy Wound Management*, 53(12):1–9, 2007.

[3] B.R. Haylen, "International Urogynecological Association (IUGA)/International Continence Society (ICS) joint report on the terminology for female pelvic floor dysfunction," *Neurology and Urodynamics*, 29:4–20, 2009.

[4] D.S. Kaufman, "Bladder cancer," *The Lancet*, 374(9685):239–250, 2009.

[5] M. Krossovich, "Pathology and management of overactive bladder," *Urinary and Fecal Incontinence: Current Managment Concepts* (3rd ed.), D. Doughty (ed.), pp. 109–165, Mosby, 2006.

[6] K. Moore, "Pathology and management of acute and chronic urinary retention," *Urinary and Fecal Incontinence: Current Management Concepts* (3rd ed.), D. Doughty (ed.), pp. 225–253, Mosby, 2006.

[7] A. Rantelli, "Treatment of female urinary incontinence," *Practice Nursing*, 20(8):384–389, 2009.

[8] P. Ward-Smith, "The cost of urinary incontinence," *Urologic Nursing*, 29(3):188–194, 2009.

Section 7

Psychiatric/Mental Health

Case 7.1 Bipolar Disorder

By Joanne DeSanto Iennaco, PhD, PMHCNS-BC, APRN

This case illustrates the complexity of caring for a patient with a psychiatric disorder who is also pregnant. Ms. D is a 25-year-old single Caucasian female who is pregnant. She has stopped her psychotropic medications due to concerns that they might be harmful to her baby. She has a history of bipolar I disorder with multiple hospitalizations over the past 5 years. In the midst of a manic episode, Ms. D got pregnant while having unprotected sex with an old boyfriend. She also has a history of substance abuse, including alcohol, marijuana, and cocaine. She lives in her own small house, which is on her parent's property. There is tension between Ms. D and her parents, who are angry that she got pregnant again.

Ms. D has a 3-year-old son, Ethan, who is placed with her parents due to her inability to appropriately care for him when she has manic or depressive episodes. Ms. D's mood is frequently labile, and she fears that her new baby will be "taken away" by her parents like Ethan was. Ms. D wants to parent her own children; being their mother is important to her.

Ethical Considerations

This case is already involved with the department of child protective services, which will be expected to continue its involvement after the birth of the child.

Clinical Case Studies in Home Health Care, First Edition. Edited by Leslie Neal-Boylan.
© 2011 John Wiley & Sons, Inc. Published 2011 by John Wiley & Sons, Inc.

ORDERS FOR HOME CARE

Patient: 25-year-old Caucasian female
Diagnoses: Bipolar disorder; pregnancy
Current medications:
- Folic acid 4 mg by mouth once a day
- Prenatal vitamin once a day
- Clonazepam 0.5 mg by mouth twice a day as needed for anxiety and insomnia

Relevant past medical history: None
Psychiatric RN: Assess and evaluate mental status and health needs; ensure that patient receives appropriate prenatal health; monitor psychiatric symptoms and use of medications to both treat patient and to protect the baby.

Reimbursement Considerations

This patient is a Supplemental Secure Income (SSI) recipient and has Medicaid (Title XIX) coverage to pay for her care, provide her with a small amount of monthly income, and provide prescription drug coverage. In high risk maternal-child health situations like this, home visits to monitor prenatal care can be provided. In addition the Medicaid coverage she has covers home visits for symptoms and medication management that will aid in preventing her need for hospitalization.

THE HOME VISIT

Ms. D lives in a small 4-room ranch house on a rural road, about 45 minutes from the nearest city (where she is being followed by a high-risk obstetrician and a psychiatrist). The yard is neatly cared for; and the interior of the house is well cared for, as well. The nurse visits with Ms. D who was tapered off of lithium 600 mg twice a day and risperidone 1 mg by mouth twice a day last month. She is now in her eighth week of pregnancy and has been doing well with her pregnancy. She tells the nurse that the plan for her symptom management during her pregnancy is to remain off of mood stabilizers and antipsychotics unless she experiences a full exacerbation and mood episode. She has discussed using a conventional antipsychotic (Haloperidol) to manage symptoms of mania if they recur. She realizes she may need to be hospitalized at some point if she has a full-blown manic or depressive

Cultural Competence

This patient lives in a rural area, which means that she travels more than 45 minutes each way to access her prenatal and psychiatric care. Other aspects of rural life that might be considered are the resources the patient has in the area (family, friends, and other support systems), including availability of community mental health supports. Individuals living at or below poverty level in these areas may also have difficulty obtaining transportation to stores for shopping and obtaining other resources.

episode. She is hopeful that she will not have one as her mood was stable in her first pregnancy.

She tells the nurse that she has not used alcohol or drugs since realizing she was pregnant about a month ago. She has also tapered back on smoking and limits herself to less than half a pack per day. She says that she smokes outside to help her to limit the amount she smokes and to keep her home smoke free. She describes a positive relationship with her family who provides her with housing next door to them, but she has felt tension in the relationship since she realized she was pregnant.

Ms. D describes a history of both manic and depressive episodes. She tends to have more hypomanic episodes than full blown mania. She had been somewhat consistent in taking her psychiatric medications prior to the pregnancy, although she relates that her past two hospitalizations (in the past 2 years) have been after "forgetting" to take her medications regularly. She says that she knows when she is getting more symptomatic by changes in her sleep pattern (staying up late, not falling asleep, not needing sleep), "moodiness" and irritability, going out too much and partying with friends, getting much more talkative and "hyper," having difficulty concentrating, and forgetting to take care of herself. She sometimes has auditory hallucinations and focuses too much on religious ideas.

Ms. D denies current suicidal ideation or intent and says that she "wouldn't do that," particularly because it would hurt her children. She does say that, although she has never attempted suicide, she thought about it when she was told that the state was taking her son Ethan away from her 2 years ago. Now that she is pregnant, Ms. D says that she stays home more and tries to be more settled down. She reports that she has not had to take the clonazepam at all and has faithfully taken her folic acid and prenatal vitamin once a day.

Ms. D says that she has already talked with the department of child and family services who is concerned about her ability to care for a

---

> **Relevant Community Resources**
>
> Referral to the local mental health center that offers group, vocational, and social activities will improve Ms. D's quality of life. Lamaze classes, 12-step groups to maintain abstinence from substances, local community mental health center for peer support, local community resources for parenting support group, food pantry (she has limited funds with SSI), State NAMI chapter for support group, and local resources.

new baby given her psychiatric illness and her history with Ethan, who is now being cared for by her parents. She has a caseworker who will be part of her care during the pregnancy. Her goals are to have a healthy baby and to be allowed to care for the baby after delivery.

The nurse and the patient decide on a plan with Ms. D to visit 2 times per week during her pregnancy. Mutual goals would focus on:

- Monitoring and managing psychiatric symptoms and medications
- Promoting physical health during the pregnancy

The maternal role is important to Ms. D. She would like to prove herself a capable mother, which has produced conflict with her family who doesn't think Ms. D has settled down enough to care for her own child. They are angry with Ms. D for getting pregnant and believe this is evidence to them of her lack of responsibility as a parent. This is of course an area of important consideration for the nurse. The nurse is required to report concerns about abuse or neglect of a child and will likely be asked to provide some kind of status report on how Ms. D is doing during her pregnancy.

There are several potential conflicts in this situation: The nurse's role is to support her patient; and this may pose potential conflicts related to working effectively with the patient, the family, and other agencies involved in the case. For this reason the nurse decides to broach these issues directly by raising the topic during the following visits before the nurse has been contacted by either the parents or the state agencies involved. By being up front with the patient about her role and responsibility in the care of both Ms. D and her unborn child, the nurse sets a precedent of honest disclosure.

As a young adult, it is currently of importance to Ms. D to gain independence from her family of origin; and beginning her own family and taking on the role of mother are important aspects of this developmental stage.

Neal Theory Implications

The Stage 3 nurse may have engaged in family and parenting sessions with the patient where her son was involved and provided direct assessment of the ability of the patient to parent.

The nurse in this case exhibits Stage 2 behavior: She collaborates with others in caring for the patient, and she assists the patient to cope and manage her needs in the home setting.

A Stage 1 nurse would focus her care strictly on assessing the patient and may not become involved in meetings where collaborative problem solving is required.

CRITICAL THINKING

1. How should the nurse handle Ms. D's questions regarding use of medications during her pregnancy?
Answer: During pregnancy, many women feel very strongly, as Ms. D has, about taking medications that could potentially harm their babies. For women with bipolar disorder, there is a high rate of recurrence of mania or depressive episode during pregnancy. One reason for the close monitoring with home care for Ms. D is to provide support and to closely manage Ms. D and her bipolar disorder to help her accomplish her wish to be medication free during pregnancy. The best approach for the nurse is to partner with Ms. D in her goal to be medication free, while teaching her that women are managed on both antipsychotic and mood stabilizer medications during pregnancy. With this patient, the prescribing psychiatrist has provided Ms. D with an as-needed dose of clonazepam for anxiety and to help with her sleep as needed. The dose of this agent is low, and Ms. D is encouraged to use it intermittently as needed to minimize risks. However, she should also be educated regarding the greater risk of a mood episode recurring if she does not have adequate sleep.

BACK TO THE CASE

The nurse visits Ms. D 2 days a week to monitor her psychiatric symptoms and provide education and support regarding her pregnancy.

Ms. D has some minor ups and downs in her mood, but nothing severe enough to cause a need for a change in medication. Over this time period, she has been getting along better with her parents, who allow her to have visits with Ethan while they are present. Ms. D is grateful for her parents taking care of Ethan and is glad they are raising him.

At her sixth month of pregnancy, the state agency involved contacts Ms. D and sets up a meeting to review how she is doing and to discuss plans for the birth of the child. The nurse and social worker from the agency are invited, as are Ms. D's parents. Ms. D is extremely anxious and tearful about the meeting, raising concerns that the state will tell her they plan to take her baby after the birth. At the meeting, the question of Ms. D's ability to parent her child is raised. When the nurse is asked, she describes the relative stability of mood over the past months and the positive steps Ms. D has taken to have a healthy pregnancy including cutting down on smoking, walking, exercising daily, and avoiding alcohol and substance use. Her parents concur that Ms. D has been doing extremely well, although they find her short tempered with Ethan when she cares for him; and they express a desire for Ms. D to have parenting support.

The state workers ask the parents if they are willing to provide care for the new baby if needed after delivery, and the parents agree that if needed they will take the baby in. The worker suggests that Ms. D attend a weekly parenting group, but explain that her attendance is not meant to suggest that she will be able to keep the baby after delivery. Ms. D is upset about this, but she agrees with the class.

❓ CRITICAL THINKING

1. How should the nurse have answered the questions about Ms. D's ability to care for her new baby?
Answer: The nurse's role in this case is not to assess the parenting skills of the patient. The nurse's role is to assess the mental health needs of Ms. D and her health during her pregnancy. For this reason, the nurse's response was to speak to the psychiatric stability of the patient, which is why she is involved in this case.

BACK TO THE CASE

On the next visit with Ms. D, she is angry and upset about the meeting. She feels she is in limbo about the baby after trying so hard the past months to do well. She reports that she has not been sleeping well and has been having difficulty concentrating. She reports feeling depressed and anxious, thinking over and over again about the meeting and worrying that the baby will be taken from her. The nurse discusses her concerns about the changes in symptoms that Ms. D has been having, and during the visit discusses the changes with the psychiatrist who suggests that Ms. D move to taking the clonazepam 0.5 mg by mouth twice a day for the next week to be sure that this does not progress to a manic or depressive episode. Ms. D is agreeable to the medication change and the nurse's visits are increased to daily to monitor the mood changes more closely.

During the next few weeks, Ms. D talks through her concerns and comes to a better frame of mind regarding her parents having to care for her baby. She decides that there are some positives in that arrangement. As a single mom she will have help caring for her baby. Her parents will allow her to sleep in their house for the first few months as long as Ms. D does not smoke in the house. Ethan will be with her and the baby. After the first week, Ms. D is able to decrease her use of the clonazepam back to an as-needed basis; and within three weeks she no longer needs to take the medication. She continues to cut back on her smoking, exercises daily, and has not used substances or alcohol since realizing she was pregnant. She is also attending the parenting class and feels hopeful that it will help her in her relationship with her children.

Interdisciplinary Care Plan

Problem	Goal/Plan	Intervention	Evaluation
High risk pregnancy, knowledge deficit regarding pregnancy and parenting	Patient will identify expected changes in next stage of pregnancy and fetal development. Patient will identify needs and goals related to support with parenting skills.	Assess for changes at each stage of pregnancy. Educate patient related to expected changes and problems that may occur with information regarding how to follow up to obtain care if needed. Discuss needs and concerns related to parenting, need for support, and available resources. Encourage attendance at parenting support group. Encourage patient to develop goals related to parenting strategies and skills.	Patient will identify expected changes with pregnancy. Patient will attend parenting support group.

(Continued)

Problem	Goal/Plan	Intervention	Evaluation
Potential for mood instability due to discontinuation of psychiatric medications	Patient will report symptoms of changes in mood stability (moodiness, irritability decreased need for sleep) in next 2 months. Patient will report use of as-needed medication to improve sleep.	Assess for changes in mental status, mood, and symptoms of psychosis. Assess for suicidal ideation and intent. Educate patient regarding methods to cope with stressors. Connect patient with appropriate mental health clinic resources to support.	Patient will report absence of suicidal ideation/ intent and safety plan to manage if thoughts recur. Patient will report stable mood and use supports to decrease anxiety and stress.
History of substance use and abuse (including tobacco, marijuana, and cocaine)	Patient will smoke <½ pack per day within 4 weeks. Patient will develop plan for support in abstaining from alcohol and substance use.	Assess patient's use of substances weekly. Assist patient to identify community resources she can use to aid in abstaining from substance use. Encourage use of healthy coping mechanisms with stress and increasing anxiety symptoms.	Patient will report decreasing use of tobacco. Patient will report success in abstaining from marijuana and cocaine use.

REFERENCES & RESOURCES

[1] American Psychiatric Association, *Diagnostic and Statistical Manual of Mental Disorders* (4th ed.), *Text Revision: DSM-IV-TR*. American Psychiatric Association, 2000.

[2] Y. Hauck, D. Rock, T. Jackiewicz and A. Jablensky, "Healthy babies for mothers with serious mental illness: A case management framework for mental health clinicians," *International Journal of Mental Health Nursing*, 17(6):383–391, 2008.

[3] M. Lagan, K. Knights, J. Barton and P.M. Boyce, "Advocacy for mothers with psychiatric illness: A clinical perspective," *International Journal of Mental Health Nursing*, 18:53–61, 2009.

[4] A.C. Viguera et al., "Risk of recurrence in women with bipolar disorder during pregnancy: Prospective study of mood stabilizer discontinuation," *American Journal of Psychiatry*, 164(12):1817–1824, 2007.

Case 7.2 Personality Disorders

By Debra Riendeau, MN, APRN, BC, PMHNP-BC

This case study illustrates the complexity of providing nursing care to individuals. This patient was involved in a motor vehicle accident 1 year ago in which she sustained a crush injury to her right knee. Less invasive therapies for her knee have been attempted; however, the injury recently required a total knee replacement. Her family is located on the other side of the country. She lives alone in an apartment with her cat. She had to leave her job as a waitress due to her injuries and medical care. Her income includes monthly settlement payments from the insurance company of the driver deemed at fault for the motor vehicle accident.

As a result of the changes in her life, she has lost contact with her previous friends. The medical providers have become her primary social contacts. At the end of the first week, the wound was healing without infection and the discharge was on schedule. When she learned that the daily visits were being decreased to every other day starting in the second week, the patient called the agency after hours to report an open wound with active bleeding. This call triggered an unplanned, unscheduled home visit by the primary nurse first thing Monday morning. The primary home health nurse contacted the insurance company for approval for additional home visits.

Application of the understanding of the psychopathology of psychiatric disorders and the use of both the therapeutic relationship and the therapeutic communication techniques are key to navigating this patient towards successful resolution of the termination phase of the nurse-patient relationship, as well as the goal of successful wound healing.

Clinical Case Studies in Home Health Care, First Edition. Edited by Leslie Neal-Boylan.
© 2011 John Wiley & Sons, Inc. Published 2011 by John Wiley & Sons, Inc.

Reimbursement Considerations

The private insurance company has authorized payment for the rental of one type of durable medical equipment (continuous passive motion machine) to be used by the patient and their provider. A specific number of visits that incorporates skilled nursing visits and venipunctures is designated. The nurse, as case manager on this case, will need to negotiate with the insurance case manager for visits beyond those originally authorized.

 ORDERS FOR HOME CARE

Patient: 37-year-old Caucasian female

Diagnoses: Right total knee replacement; borderline personality disorder

Current medications: Warfarin 1 mg once a day at 4 p.m.

Relevant past medical history: The patient has no history of other illnesses or injury.

Durable medical equipment: Continuous passive motion (CPM) machine

RN: Skilled nursing assessment and evaluation. Weekly laboratory draws for prothrombin times with international normalized ratio (PT/INR). The insurance company authorized daily nursing visits for the first week, then visits every other day for the second week. By the third week, the patient was to be seen 2 times, then discharged by the end of the third week. There is authorization for 1 emergency skilled nursing visit.

PT: Evaluation, assessment, and teaching related to the use of the continuous passive motion (CPM) machine.

 THE HOME VISIT

On a Friday afternoon, the patient was admitted to home health services upon discharge from an orthopedic unit in a local hospital. Due to the location of her injury and subsequent surgery, the patient could not drive. Initially, the nurse opened the case. The nurse was authorized to perform a skilled nursing assessment of the wound as well as venipunctures weekly to monitor the PT/INR in relationship to warfarin administration. It was anticipated that the wound would be healed without infection in 21 days. This discharge outcome was reviewed with the patient. The physical therapist performed their initial evaluation after the nurse completed the admission assessment.

Neal Theory Implications

Stage 3: The professional in this stage collaborates with other disciplines both within and outside of home care and is autonomous with the clinical aspects of the case and the logistical aspects of working with the agency. The nurse in this case demonstrated autonomy by recognizing the mental health disorder that is interrupting the process of healing in this case and took appropriate action immediately to guide the case to a successful closure. The nurse recognized the underlying problems that the patient was experiencing (social isolation, ineffective social interactions, and fear of abandonment) and took action to diminish the effect of these issues in the treatment plan.

Stage 2: The professional in this stage will demonstrate more comfort in dealing with health care issues and the complexity of the home care environment. There is still a need to seek the experience of other health professionals to problem solve and negotiate the care needs of the patient. The nurse may be familiar with the medical issues of healing, but may unaware of the severity of the mental health disorder that has arisen. The nurse may be hesitant to employ a psychiatric nurse as a consultant in ways to deal with the behaviors being demonstrated by the patient in this case.

Stage 1: The clinician in this stage will assess the patient and recognize the need for assistance with the case but may be unsure as to how to proceed in the home setting. The nurse will need to ask questions and require assistance in managing the patient's care and treatment plan. The nurse may not realize the severity of the behaviors demonstrated by the patient in this case. The nurse may focus mainly on the wound care and recovery process of the total knee replacement. The nurse may not realize that a referral to a psychiatric nurse is indicated.

? CRITICAL THINKING

1. What is the nurse's priority goal for the care of this patient?
Answer: Initially, the nurse would focus on establishing trust and building a therapeutic working relationship with the patient. A

therapeutic relationship provides the foundation for a collaborative agreement with the patient to establish reasonable goals for care. In this case, these include the goal of the right knee incision healing without infection and discharge from home health services as soon as possible to be least disruptive to the patient's normal life.

2. What factors can interfere with achieving these goals?
Answer: Environmental factors such as the availability of clean water to maintain wound cleanliness and nutritional factors, such as a well-balanced diet providing additional protein for wound healing, are necessary. Psychosocial factors such as a patient's personality traits can also interfere with goal or outcome attainment.

3. What will the physical therapist (PT) do upon arrival at the home?
Answer: The PT will evaluate the patient, educate the patient on the proper use of the continuous passive motion (CPM) machine, and set up a plan to gradually increase the amount of flexion prescribed by the physician.

 BACK TO THE CASE

The patient was seen daily over the weekend by both the physical therapist and skilled nurse. The following week, the physical therapist assessed the patient for compliance with the use of the CPM machine, as well as monitored for the increases in flexion ability of the patient to coincide with the physician's prescribed goal for the degree of flexion available to the knee replacement hardware. This patient actively participated in all aspects of physical therapy and complied with the use of the continuous passive motion machine. The degree of flexion ordered by the physician began at 40 degrees (which had been obtained in the hospital) and progressed as tolerated by 10 degrees every day. The nurse performed skilled nursing visits every day to assess vital signs, monitor the wound for signs and symptoms of infection, and reinforce teaching related to warfarin.

During these daily visits, the patient was friendly, and cheerfully stated that the daily nursing visits are "the best part of my day." Additionally, she informed the primary nurse that she is the "best" nurse she has ever met. The daily skilled nursing visits were lasting longer as the patient shared more details and stories of her life. The nurse was experiencing difficulty managing the length of the visit because she would often have to cut off the conversation in order to follow her schedule to see her other patients scheduled for that day. The rehabilitation process was proceeding as expected. The physical therapist discharged off the case when the patient successfully reached the flexion goal of 110 degrees.

Rehabilitation Needs

Physical therapy is needed to educate the patient in the use of the continuous passive motion (CPM) machine and oversee the increase in knee flexion ordered by the physician.

? CRITICAL THINKING

1. From the statement the patient is making, what psychological/emotional factors could the patient be experiencing from the daily visits from the nurse?
Answer: This patient is experiencing primary gain from the daily in home visits. Primary gain is the relief from emotional conflict or tension provided by neurotic symptoms or illness. The patient is gradually increasing the length of the visits in order to escape the loneliness that is often experienced by patients with this diagnosis. The more the patient talks, the longer the nurse stays with her. Allowing the patient to extend the conversations in length reinforces the patient's storytelling. The nurse is rewarding the patient with positive attention the longer she stays.

2. What actions can the nurse take to block the establishment of detrimental primary gain?
Answer: The nurse can establish an anticipated length of visit during the initial admission process. This outlines the parameters of the therapeutic relationship. The nurse should list the skilled nursing activities that will be performed in each visit while demonstrating unconditional positive regard. For example, "During each visit, I will perform a general assessment, obtain your vital signs, assess your wound for signs and symptoms of infection, provide teaching as needed, and answer any questions that you have. This should take me about 40 minutes." This provides structure for each visit and allows the nurse to maintain professional boundaries.

BACK TO THE CASE

After completing the skilled nursing visits on Saturday and Sunday, the weekend per diem nurse informs the patient that nursing visits will be decreasing to every other day for the second week. Since the patient was seen on Sunday and there were no medical issues pending, a home health skilled nursing visit was not scheduled for Monday, but rather for Tuesday. On Monday, the primary nurse came to work to discover that this patient had left 3 frantic messages on her voicemail requesting the primary nurse to come today because her wound is now open. Subsequently, the primary nurse makes this patient her first priority visit to assess the wound. When the nurse arrives, she is greeted by an anxious patient who states, "I am so happy to see you; I wish you had to work weekends, too." The nurse inspects the wound to see that the distal portion of the wound now has a 0.5-cm open area. The patient states the scab was itchy and she picked off the scab. She states, "Now that it is open, will you have to be here every day?" She then proceeds to recount a detailed version of how she spent the weekend including the visits from the weekend nurse who she states is "not as good a nurse as you are."

Relevant Community Resources
Notification of the fire department and police department that she is homebound and unable to drive

? CRITICAL THINKING

1. Which statements and actions of this patient are indicative of a patient with a personality disorder?
Answer: Patients with this type of personality disorder experience feelings of abandonment (real or imagined). When the weekend nurse reviewed the care plan to decrease the number of visits per week with this patient, the reaction of the patient demonstrated her interpretation of the normal course of a successful rehabilitation as her nurse abandoning her. The patient's statement comparing the primary and weekend nurses' levels of abilities is reflective of a behavior known as "splitting." Splitting is defined as "the primary defense or coping style used by persons with borderline personality disorder" reflecting "the inability to incorporate positive and negative aspects of oneself or others into a whole image" (Varcarolis, 2010, p. 437). This is also an example of "all or none" or "black or white" thinking.

2. What course of action by the nurse will be therapeutic for this patient?
Answer: Patients exhibiting these behaviors may often be labeled difficult patients. By empathizing with the patient concerning her situation (living alone, social isolation, and unemployment) the nurse can support the patient and empower her to identify and verbalize her feelings. The nurse should ignore the comment about the differences in abilities between the nurses. Without positive reinforcement, the behavior of splitting will then extinguish. The statement by the patient asking if the nurse will now need to come every day due to the open

wound is reflective of the underlying fear of abandonment which is a hallmark of the patient's psychiatric diagnosis. By opening the knee incision, the patient interferes with the planned schedule for discharge and delays the feelings of abandonment.

3. What actions can the nurse take to assist this patient in dealing with her feelings of abandonment and continue with the planned discharge?
Answer: Providing consistency in responses and interactions, setting clear and consistent boundaries and limits with regard to behaviors, setting goals, and the use of supportive confrontation are the most effective ways to support this patient. If behavioral problems such as those outlined in this case arise, the nurse should calmly review the therapeutic goals or outcomes with the patient. In this case, the nurse should restate the plan for decreasing visits and the anticipated discharge next week. To help the patient lower her anxiety and transition to the pending discharge date, the nurse could elect to set aside a time for the patient to call the agency for a brief check-in with the nurse in the early morning on the days that no skilled nursing visit is scheduled. This brief phone call might assist the patient with alleviating the acute feelings of abandonment, decrease the patient's anxiety, and allow her to adjust and transition to the pending discharge scheduled for the following week.

Interdisciplinary Care Plan

Problem	Plan	Interventions	Evaluation
Knowledge deficit: Surgical recovery and use of CPM machine	Patient will verbalize an understanding of the surgical recovery process in 1 visit. Patient will demonstrate proper use of CPM machine in 1 visit.	Teach the patient signs/symptoms of wound infection to report to the nurse. Physical therapist will teach patient the correct use of the CPM machine as ordered by physician.	Patient participated fully with the therapeutic care plan and verbalizes s/s of wound infection. Patient demonstrated independent use of CPM machine.
Alteration in cardiac status: Warfarin use	Patient's cardiac status will remain stable on medication throughout the recuperation period.	Teach patient dietary restrictions (foods high in vitamin K) while on warfarin therapy. Teach patient to take warfarin late in the afternoon. Teach patient about weekly blood draws for PT/INR.	Patient demonstrates understanding of foods high in Vitamin K. Patient takes warfarin at 4 p.m. each day. Patient has weekly blood draws in the early morning.

(Continued)

Problem	Plan	Interventions	Evaluation
Alteration in mobility	Patient will gradually increase activity level in 1 month. Patient does active range of motion on the unaffected leg 4 times a day while on CPM machine therapy time.	Physical therapist will teach the patient exercises for unaffected leg. Teach patient to gradually increase activity level as ordered by physician.	Patient has complied with active ROM on unaffected leg 4 times a day. Patient gradually increased activity level.
Social isolation	Patient will experience less time spent alone in her home by having family and friends visit or by joining Internet support groups/blog while recuperating at home in 1 week.	Encourage patient to interact with family and friends daily. Assist patient with finding an Internet support group or blog that she prefers.	Patient's family and friends are in contact daily. Patient is active in an online support group/blog.
Impaired social interaction	Nurse will provide consistent structure to each home health visit in first visit. Patient will identify inappropriate behavior (opening a healing wound) in 1 visit. Patient will work with nurse on appropriate ways to terminate the therapeutic relationship in 1 visit.	The nurse will provide positive attention to patient behaviors that are appropriate and productive in the termination process. Nurse will outline how each skilled nursing visit will be conducted. Nurse may offer a short 5-minute telephone conversation each morning of the days there is no skilled nursing visit as needed.	Patient acknowledges the destructive behaviors used to lengthen the course of home health treatment (opening the wound). Patient identifies and verbalizes appropriate ways to terminate the therapeutic relationship and transition to independent self-care.

Problem	Plan	Interventions	Evaluation
Ineffective coping	Patient will successfully terminate the therapeutic relationship by the end of treatment. Patient will acknowledge and verbalize feelings of loss of the therapeutic relationship in 2 visits.	Nurse will model a consistent positive pattern of interaction with the patient. Nurse will provide positive praise when patient verbalizes feelings of loss with the termination process. Nurse will lead patient through appropriate problem solving process: Define the problem. Explain alternatives. Make decisions.	Patient identifies behaviors leading to a delayed discharge from home health care. Patient demonstrates the ability to use new appropriate problem solving skills in regards to termination of the therapeutic relationship. Patient engages in each home health visit within the time frame allocated for the visit. Nurse recognizes splitting behavior as a maladaptive coping behavior.
Alteration in comfort: Pain in lower extremity	Patient will verbalize pain management to 2–3/10 in 1 visit.	Assess pain level during each home health visit. Nurse contacts orthopedic surgeon for pain not relieved to 2–3/10.	Patient verbalizes pain is consistently controlled to a level of 2–3/10. Nurse advocates with physician for adequate pain control as needed.

REFERENCES & RESOURCES

[1] J. Battaglia, "Transcend dread: 8 ways to transform your care of 'difficult' patients," *Current Psychiatry*, September(9):25–29, 2009.

[2] "Continuous Passive Motion (CPM) Machine," http://en.wikipedia.org/wiki/Continuous_passive_motion

[3] S. Driscoll and N. Giori, "Continuous passive motion (CPM): Theory and principles of clinical application," *Journal of Rehabilitation, Research and Development*, 37(2):179–188, 2000.

[4] N. Keltner, L. Schwecke and C. Bostrom, *Psychiatric Nursing* (4th ed.), Mosby, 2002.

[5] L. Neal, "Neal theory of home health nursing practice," *Image: Journal of Nursing Scholarship*, 31(3):251, 1999.

[6] E. Vacarolis and M. Halter, "Foundations of psychiatric mental health nursing; A clinical approach," *Personality Disorders* (6th ed.), Saunders Elsevier, 2010.

Case 7.3 Schizophrenia

By Joanne DeSanto Iennaco, PhD, PMHCNS-BC, APRN

This case study illustrates how the home health nurse cares for a patient with schizophrenia. John is a 24-year-old, single African American male who has a history of schizophrenia. John was recently discharged from the hospital on depot antipsychotic medications.

"Depot antipsychotic medications" refers to long-acting injectable antipsychotics that can be given every 2 to 4 weeks, usually relieving the patient of having to take medication daily or several times a day. Risperdal Consta is the form of the long-acting injectable antipsychotic risperidone. It is similar to fluphenazine decanoate (prolixin decanoate), which is an older agent. The medication is delivered as a very slow release medication over the 2- to 4-week period. Depot medications are very helpful when patients don't take their medications consistently.

He lives in a very small apartment that is located within an apartment building that his family owns. John was admitted due to being acutely psychotic, with auditory hallucinations of the command type. He believed that the devil was talking to him and telling him to run in front of a car on the busy street where he lived. Family members found him running across traffic. The police were called, and he was admitted to a psychiatric unit for stabilization and treatment. John had not cared for himself for several days; therefore, he had poor hygiene and grooming. He does not interact with his family much, feeling that they intrude on his life and judge him. He frequently becomes agitated during acute phases of illness, often becoming argumentative with passersby and family members in the neighborhood. John's family is quite anxious to be involved in his care and support him so that he does not end up in an institution or on the streets. This was John's third psychiatric

Clinical Case Studies in Home Health Care, First Edition. Edited by Leslie Neal-Boylan.
© 2011 John Wiley & Sons, Inc. Published 2011 by John Wiley & Sons, Inc.

195

hospitalization this year, and he has had multiple hospitalizations in the 5 years since he was diagnosed with schizophrenia.

Cultural Competence

John is an African American who lives in the immediate vicinity of his large family who looks out for him. This is an important support and asset that John has that enables him more stable community living than many patients with chronic psychiatric needs. With John's permission, the nurse can assist with family meetings, if needed, to help to sustain the family support without it interfering with John becoming more independent. Striking a balance between the family's desire to help John and John's perception of his family trying to "control" him is important to John's adjustment in the community.

 ## ORDERS FOR HOME CARE

Patient: 24-year-old African American male
Diagnoses: Schizophrenia; metabolic syndrome
Current medications:
- Risperidone 1 mg by mouth twice a day
- Risperdal Consta 25 mg IM once every 2 weeks

Relevant past medical history: Metabolic syndrome identified during recent hospitalization
RN: Assess and evaluate needs for psychiatric nursing and medication management

Reimbursement Considerations

John has title XIX Medicaid coverage that provides for his medical and psychiatric care. Medicaid also will cover home visits by a skilled psychiatric nurse to provide medication evaluation and management, particularly when adherence is a problem and when services can prevent rehospitalization. Medicaid coverage will pay for the administration of the depot medication John has been prescribed. Reimbursement varies by state and should be investigated in terms of the frequency of care that can be covered. John has never worked, due to his disabling psychiatric needs, and may qualify for SSI, for which the nurse and the social worker may be able to help him apply. Supplemental Security Income (SSI) would provide some income monthly for John to assist him in living more independently of his family.

THE HOME VISIT

The nurse visits John in the afternoon and finds him lying on the couch with his headphones on. The 2-room apartment has a strong odor of rotten food and cigarette smoke, and every surface is covered with clothing, used food containers, and wrappers. He tells the nurse that no one looked in on his place while he was in the hospital and allows the nurse to open the window to get some fresh air. John reports he is doing "okay" since he was discharged yesterday. He says that he is just resting and feels tired today.

He reports that he hears voices occasionally (approximately once per day) and they aren't as frightening as they were before he was hospitalized. He says that he has not had any command hallucinations. He describes his mood as "okay" and says that he never feels really good, but says he currently is not feeling depressed. His affect is flat, and he makes infrequent eye contact. He denies feeling paranoid, although he states this has been a problem in the past. He reports that he forgot to take the Riseridone during the day yesterday, so he took 2 pills last night and the 1 pill that was due this morning. When asked about his family, he says, "They just want to control me" and sounds angry with them. He says that they bug him about taking care of his apartment, taking his medication, and going to the doctor. They also bring his meals and groceries to him. He is unable to find his information from discharge that tells him when his next appointment is and states he'll call his psychiatrist tomorrow. He has a home phone but is unable to recall the name or phone number for his psychiatrist. He identifies goals of: being more independent of his family and staying out of the hospital.

Ethical and Legal Considerations

Given John's recent suicide attempt based on command auditory hallucinations, the nurse needs to be sure to assess for the status of psychotic symptoms, including hallucinations and delusions, as well as directly assessing for suicidal ideation or intent. As John is tapered off of the oral dose of medication, the nurse will monitor for changes in or increases in auditory hallucinations. John's family desires involvement in his care. However, information cannot be shared with them nor can they be directly engaged in his care if John refuses permission. Documentation must clearly identify John's safety and the absence or presence of suicidal ideation or intent.

The nurse realizes that it would be appropriate to bring in the psychiatric home health nurse for consultation on this patient's case and to perhaps take over the case. The psychiatric nurse visits the next day and identifies that he needs to assist John with meeting his goal of staying out of the hospital by assisting in medication management and psychiatric symptom management and to meet his goal of being more independent of his family by helping him with home management/ maintenance and self-care needs. The nurse helps John to put his medications in a medication box to aid him in remembering to take his dose as scheduled. He provides education regarding the patient's medications and use of the medication box and explains that the feeling of being tired yesterday may relate to taking both doses of Risperidone the night prior, as well as his regular dose in the morning. He asks about the sedation and finds that it had improved later in the day, and the nurse reinforces the need to take the dose as prescribed in the morning and evening to avoid sedation.

Rehabilitation Needs

The nurse will consult with the agency social worker regarding helping John to access entitlements, such as SSI that may help John to live independently and with greater stability.

John's most recent psychotic symptoms relate to the devil. It will be important to assess the role of religion and spirituality in his life and its expression within his acute and chronic symptoms. If John is hyper-religious, one would not encourage discussion and involvement in religious topics, as it may exacerbate the psychotic symptoms. However, the nurse does want to pay attention to the fact that a religious oriented symptom is a feature of his illness.

John is a young adult who is attempting to establish himself as an independent adult with a separate identity from his family. It will be important to engage John regarding his ability to care for his own needs, to identify vocational or avocational interests or goals, and to allow for his need for independence versus involvement of family members who might try to aid in improvement of his quality of life.

Neal Theory Implications

Stage 3: The nurse collaborates with community providers and family to support the patient, contacting them as appropriate to aid in titration of medications and reporting of changes in symptom status.

Stage 2: The nurse works with the patient and his family to assure his positive adaptation and transition to living independently. The nurse works with patient to set goals regarding managing his apartment so that he can be more in charge of his own living situation.

Stage 1: The nurse assesses the patient's psychiatric symptoms and reports them as needed to other providers.

?   CRITICAL THINKING

1. Why was home care part of the discharge plan for John? In what situations would this be preferred and reimbursable versus attending an outpatient clinic?
Answer: While John is young and physically able to attend an outpatient clinic, his symptoms are such that he is not able to organize and attend outpatient appointments consistently. His history of multiple psychiatric hospitalizations in the past 5 years attest to the instability he experiences due to his psychiatric symptoms. Home care is a viable option and may be particularly useful when there is a history of sporadic attendance at mental health services, when there are comorbidities, and when additional support is required to stabilize the ability of the patient to remain living independently in the community. In John's case there is a stable place for him to live, which is supported by his family who lives nearby. For this reason, a residential program is not the best choice, even though it might also offer a person with chronic psychiatric needs support, medication management, and other services to maintain community-based independent living. John has recently been started on a depot form of his antipsychotic, which will require some monitoring both with a tapering (and possible discontinuation) of the oral dose of the antipsychotic drug and possible dose adjustment of the depot form of medication. Having regular visits from the nurse can aid in evaluation of the day-to-day effects of the medication and provide further evaluation and identification of needs that can be met by other community services. A hoped-for outcome with John would be his decreased need for nursing services to every 2 weeks when his depot medication is administered. Eventually as John further stabilizes he may obtain his medication through the clinic where he is prescribed the medication (if they provide this service).

BACK TO THE CASE

The psychiatric nurse visits John daily at first, to be sure that John is taking his medication properly with the help of the medication box. John is able to take his oral dose of medication without a problem. The nurse decreases his visits to twice a week the next week to monitor the patient's symptoms as the prescriber has decreased the Risperidone to 1 mg by mouth once a day. John is doing well and has had no increase in his auditory hallucinations. His mood is good, he is not feeling sedated, and he is taking better care of his apartment by throwing away the containers and food wrappers from his meals.

> ### Relevant Community Resources
>
> Referral of John to services that would assist him in independent living include:
> Referral to the local mental health center that offers group, vocational, and social activities that will improve John's quality of life.

At the start of the following week, the nurse administers the depot Risperdal Consta injection and completes her assessment. John will remain at his current oral dose of risperidone, and the nurse guides John in filling his med box for the week. John has started taking a daily walk in the neighborhood in the afternoon and is considering whether he will try to quit smoking. He remains overweight, but his weight has been stable since his admission to care. He is "thinking about" attending a health concerns group at the mental health center, but he hasn't followed through on that referral yet. He will meet with his psychiatrist this week at the clinic. The nurse and John discuss a plan to visit weekly for another month, then decreasing visits to every 2 weeks after that time if his symptoms remain stable.

Interdisciplinary Care Plan

Problem	Plan	Interventions	Evaluation
Psychosis (evidenced by auditory hallucinations, paranoia)	Within 2 weeks, patient will report a decrease in frequency of auditory hallucinations to weekly.	Assess for symptoms of psychosis. Discuss ways to decrease stimuli or use other stimuli to distract from auditory hallucinations.	Patient will report absence of command hallucinations and lower frequency of auditory hallucinations.

Problem	Plan	Interventions	Evaluation
	Within 2 weeks, patient will take daily medications correctly.	Discuss coping methods to decrease anxiety and symptoms. Educate patient about related use and effects/side effects of medications.	Patient will take daily medications correctly.
Difficulty managing home environment	Patient will discard daily trash and clean kitchen area of apartment within 4 weeks.	Assess for needs for assistance with management of apartment. Assist patient in setting realistic goals related to caring for apartment.	Apartment will be free from garbage.
Difficulty managing own self-care	Patient will attend to daily hygiene. Patient will make an appointment with primary care provider for physical exam within 4 weeks.	Assess for physical health needs. Assist patient to connect with primary care provider. Educate patient related to health promotion.	Patient will wear clean clothing and shower weekly. Patient will report attending the appointment with primary care provider.

REFERENCES & RESOURCES

[1] American Psychiatric Association, *Diagnostic and Statistical Manual of Mental Disorders* (4th ed.), *Text Revision: DSM-IV-TR*. American Psychiatric Association, 2000.

[2] K. Edward, B. Rasmussen and I. Munro, "Nursing care of patients treated with atypical antipsychotics who have a risk of developing metabolic instability and/or type 2 diabetes," *Archives of Psychiatric Nursing*, 24(1):46–53, 2010.

[3] N. Katakura, N. Yamamoto-Mitani and K. Ishigaki, "Home-visit nurses' attitudes for providing effective assistance to patients with schizophrenia," *International Journal of Mental Health Nursing*, 19:102–109, 2010.

[4] "National Alliance for the Mentally Ill (NAMI) Consumer Web Site," http://www.nami.org/template.cfm?section=Consumer_support

[5] A. Rudnick and J. Martins, "Coping and schizophrenia: A re-analysis," *Archives of Psychiatric Nursing*, 23(1):11–15, 2009.

Case 7.4 Schizoaffective Disorder

By Joanne DeSanto Iennaco, PhD, PMHCNS-BC, APRN

This case illustrates how the home health nurse cares for a patient with psychosis and mood symptoms (schizoaffective disorder). Rob is a 29-year-old, single male who is referred to home care post pneumothorax from a rib puncture and surgery to repair a broken radius, after a "fall from a height." Rob has a history of psychotic symptoms as well as mood symptoms that have troubled him since the age of 16. He reports that at 16 his family decided to kick him out of the house because he "was more trouble than he was worth."

Rob has a history of substance abuse, including alcohol, marijuana, cocaine, and "whatever is available." Rob is an active smoker. He has been homeless off and on for the past 2 years, since moving to the state. He has one friend he "can count on" with whom he frequently is able to stay. However, the friend is unemployed, has substance abuse problems, and is known to hang around with drug dealers and other addicts.

On the initial phone contact with Rob, he is abrupt and does not commit to being at home for the planned visit. He does not identify a time that would be good to visit and asks, "What the hell do you want to come to my house for anyway?" The nurse explains the need to follow up on both his mental health as well as medical needs, and he tells the nurse he has a doctor for that. The nurse explains that the role of the nurse is to help him manage his day-to-day health needs between doctor visits, and particularly now to be certain that his wrist is healing well. He states he does have some pain and "If you can help with that, I'll be here." The nurse reviews the medications and instructions provided by the hospital upon his discharge and discusses the importance of using his pain medication in a scheduled way if the pain is intense.

Clinical Case Studies in Home Health Care, First Edition. Edited by Leslie Neal-Boylan.
© 2011 John Wiley & Sons, Inc. Published 2011 by John Wiley & Sons, Inc.

The nurse ends the conversation with confirmation of a visit to Rob at 3:00 p.m. that afternoon.

Cultural Competence

Rob ends up homeless, which presents a variety of special needs different from patients in stable housing in the community. To start with, his homelessness makes it difficult for him to receive home care. Most individuals who are homeless are also living below the poverty level and have inadequate resources to support them when housing is unstable. Scheduling appointments with Rob and visiting Rob will be difficult unless his lack of housing is addressed as a priority.

 ORDERS FOR HOME CARE

Patient: 29-year-old, single Caucasian male

Diagnoses: Fall from height: rule out suicidal ideation or intent; status post pneumothorax after rib puncture; right radius fracture; status post open reduction and internal fixation; schizoaffective disorder; polysubstance abuse; rule out dependence

Current medications:
- Tylenol #3 1–2 tabs by mouth once every 4–6 hours
- Risperidone 3 mg by mouth twice a day
- Lithobid 600 mg by mouth twice a day

Relevant past medical history:
- Schizoaffective disorder
- Polysubstance abuse (alcohol, marijuana, cocaine)
- Long history of both inpatient and outpatient mental health treatment. Patient is known to "disappear" for long periods of time and reappear with full psychotic symptoms. Mood becomes hypomanic/irritable, with grandiosity, auditory hallucinations, and delusions. Intermittently becomes depressed per report of psychiatrist.

Referred to home care at hospital discharge by the orthopedic surgeon for followup, prevention of complications post pneumothorax and surgical reduction of radius fracture, and monitoring of psychiatric status.

RN: Assess and evaluate needs post pneumothorax and wrist surgery and assess mental health needs

OT: Assess and evaluate right arm mobility post surgery

Rob may have multiple spiritual concerns. Many patients with psychotic disorders have become disenfranchised with their friends and families. They often have considerable difficulties with disorganization and lack effective goal setting, initiative, and motivation to meet goals. This may result in a lack of purpose or meaning.

Rob is an adult who supports himself on Social Security Disability payments. He has not been successful in meeting usual developmental goals including establishing significant interpersonal relationships and establishing vocational or avocational interests and goals. His mental health problems have created instability due to frequent emergence of symptoms and transient relationships that often are not mutually fulfilling.

Reimbursement Considerations

Rob receives Supplemental Security Income (SSI) and thus is eligible for Medicaid coverage for his health needs. Medicaid provides for in-home care to those eligible. Medicaid does provide for in-home visits by a nurse and for medication management for those with psychiatric needs. Individual state requirements may vary, and the nurse should investigate the rules and requirements for the locale in which she works. Most states will provide for psychiatric home care services, given the need of the individual for in home services. It would be expected that Rob would qualify for assessment and prevention of medical/surgical complications and assistance in the stabilization of psychiatric needs and the transition home.

? CRITICAL THINKING

1. What factors make Rob at risk for not stabilizing and transitioning well to the home environment?

Answer: Rob has multiple needs during the acute recovery from his injury and broken wrist, as well as psychiatric needs that require stabilization. His lack of a stable home situation is a major risk factor, as are his mental health problems, given his prior symptom instability and lack of medication adherence.

THE HOME VISIT

The nurse visits Rob later that day to complete the admission assessment. The apartment where Rob is staying is in an impoverished neighborhood that has a great deal of drug related activity. The building looks abandoned. After ringing the outside bell several times, the nurse is buzzed in and proceeds upstairs to the second floor apartment. Rob is standing, looking out the door as the nurse comes up the stairway. The lock on the door appears to have been partly broken.

Rob is anxious, irritable, and appears to be in pain. He is tall and very thin and appears disheveled. His arm is in a closed cast, and he says that he has a bandage over his chest wound. Initially, he stands in the doorway to the apartment and refuses to let the nurse enter, stating that it isn't his place. The nurse asks him to check with his friend to see if it is okay for the nurse to come in. He allows the nurse to enter; and his friend, Tony, also greets the nurse.

His friend says that he is moving in a few weeks, and that's why there is no furniture. The air is heavy with smoke inside the apartment, and the room is nearly bare except for a mattress on the floor in the corner where Rob indicates he has been sleeping. Both the patient and the nurse move to the kitchen where there is a table and two chairs. The cabinets do not have doors so it is possible to see that there is no food. Rob moves very slowly and appears weak.

The nurse begins the assessment of Rob, starting with the observation that it appears that he is in pain. He says that he was discharged with a 3-day supply of pain medication and that he has been waiting until the pain is really bad to take them. He has not taken any since last night. He is knowledgeable about the purpose of his psychiatric medications and explains that he has been prescribed this combination for nearly a year. He reports that he often "gets messed up" taking them every day. He says that the best he did with taking his medications was several years ago when he got a shot, but he doesn't like needles.

The nurse assesses his respiratory status and finds that his lungs are clear to auscultation and his dressing is dry and intact. He denies alcohol or illicit substance use since his discharge from the hospital yesterday. Rob says that he usually sees his therapist every other week, but he doesn't remember whether his appointment is this week or next. He has a guardian who helps him with his finances, but he hasn't been in contact with that guardian in several months.

He admits that he does not feel well enough physically to get to the mental health clinic this week. Rob is scheduled for a follow-up appointment with his orthopedic surgeon in 1 week. Rob says that his last meal was at the hospital yesterday. It is the last week of the month, and Rob is out of money until his SSI check comes in next week.

Neal Theory Implications

Stage 3: The nurse in this case was a stage 3 nurse. She is experienced and able to autonomously determine the best action given the circumstance that now Rob is homeless and cannot be provided with in-home care. She contacts the ACT team, to provide some continuity in his care.

The stage 2 nurse would have knowledge of the community resources and appropriate possibilities for continuity of care, but may need assistance in making the referrals required.

A stage 1 nurse would recognize the problems inherent in Rob's homelessness, but would not be able to proceed to identify the appropriate community resources that could pick up with Rob's care at this time.

? CRITICAL THINKING

1. What are the priorities of assessment with Rob?
Answer: Whenever there is a safety concern, it is important to assess for the current presence of suicidal ideation and intent. Safety concerns also exist in this situation in terms of the safety of Rob's home environment. He lives in a dangerous neighborhood, and the lock to his apartment seems to be broken. It is unclear how he might contact help if he needed it, although Rob says that he has access to his friend's cell phone.

 ## BACK TO THE CASE

The admitting nurse has brought the psychiatric nurse into the case, and it is the psychiatric nurse who sees Rob for the remainder of his visits, along with the OT. Rob reports that, when his mental illness gets worse, he is irritable and tends to feel paranoid. He often is more active than normal and can go long periods without needing sleep. He states that it is those times when he is most likely to use substances, including cocaine and marijuana. He admits that he sometimes has depressive feelings and that he was feeling very down when he fell and broke his arm. He denies suicidal thoughts or intent currently, but states that when he fell he was hoping he'd "land on his head and end it all." He claims he didn't jump off the second floor landing that he fell from; but he says that he was pushed by a friend he was partying with and that it was a mistake. He says that he has had suicidal thoughts in the past but hasn't tried to kill himself in the past. He denies ever planning to kill himself.

Rob currently denies auditory hallucinations, although he reports that he experiences them when he misses his medications or is under a lot of stress. He often hears a male voice that tells him that others don't care about him or that he is not safe around certain people. He reports difficulty managing his anger and frequently getting into verbal and sometimes physical altercations with others. He reports that these problems have been less of a concern since he was in the hospital for this injury where got his medications regularly and didn't have to worry about where to live or get his next meal.

Rehabilitation Needs

Occupational therapy (OT)

His goals are to:

- Get his own apartment
- Pain relief in his arm

Based on the history and physical assessment the nurse's concerns in treating Rob include:

- Pain from wrist surgery
- His unstable housing situation
- Potential for exacerbation of psychiatric symptoms

The nurse has the following additional goals for her care of this patient:

- To monitor for mood instability
- To monitor for suicidal ideation and intent
- To monitor for substance use
- To assist in managing the medication regime to enhance adherence
- To connect the patient with community resources including Meals on Wheels, ride/transportation to the next clinic appointment, and housing options.

? CRITICAL THINKING

1. Are there other providers that should be called to assist with the case?
Answer: Yes, once the pain has subsided and the cast has been removed, an occupational therapist (OT) could be called in to assist with exercises

to ensure that Rob regains function in his hand and arm. In all likelihood, if Rob is adherent to his medications, he can probably attend an outpatient rehabilitation center to see an OT. The MSW can work with Rob to assist him in finding more suitable housing.

2. Are there any interventions required prior to leaving Rob's residence today?

Answer: Rob should be assisted to get engaged with community resources such as Meals on Wheels and to reconnect with the mental health clinic to determine his next appointment. If he is unable to walk or take the bus to this appointment, medical transportation can be arranged for him. Rob should also be instructed to contact either the nurse or the mental health clinic if he is feeling unsafe and having suicidal thoughts or having a return of other mental health symptoms. He should be helped to organize his medications and be provided with information about each medication.

 BACK TO THE CASE

Prior to leaving today, the nurse assists Rob by calling and referring him to Meals on Wheels; and he contacts the local community mental health center clinic where he attends therapy to determine when his next appointment is. The nurse sets up his medications in a medication box to assist him in taking them regularly. She also instructs him on the need to take the pain medication when he starts to notice it, before the pain becomes intense and discusses how this will help to prevent him from ending up in as much pain as he is in currently.

Relevant Community Resources

Food pantry
Homeless shelters

The nurse arranges to visit Rob again before the end of the week to reassess his wound, and to reevaluate how he is taking his medications. She provides the contact number for the agency should he need a visit sooner or have further questions. In planning for the case with the social worker, a plan is made for Rob to be referred to a community residential treatment center to attempt to break the cycle of housing instability. He can also attend Alcoholics Anonymous and other 12-step groups at the local clinic to support him in not abusing alcohol and other substances. Referral to local support programs for mental health patients that offer recreational and other activities will also aid in Rob's recovery.

Unfortunately, when the nurse contacts Rob to arrange a time for the follow-up visit, his friend Tony informs the nurse that they both got kicked out of the apartment where they were staying yesterday. They are both homeless right now and spent last night at a local shelter. Tony says that the nurse can probably find Rob at the park near the center of the city or at the shelter if it is after 4:00 p.m.

Ethical and Legal Considerations

Caring for Rob may pose several ethical concerns, including:

- Providing care to individuals who do not perceive a need for care
- Appropriate management of his pain medication given his history of substance abuse
- Safety of the nurse while providing care to Rob in a setting of drug addicts and dealers

It will be important for the nurse to document whether Rob currently suffers from suicidal ideation or intent. It is unclear whether the fall he experienced was due to jumping from a height or a fall.

? CRITICAL THINKING

1. What should the nurse do now?
Answer: To be able to receive home care, individuals generally need an address at which they can be visited. In the case where individuals do not have housing and are homeless, often they can be referred to the local Assertive Community Treatment (ACT) team, which has mobile clinicians who can follow Rob in the community. The nurse tells Tony to have Rob call her when he next sees him in case she is unable to find him today. The nurse considers referral to the ACT team, and stops by the park to attempt to follow up with Rob and discuss the referral to the ACT team with him.

Rob is in the park, and the nurse and Rob discuss the change in Rob's living situation. Rob tells the nurse that the pain is much better since earlier in the week and that he hasn't needed medication today. He says that he took the medication and shows the nurse the medication box that confirms this. Rob is agreeable to meeting with the ACT team, and the nurse helps him locate the nearest soup kitchen for lunch. Before leaving Rob, the nurse calls the ACT team, provides some referral information, and puts Rob on the line so they can arrange to meet later that day.

Interdisciplinary Care Plan

Problem	Goal/Plan	Intervention	Evaluation
Potential for infection and altered respiratory status due to status post pneumothorax and surgery for wrist fracture	Chest wound will heal and be free of infection within 1 week.	Assess for wound healing. Assess respiratory status. Encourage coughing and deep breathing. Educate patient regarding hygiene surrounding the wound. Educate regarding signs/ symptoms of wound infection or respiratory infection.	Patient will have lungs clear to auscultation. Wound will remain clean with dry sterile dressing and without signs/ symptoms of infection (redness, swelling, drainage).
Pain in arm/ wrist and chest wall due to fracture	Patient will report reduced pain within 1 week.	Assess for level/ degree of pain. Assess for change in ability to move freely and use arm. Educate patient regarding appropriate use of pain medication. Educate patient regarding splinting chest wall when coughing.	Patient will state pain is a 2/10 or 3/10 on pain scale.
Instability of mood and psychotic symptoms	Patient will report stable mood, and decreased psychotic and other symptoms (auditory hallucinations, paranoid ideation, anger) within 4 weeks. Patient will report plan to call crisis line or mental health clinic if he has recurrence of suicidal thought or intent in 1 week.	Assess for changes in mental status, mood, and symptoms of psychosis. Assess for suicidal ideation and intent. Educate patient regarding methods for coping with stressors. Connect patient with appropriate mental health clinic resources for support.	Patient will state decrease in auditory hallucinations and paranoid thinking, angry outbursts. Patient will report lack of suicidal ideation/intent and plan to safely manage if those thoughts recur.

(Continued)

Problem	Goal/Plan	Intervention	Evaluation
Need for symptom and medication management	Patient will identify new strategies to manage angry feelings within 1 month. Patient will correctly self-administer medications daily within 2 weeks.	Assess for effects and side effects of medications. Discuss positive methods to cope with angry feelings. Orient patient to medication box and educate related to correct self-administration of medications. Educate patient related to effects and side effects of medications.	Patient will state use of 1 new strategy to manage angry feelings. Patient will correctly take medications.
History of substance use and abuse (tobacco, marijuana, cocaine)	Patient will attend self-help group to aid in avoiding substance use.	Assess patient's substance use each visit. Help patient locate and connect with resources for treatment of substance abuse. Educate patient related to negative effects of substance use and abuse on health and mental health.	Patient will report no use of illegal substances.
Housing instability and lack of community support systems	Patient will report stable housing has been attained within 1 month. Patient will report reconnection with community mental health services.	Assess needs related to community mental health services. Assist patient to locate community resources related to safer housing in the community. Educate patient related to programs and entitlements that he may be eligible for and that will assist in search for stable housing.	Patient will report plan to move to safe housing situation. Patient will report attendance at community mental health clinic.

REFERENCES & RESOURCES

[1] American Psychiatric Association, *Diagnostic and Statistical Manual of Mental Disorders* (4th ed.), *Text Revision: DSM-IV-TR.* American Psychiatric Association, 2000.

[2] E.L. Meerwijk, B. van Meijel, J. van den Bout, A. Kerkhof, W. de Vogel and M. Grypdonck, "Development and evaluation of a guideline for nursing care of suicidal patients with schizophrenia," *Perspectives in Psychiatric Care,* 46(1):65–73, 2009.

Section 8

Musculoskeletal

Case 8.1 Muscular Dystrophy

By Sharron E. Guillett, PhD, RN

This case study illustrates how the home health nurse works with the patient and family to promote physiologic functioning and to promote the patient remaining at home. The patient is a 40-year-old female who was born with type 1 spinal muscular atrophy (SMA). Type 1 is the most severe form of this disease that destroys the anterior horn cells of the spinal cord. Type 1 children never learn to crawl, sit, or walk; have difficulty holding up their heads; and are in constant danger of respiratory arrest. Remarkably, Ms. R has lived past all expectations with minimal sequelae. This is due in large part to the constant care she has received from her family, especially her sister who has lived with and cared for her for the past 20 years. Ms. R has just been released from the hospital following an upper respiratory infection that compromised her respiratory system. While hospitalized, she was also treated for an impacted bowel. The nurse will need to collaborate with a variety of disciplines to promote physiologic functioning and support vital organ systems.

 ## ORDERS FOR HOME CARE

Patient: 40-year-old Caucasian female
Diagnoses: SMA type 1, osteoporosis, diabetes, hypertension, sleep
    apnea, severe depression, gastroesophageal reflux disease (GERD)

Clinical Case Studies in Home Health Care, First Edition. Edited by Leslie Neal-Boylan.
© 2011 John Wiley & Sons, Inc. Published 2011 by John Wiley & Sons, Inc.

Current medications:
- Protonix 40 mg once a day
- Celexa, 20 mg once a day
- Lotensin 20 mg once a day
- Lipitor 10 mg at bedtime
- Ambien 5 mg once a day
- Diazepam 5 mg 1–2 tabs daily as needed
- OxyContin 40 mg every 4 hours
- Avandia 8 mg once a day
- Colace 100 mg as needed
- Caltrate once a day
- Lexapro 20 mg at bedtime

Relevant past medical history:
- Congenital SMA
- Adult onset noninsulin-dependent diabetes diagnosed at age 30
- Sleep apnea for past 5 years
- Recently diagnosed hypertension

RN: Assess and evaluate.
OT: Assess and evaluate.
PT: Assess and evaluate.
RT: Assess and evaluate.
MSW: Assess and evaluate.

Cultural Competence

Ms. R is a middle-aged Caucasian woman. It is important for her to have some control over her environment and to make decisions regarding her plan of care.

 THE HOME VISIT

The nurse arrives at the apartment building, which has a secured entry system, and pushes the buzzer by the patient's name. After identifying herself, the nurse is buzzed in by someone with a female voice. The entry area of the building is clean and very well appointed. The apartment is on the third floor. The nurse is greeted by a pleasant young woman who identifies herself as the patient's sister. She lives with and cares for the patient. Ms. R is in the living room watching TV. She is tetraplegic. The only body part she can move independently is her thumb, which she uses to control her powered wheelchair. The chair has a head support, tray table to support her arms, and a custom seating system. Ms. R is alert, talkative, and engaging. She is breathing without assistance and is not using oxygen although there are discernible marks on her face that suggest she has been using oxygen. Ms. R is sipping coffee from an elongated straw which frequently escapes her mouth and needs repositioning. Her sister is never more than an arm's length away during the interview.

The sisters share great affection for each other and are obviously a team committed to extending Ms. R's life and its quality. Ms. R is very knowledgeable about her illness and realizes that she has lived longer than most people with her illness. This makes her afraid that she is dying. She has explored many alternative therapies and metaphysical approaches to life and is frustrated by her inability to use her mind to its fullest because of her physical limitations. She has a voice-activated phone and computer system and does "counseling" for other people like herself. Her sister describes her as hypervigilant about her body and body functions and says she wakes up every morning in a panic that she is "running out of time." The patient agrees that she has trouble calming her thoughts in the morning. As the day wears on, she is able to use self-talk and meditation to calm herself. She believes in alternative therapies and the healing nature of positive thought, essential oils, certain gems, prayer, and meditation. She is open to many world views.

The patient is chronically constipated and is on a bowel regimen. The sister is always looking for natural cathartics to promote bowel function. She acknowledges that the patient takes a great deal of OxyContin which contributes to the constipation. The patient somewhat defensively explains that she is in a great deal of pain most days and that the OxyContin "barely touches it." She describes the pain as a constant boring pain that the medication keeps at level of 3 or 4. The patient also takes Valium regularly. The patient and her sister agree that the goals for care are aimed at preventing physiologic decline:

- Provide respiratory support at night.
- Promote adequate nutrition without compromising the patient's airway.
- Manage pain with least amount of medication possible.
- Promote bowel function.
- Increase independence/self-actualization.
- Prevent injury/skin breakdown.
- Prevent caregiver burnout.

Physical exam reveals a woman with a "cushingoid" appearance (round face, truncal obesity, atrophied limbs) in no acute distress. Her vital signs are within normal limits. Her lungs are clear, although she struggles to take a deep breath. The sister reports that the patient has no trouble breathing during the day but uses Bi-PAP at night (explaining the marks on her face). The nurse notes that the patient lists a little to the side and learns that they are in the process of getting a new seating system that provides more support and less effort to manipulate. The patient's skin is dry and intact, although there is evidence of a healed ulceration on the left earlobe. The patient is well groomed with manicured fingernails and toenails. Both feet and hands are edematous. Edema is nonpitting and does not change with position of the limbs. The abdomen is difficult to assess, but bowel sounds are present.

Neal Theory Implications

Stage 3: The professional in this stage is confident and comfortable collaborating with other disciplines and agencies. The nurse recognizes the need to take the lead role in case management even though the patient's skilled nursing needs may be resolved in a few visits. The nurse at this stage knows that the patient's quality of life will depend on how well the services are coordinated. The nurse is also aware of the need to incorporate the sister into the plan of care and assesses the sister's well-being and ability to continue to provide the level of care required.

Stage 2: The nurse at this stage is capable of assembling the appropriate team. However, that nurse may believe that her job is done once the team is assembled. The nurse at this stage correctly focuses on physical and safety needs but may overlook the need the patient has for self-actualization, as well as the respite needs of the sister.

Stage 1: The clinician in this stage will assess the patient and may believe that she and her sister are managing well and just respond to the needs they express. The nurse at this stage may not be comfortable probing further or asking the sister to demonstrate care activities to see if there is potential to improve independence, nutrition, mobility, or strength with the addition of other disciplines.

Based on the history and physical examination, the nurse discovers the following data:

- Ms. R is wheelchair bound but is able to move about home.
- Ms. R is incontinent of bowel and bladder and wears Depends.
- Ms. R is totally dependent for activities of daily living (ADL) and instrumental activities of daily living (IADL).
- Ms. R is frightened of dying.
- Ms. R could not summon help or exit the apartment in case of emergency.
- Ms. R takes high doses of pain medications and tranquilizers without blunting her affect or cognitive abilities.

- Ms. R believes in the healing properties of prayer, essential oils, meditation, gem stones, and herbs.
- Ms. R's current seating system does not provide proper alignment and support respiratory efforts.
- Ms. R is both depressed and anxious.
- Ms. R is not sexually active.

Rehabilitation Needs

Physical therapy
Bowel program
Respiratory therapy
Vocational therapy

? CRITICAL THINKING

1. What is the priority for care for Ms. G?
Answer: The priority is safety. Clearly Ms. R cannot be left alone for any length of time; but beyond that, she is always at risk for respiratory compromise or failure. The apartment has been adapted for safety and accessibility, but there is no way that Ms. R could exit in case of fire or other emergency. Suppose the sister is taken ill and cannot summon help—How would Ms. R get help? A simple medical alert system needs to be installed, connecting them to someone in the building and or the fire department or rescue squad. The respiratory therapist (RT) needs to evaluate respiratory function and make recommendations regarding pulmonary toilet positioning and ventilator support/alarms at night. The respiratory therapist can also teach the sister how to help the patient clear secretions, protect the airway, and do quad coughs.

2. What will the physical therapist (PT) do when he/she arrives at the home?
Answer: The PT will assess the seating system and recommend assistive devices to maintain proper body alignment. The PT will also assess the extent of muscle atrophy in the limbs, suggest passive range of motion (ROM) exercises, and assess the need for orthotics to promote proper positioning.

3. Who should take the leadership role in this case?
Answer: The registered nurse (RN) is in the best position to lead the team as she has the big picture and can manage the patient's plan of care holistically. Ms. R has numerous physiologic needs, but she and her sister also need a great deal of psychosocial support. A single point of contact will simplify the process of getting needed services, integrate

care, and ensure appropriate followup. This will decrease Ms. D's anxiety. The nurse is also in the best position to evaluate how the sister is coping with the stress of caregiving.

BACK TO THE CASE

Reimbursement Considerations

The patient is too young to be eligible for Medicare; but she does qualify for Social Security benefits, Medicaid, and 35 hours per week of Medicaid-supported home care.

Her sister is paid to provide her care through a Medicaid waiver.

The nurse praises Ms. R and her sister for how well they have done in caring for each other. The nurse encourages Ms. R to pursue her intellectual interests and try to focus her concerns outward. She suggests that they think about sharing their strategies for success with others. Ms. R likes this idea. The nurse discusses the medication regime with the sisters, and both are adamant that the pain medications are essential. The nurse suggests that they talk to the doctor about an alternative for Valium since it can be habit-forming. They agree to at least discuss it. The nurse suggests a medical alert system, which seems to increase Ms. D's anxiety. She says her sister never leaves her unattended. The nurse gets them to agree to let the fire department and rescue squad know that she is disabled and provide the location of her bedroom. She will continue to pursue a life alert system in subsequent visits.

The nurse discusses the bowel management program and discovers that the sister actually physically massages the patient's abdomen daily to move stool through the colon. The nurse provides a bowel management booklet and orders enema sets for periodic use. She also provides a list of laxative producing foods.

Relevant Community Resources

Notification of the fire department and police department that she is disabled

Transportation for shopping and socialization

Respite care

The nurse contacts the primary care provider (PCP) and requests a prescription for Ativan, which the PCP provides.

? CRITICAL THINKING

1. Should the nurse request a psychiatric consult?
Answer: The patient is depressed and fearful. She is currently relying on a number of medications to manage her thoughts and emotions. Because the patient has studied counseling herself, it is a topic that could be discussed easily. One approach is for the nurse to ask if the patient has considered seeking some help from a counselor or religious leader. Regardless of the answer, the groundwork is laid for a more in-depth discussion of the benefits of receiving this type of help. The nurse could point out that at the very least a review of the antidepressants, tranquilizers, and mood elevators she is on might be beneficial.

2. What should the nurse do about Ms. R's use of alternative therapies?
Answer: Ms. R is very bright, and she can research the benefits of alternative therapies herself. The nurse can encourage her to use trusted web sites such as the NIH to examine the research that is available. The patient should not take St. John's Wort or any substance with Chinese herbs as these affect clotting and blood pressure. The patient should also be advised to let the caregiving team know any alternative therapies that the patient is using so that they can be incorporated into the plan of care.

Interdisciplinary Care Plan

Problem	Goal/Plan	Intervention	Evaluation
Potential for airway compromise	Patient will not aspirate or experience atelectasis, will be free of congestion, and will use measures to support ventilation at night.	RT will teach pulmonary hygiene techniques and assure proper care and use of Bi-PAP equipment. RN will teach feeding strategies and positioning for eating. PT will make recommendations for seating system that allows optimal lung expansion.	Sister performs quad cough twice daily. Patient sleeps comfortably and does not awake with headache from oxygen deficit. Pulse oximetry on room air remains within normal limits.

(Continued)

Problem	Goal/Plan	Intervention	Evaluation
Chronic pain	Patient will manage pain without increasing pain medications	Encourage patient to use meditation and other strategies to decrease pain levels.	Patient is able to manage pain on current medication regime.
Anxiety related to perceived decline in condition	Patient will verbalize her concerns and attempt to find appropriate coping strategies.	Listen actively to patient fears and worries. Encourage patient to engage in activities that allow her to express herself and feel that she is contributing to her care. Refer to counseling if symptoms become overwhelming.	Sister reports that panic attacks are less severe. Patient is able to control morning outbursts. Patient is able to discuss fears openly and plan for end of life. Patient engages in social activities.
Chronic constipation	Patient will not become impacted.	Recommend strategies for keeping stool soft and review bowel management program with sister.	Patient will be able to evacuate bowel according to her normal pattern.
Caregiver stress	Sister will maintain health and outside relationships.	Encourage sister to spend some time away from caregiving responsibilities. Teach sister lifting and moving techniques to decrease risk for injury. Recommend equipment to ease caregiving burden.	Sister engages in activities outside of the home weekly. Sister and patient allow each other private time and space daily. Patient is able to obtain lifting equipment.

REFERENCES & RESOURCES

[1] "Fight SMA," http://www.fightsma.org
[2] National Insitutes of Health, "Eunice Kennedy Shriver," National Institute of Health & Human Development. http://www.nichd.nih.gov/

Case 8.2 Cerebral Palsy

By Sharron E. Guillett, PhD, RN

This case study illustrates how the home health nurse works with the patient and family to promote quality of life. The patient is a 27-year-old female who has had cerebral palsy, specifically spastic quadriparesis, since birth. She is in a wheelchair, has very little use of her right side, is cognitively delayed, and lives with her parents who are both in their late 50s and who are employed full time outside of the home. The patient has been in school or a sheltered environment during the day since the age of 3. She has now "aged out" of the educational system. Her parents had pieced together a system of caregiving relying on family, friends, and neighbors until the patient had a fainting spell and a subsequent lab test revealed a blood sugar of 45. The family no longer feels that the patient can be left alone; but, financially, both parents need to work. The patient recognizes the need for help and is accustomed to having someone assist her with activities of daily living (ADL) and instrumental activities of daily living (IADL) but resents having someone in the house "following her around" all of the time.

The nurse case manager will need to assemble a team that protects the patient from harm while supporting the patient's need for independence and privacy.

Cultural Competence

Ms. T is a young Caucasian woman. The law provides for her to have age-appropriate care, but that is difficult to arrange. She is too old for most community-based athletic groups and younger than most of the care providers available. It is important for her to associate with her peers. The nurse can encourage her parents to support efforts at making and maintaining these associations and friendships.

Clinical Case Studies in Home Health Care, First Edition. Edited by Leslie Neal-Boylan.
© 2011 John Wiley & Sons, Inc. Published 2011 by John Wiley & Sons, Inc.

ORDERS FOR HOME CARE

Patient: 27-year-old Caucasian female
Diagnoses: Cerebral palsy, hypoglycemia
Current medications:
- Lisinopril 10 mg three times a day
- Carbamazepine 60 mg twice a day
- Claritin 10 mg once a day
- MVI 1 once a day

Relevant past medical history:
- Seizure disorder controlled with medication
- Multiple surgeries to release tendons and correct hip positioning
- Eczema/urticaria

RN: Assess and evaluate.
OT: Assess and evaluate.
MSW: Assess and evaluate.

Reimbursement Considerations

The patient is too young to be eligible for Medicare, but she does qualify for 30 hours per week of Medicaid-supported home care and has received Social Security since she was 18 years old. She is also covered by private insurance for routine medical care. The nurse, as case manager on this case, will need to work with social services to establish Medicaid supported home care and respite care for the hours not covered by Medicaid.

THE HOME VISIT

The nurse is the first to enter the home, which is a 2.5-story single home. The home is clean, uncluttered, and well organized. A woman who introduces herself as Ms. T's mother meets the nurse at the door. Ms. T is waiting at the kitchen table. She is seated in a wheelchair with contoured seating. She appears frail and much younger than her stated age. She is clean and well groomed, without make up or jewelry. The nurse introduces herself and begins to do the admission assessment.

Ms. T is pleasant and cooperative. The nurse notes that the patient startles easily, has disconjugate gaze and pulls away when touched. Ms. T states that she is tactile defensive and that loud noises or sudden moves make her jump. The nurse asks the patient what she can do for herself and the patient replies "not much." The patient's mother indicates that the patient tries to do what she can for herself and does assist with dressing, brushing her hair, and brushing her teeth. She can also feed herself but needs help cutting up food and pouring liquids. She has adapted silverware and contoured plates. She is basically dependent in all ADL and IADL. She is not able to sit or stand independently or transfer due to lack of balance, and she is very frightened of falling. Ms. T has good language skills, although she sometimes perseverates. She enjoys music and spends a lot of time on the Internet. She cannot do simple math, cannot figure out time without a digital clock, and has trouble spelling. She can print with varying degrees of legibility. She has a cell phone and knows how to summon help, but mental processing is scattered.

The home is equipped with a full-size elevator that provides access to all 3 levels of the house. However, access to the elevator is situated differently on upper and lower levels so that the patient can enter the elevator independently but cannot exit without help. The patient's living area is on the second floor. Her room and bathroom are spacious and adapted for use and safety. She has a computer and television in her room. Since she had the fainting episode, a small refrigerator has been placed in the adjoining room. It is stocked with candy, pudding, and applesauce. Ms. T's mother and father prepare her meals and bring them to her room when she does not feel like joining them for dinner.

The nurse learns that the patient knows the importance of taking her medications on time and that her parents mix them with pudding and administer them to her. She denies seizure activity but states she sometimes blacks out. The parents state they have not witnessed any blackouts. The nurse wonders if perhaps the patient is experiencing absence seizures.

The nurse examines Ms. T and finds that she has severe lordosis and a small C curve at her upper thoracic spine. She maintains her balance by constantly grasping the right armrest of her wheelchair; and as a result, she has an overdeveloped right bicep. Her patellae are slightly higher than normal due to her spasticity, and she is most comfortable with her legs slightly extended. She is able to take a few steps if supported but is easily fatigued. The nurse notes fasciculation in the right quadriceps. Ms. T denies problems with continence as long as someone can get her to the bathroom. She has a boyfriend but they rarely see each other. She is not sexually active. When questioned about her goals for care she states, "I just don't want people to bug me." Ms. T's mother identifies the following goals for her daughter.

- To remain safe
- To maintain adequate nutritional intake

- To prevent contractures, skin breakdown
- To increase independence with ADL and IADL
- To participate in activities outside of the home
- To develop skills leading to employment

Neal Theory Implications

Stage 3: The professional in this stage collaborates with other disciplines both within and outside of home care and is autonomous with both the clinical and reimbursement aspects of the case and the logistical aspects of working with a variety of agencies.

Stage 2: The professional in this stage may not feel comfortable requesting orders for other disciplines or working within the patient's environment to manage care. The professional in this stage may also have trouble discriminating between services provided as part of this episode of care and those provided as a result of the patient's disability status.

Stage 1: The clinician in this stage will assess the patient; and seeing that she is very communicative and engaging, the clinician may not recognize the true level of assistance needed.

Based on the history and physical examination, the nurse discovers the following data:

- Ms. T is wheelchair bound but is able to move about the home.
- Ms. T has poor balance and no protective reflexes and cannot sit or stand independently.
- Ms. T has limited use of right hand.
- Ms. T has exaggerated startle reflex.
- Ms. T has cognitive delay and is at risk for caregiver abuse.
- Ms. T has been receiving assistance with all of her ADL.
- Ms. T denies pain but occasionally has headaches.
- Ms. T has no history of depression but is often saddened by her inability to do things that other people do.

Rehabilitation Needs

Physical therapy (PT)
Occupational therapy (OT)
Vocational therapy

| ? | **CRITICAL THINKING** |

1. What is the priority for care for Ms. T?
Answer: The priority is safety. Maintaining a safe environment is complex in this case, because the patient appears to be capable of caring for herself and her cognitive delays are not readily ascertained. She also fabricates stories, which makes it difficult to discern real from imagined experiences. This makes her especially vulnerable to people who take advantage of individuals with limited intellectual capacity. Ms. T's parents need to be cautioned about screening companions and home health aides (HHAs) as well as being vigilant for indications that their daughter is being manipulated.

All rooms in the house have been adapted for safety and accessibility, but there are still some areas of concern such as ungated stairways. Also, there is no way for the patient to get out of the house from the second floor in case of fire or intrusion. A medical alert system might be useful. The physical therapist (PT) and the occupational therapist (OT) will make recommendations regarding keeping the home uncluttered, installing grab bars in the shower, installing smoke and carbon monoxide detectors, and insuring that the patient can reach the phone and the light switches in each room.

2. What will the OT do when she/he arrives at the home?
Answer: The OT will do an ADL assessment to determine ways to promote independence and make recommendations regarding adaptive equipment. The OT will also assess upper-extremity and hand strength and teach Ms. T exercises to maintain function. Although Ms. T is very good with the computer, she only uses one hand; therefore, sending emails is very time consuming for her. The OT is able to obtain computer adaptations that will help Ms. T work more efficiently, as well as prepare her for opportunities to work from home.

3. What is the role of the medical social worker (MSW) in this case?
Answer: The MSW evaluates the needs and financial resources of the patient to determine eligibility for state and federal support. Ms. T currently receives full Social Security benefits due to her disability. She also has a Medicaid number; but since he is covered on her parents' insurance, she can only use her Medicaid monies for services not otherwise covered. The MSW ascertains that Ms. T is eligible for a Medicaid supported HHA and provides a list of approved home health care agencies in the area. The HHA will visit Ms. T daily to assist her with ADL. The HHA will assist her with grooming and oral care, prepare her meals, assist her with toileting, get her in and out of her wheelchair, and assist her with her exercises. The HHA will also do Ms. T's personal laundry, make her bed, and clean her room. Although the home health aide hours provided as part of this plan of care are limited, once

this episode is resolved, Ms. T is eligible to have a home health aide on daily basis by virtue of her disability. The MSW will work with Ms. T to find community resources to help her with transportation for shopping and appointments.

BACK TO THE CASE

The nurse explains to Ms. T and her mother that she can stay at home safely if a suitable HHA can be found. The nurse praises Ms. T for her desire to be independent and assures her that she can have a helper and still maintain privacy and control over her life. The nurse recommends that a "lifeline" system be established and that local police and fire departments be made aware of Ms. T's disabilities and the exact location of her bedroom. This is especially important since evacuation in case of a fire would be impossible without help. The patient reluctantly agrees to try an agency but expresses concern over being either hurt or interfered with.

Relevant Community Resources

Notification of the fire department and police department that she is disabled
Transportation for shopping and socialization
Therapeutic sports/recreational groups

The nurse calls the primary care provider (PCP) and requests an order for a drug level for carbemazapine, a PT evaluation and a one time visit from a registered dietician to assess, evaluate and provide a diet plan to address the hypoglycemia. The physician agrees to the plan.

CRITICAL THINKING

1. What can the family do to protect the patient from unscrupulous caregivers?
Answer: Before allowing any caregiver into the home, the family needs to be sure that the agency has been vetted by the county department of social services. Additionally, the family should check that the home health aide had a criminal background check done by the home care agency and was cleared to provide care. Ms. T should be cautioned

against discussing finances or where money or other assets are kept. Money and jewelry should not be left in the open. Duplicates of home and car keys should be stored safely. Ms. T should also be encouraged to report any rough or inappropriate physical contact or inability to get help when summoned. Having friends and neighbors call or stop by periodically is also helpful.

2. Why did the nurse decide to involve a dietitian?
Answer: The patient is undernourished and frail in appearance. Her estimated weight is 70–75 pounds. The patient states she eats a lot, but her parents report that she does not eat breakfast and eats very small portions at lunch and dinner. She likes crunchy snacks before bedtime. Her personal refrigerator is stocked with simple sugar sources, which will only exacerbate hypoglycemia. A dietitian will be able to assess Ms. T's caloric needs and work with her to develop a diet plan that contains nutrient-dense foods and snacks to address the hypoglycemia.

3. What can the nurse do to promote a high quality of life for Ms. T?
According to the Canadian Health Model (1998), quality of life is the ability to enjoy the self defined important aspects of one's life. The nurse promotes this quality of life by first determining what it is that matters to Ms. T and then helping her attain that. For example, if walking is not something that Ms. T feels is important to the quality of her life, the nurse should not focus on walking no matter how strongly the nurse believes it will make a difference in Ms. T's life.

In this case, Ms. T values her independence and her ability to spend time with her friends. Therefore, her quality of life will be enhanced if the nurse can put together a team that will increase Ms. T's ability to carry out her ADL independently and manage her toileting needs and her blood sugar when out in the community.

Interdisciplinary Care Plan

Problem	Goal/Plan	Intervention	Evaluation
Knowledge deficit regarding hypoglycemia	Patient and family will verbalize understanding of factors contributing to hypoglycemia and dietary patterns to correct it.	Teach patient and parents about the importance of eating protein or complex carbohydrates every 2 hours.	Patient will stock personal refrigerator with boiled eggs, cheese sticks, or peanut butter snacks.

(Continued)

Problem	Goal/Plan	Intervention	Evaluation
Self-care deficit	Patient will be able to dress upper body and perform grooming without assistance.	Purchase clothing that is easy to pull on over the head, with easy fasteners. Teach patient to use assistive devices to retrieve clothing. Purchase adapted toothbrush for easy grip and angle that supports hand motion.	Patient performs morning and bedtime grooming with minimal assistance. Patient puts on shirts and tops with minimal assistance and minimal frustration.
Weakness in extremities	Patient will have increased strength in all extremities within 2 months.	Teach patient strengthening exercises. Encourage ambulation.	Patient is able to participate more in self-care related to increased strength. Patient is able to stand and ambulate from bathroom to bed without fasiculations or fatigue.
Diminished quality of life related to lack of independence	Patient will express satisfaction with home care arrangements and ability to socialize.	Be sure that patient is allowed ample time alone for privacy needs and is given time to carry out ADL independently.	Patient reports that caregivers provide privacy, assist the patient as requested, and respect her need for independence.
Risk for injury	Patient will not incur any injury.	Home health aide will be present when parents are at work. Caregiver will be alert to changes in condition consistent with low blood sugar or seizure activity.	Patient will not experience blackouts or fainting spells.

Problem	Goal/Plan	Intervention	Evaluation
Social isolation	Patient will verbalize satisfaction with social relationships within 3 months.	Improve patient's strength and mobility. Obtain adaptive devices and equipment that will enable patient to participate in activities outside of the home.	Patient is able to meet friends at the shopping mall.

REFERENCES & RESOURCES

[1] R. Renwick and I. Brown, "The Centre for Health Promotion's conceptual approach to quality of life: Being, belonging, and becoming," *Quality of Life in Health Promotion and Rehabilitation: Conceptual Approaches, Issues, and Applications*, R. Renwick, I. Brown and M. Nagler (eds.), pp. 75–88, Sage, 1996.

[2] "United Cerebral Palsy," http://www.ucp.org

Case 8.3 Osteomyelitis, Decubitus Ulcer, and Paraplegia

By Linda Royer, PhD, RN

This case illustrates the complexities of spinal cord injury (SCI) and its consequences to young adults, as well as the many-faceted aspects of service required of the home health agency to improve and maintain function and productivity in the patient.

Mr. Q is a 29-year-old Caucasian male living alone in a 6-story apartment building in a medium-size city. He is divorced and has an 11-year-old son; custody of the child is shared with his ex-wife. Relations between the parents are cordial but distant. The patient graduated from college and established his own computer programming and web management business, which he operates from his apartment. He is covered by his company's insurance plan. His SCI was a result of a fall of 30 feet while mountain climbing at age 18 years. He sustained injury at the C-7 junction and is paralyzed in the lower extremities and unable to voluntarily control elimination functions. He has upper-extremity strength for mobility and moderate fine muscle control. He uses a hand-powered wheelchair, drives his own car modified with hand controls, and enjoys activities on his all-terrain vehicles kept at his parents' farm. He has a history of hospitalizations for recurrent decubitus ulcer breakdowns.

Mr. Q has been referred to the home health agency by the medical center where he has been treated for the past 7 days for a decubitus ulcer over his right ischial tuberosity, this time stage IV with osteomyelitis and methicillin resistant *staphylococcus aureus* (MRSA) infection. His wound was debrided and oxygenation-driven wound vacuum treatment begun as well as an intravenous (IV) antibiotic. (Refer to Box 8.3.1).

Clinical Case Studies in Home Health Care, First Edition. Edited by Leslie Neal-Boylan.
© 2011 John Wiley & Sons, Inc. Published 2011 by John Wiley & Sons, Inc.

Box 8.3.1 CA-MRSA Fact

"In general, CA-MRSA has far less risk of any complications than HA-MRSA as long as the patient does well with treatment and does not require hospitalization. However, people that do get complications generally have a chance for a worse outcome, as organ systems may be irreversibly damaged."

Source: http://www.medicinenet.com/mrsa_infection/article.htm

In Mr. Q's case, pneumonia is a threat. He was hospitalized due to his overall condition and deficits of paraplegia and received effective treatment in a timely fashion. He was discharged to restrictive activity to his home.

ORDERS FOR HOME CARE

Diagnoses: Recurrent decubitus ulcer, stage IV, with methicillin-resistant *staphylococcus aureus* (MRSA); paraplegia due to spinal cord injury (SCI) for 11 years

Current Medication: Vancomycin 1230 mg intravenously (IV) every 12 hours; maintain PICC line

RN: Assess and evaluate. Physician's orders include care of PICC line and administration of IV antibiotic, Vancomycin, 1230 mg every 12 hours, as well as continuance of wound protocol (negative pressure wound pump) except for off periods of 4 hours twice per day.

Reimbursement Considerations

Mr. Q has a reliable insurance plan that has covered him since he became emancipated. He states he has good rapport with his agent and has been assured he will have coverage for needed home care services.

THE HOME VISIT

The home health nurse is familiar with Mr. Q because he first managed his case in the community after the accident. Mr. Q has experienced 2 other episodes of skin breakdown, but this is the first time the site has become seriously infected. It has been disappointing to see him return to the hospital repeatedly over these intervening years, because it seems he can never get Mr. Q to take full responsibility for his self-management status. That is due partly to several intervening factors: his zest for adventuresome activities and his bent for traveling, his casual attitude of disregard for self, long hours in his chair working at the computer, and an apparent deficit sense of self-worth. The nurse hopes that this time he can make an impact on Mr. Q's spirit and instill a more responsible regard for his own safety. Because Mr. Q is now battling MRSA, the nurse's concern is heightened regarding successful treatment and prevention of further spread of the disease among his family, friends, caregivers, and the community.

Ethical Considerations

Ethical concerns beyond consent for treatment were discussed at the beginning of the visit, and the patient signed documents for the home health agency and a HIPAA acknowledgement form. Of primary importance is the appropriate handling of the knowledge that he has been infected with CA-MRSA. On questioning him, he states that his friends and family know that he is infected; and they were educated in various ways about the importance of limiting transmission through wound precautions, handling of linens and clothing, and frequent hand washing.

Mr. Q has been discharged to his own apartment with the provision that a family member visit him twice daily to assist with his wound care and activities of daily living (ADL). The other option was for him to go to his parent's farm for several weeks until his decubitus healed to a stage II status; however, Mr. Q wanted to get back to work in his home office as soon as possible to complete jobs for his current customers. When the nurse arrives at this first visit, he brings a nursing student with him and meets Mr. Q's mother, Ann.

They find the apartment orderly, clean, and airy. The home care supplier has already delivered equipment and supplies, such as a hazardous waste disposal can with lid, small oxygen tank and wound vacuum apparatus, and dressings. The IV administration division of the home care agency had just delivered the IV pump and administration supplies. The pharmacy courier had delivered the antibiotic (Vancomycin).

Mr. Q is lying on his futon prone and propped with pillows. Rapport is reestablished between the nurse and the patient and his mother; the nursing student is welcomed. The nurse explains agency policies, some of which have changed as a result of new regulations of the Health Care Affordability Act; papers are signed and insurance information is documented in the agency software on the nurse's laptop. Because this will be a lengthy visit with much ground to cover regarding treatment and education, the assessment is begun.

In addition to information above about his SCI, Mr. Q's health history reveals a normal upbringing in a loving rural family with 3 other siblings, all of whom are in good health. It is unclear where he contracted MRSA, but is suspected that it was community acquired (CA-MRSA) due to exposure through a friend whom he often visits who had a boil on his leg that he had ignored for some time.

The student conducts the assessment under the nurse's supervision and with Mr. Q's permission. Before approaching the patient, the nurse and the student don gloves. Vital signs are normal; however, they will continue to be concerned about Mr. Q's temperature and urge him to check it and record it every morning and evening. Heart sounds are normal; and his lungs are clear throughout, though respiration excursion is shallow. Pulses in all extremities are evaluated by palpation and auscultation and by Doppler on the lower extremities. Inspection of Mr. Q's skin for turgor and intactness reveals a dry condition with weak turgor, but generally with adequate venous return upon blanching. Toenails need trimming. Daily emollient treatment to his skin will be necessary. There are no signs of scarring or disfigurement of skin tissue on his body, in spite of sensation deficits. There is a PICC line in his left antecubital space with a transparent dressing intact. The site is free of redness or streaking.

Finally, with aseptic technique, they examine Mr. Q's right ischial decubitus ulcer, covered by a flexible hydrocolloid dressing. Over the 7 days in the hospital the wound was treated continuously with the wound vacuum, absorbing sponges, and periodic normal saline flushes. The wound bed is bright red, which is a typical result of this organism [3]. Of concern, however, is the exposure of approximately 2 cm of the ischial osteum in the bed of the wound and the thick yellow exudate. They are happy to see evidence of epithelialization—the forming of granulation tissue. The wound is approximately 8 cm. across. While the wound is exposed, the wound vacuum apparatus is set up for continuous vacuum. Mr. Q's mother is taught how to operate it. Mr. Q has been managing the equipment in the hospital; but, in this case, it is important for the caregivers to also be proficient in its use and importance (Refer to Box 8.3.2).

Box 8.3.2 Negative Pressure Wound Evacuation

The wound pump consists of a nonadherent, porous dressing, and a drainage tube inserted into a port in the dressing and connected to an electric vacuum pump that supplies negative pressure to the wound. Some pumps have a sponge-like item that rests on the wound, soaks up the exudate, and disperses the pressure gradient. Suction levels of –125 to –150 mmHg are usually applied. A clear plastic dressing covers the area. The pump promotes healing by: (1) increasing tension on the tissues and thus stimulating mitotic cell division, (2) increasing blood flow in the local capillary bed, and (3) evacuating the exudate so that granulation tissue may form.

Because bleeding could occur as a complication, the practitioner and the user must be vigilant in observing the site of treatment. It is applied intermittently once exudate has reduced to a manageable volume.

Sources:

Institute for Clinical Systems Improvement. *Health Care Protocol: Pressure Ulcer Prevention and Treatment Protocol.* (April, 2006).

Miller, S., Ortegon, M., and Serena, T. (January, 2006). Negative pressure wound therapy: An option for hard-to-heal wounds. *Nursing Homes.* Retrieved on 8/8/10 from http://www.thefreelibrary.com/Negative+pressure+wound+therapy:+an+option+for+hard-to-heal+wounds-a0141755736

Agency for Health Research and Quality (AHRQ) has published technical guidelines for wound care and posted them on their website at http://www.ahrq.gov/clinic/ta/negpresswtd/npwtd02.htm.

Mr. Q persists in an undernourished condition; he is of slight build, but about 10 pounds underweight. He lacks enthusiasm for cooking and planning meals for himself. He eats out once per day. On his occasional stays at his parents' home, his nutritional status improves for awhile because of his mother's attention and good cooking. He also eats well when he visits his buddies (Refer to Box 8.3.3).

Box 8.3.3 Specific Nutritional Needs

For wound healing: Foods high in protein and antioxidants to aid in the production and work of neutrophils, lymphocytes, macrophages, and fibroblasts.

Protein: ½ the patient's weight in grams. (Patient weighs 110 pounds; therefore, 55 grams.)

Carbohydrates (with limited added sugars) and fats (unsaturated and not trans fat)

Vitamin C: At least 60 mg per day

Zinc: 12–15 mg per day

(Continued)

> Typical daily food components: Grains—7 ounces.; Vegetables—
> 3 cups; Fruits—2 cups; Milk—3 cups; Meat and/or beans
> (legumes)—6 ounces; 6 tsp. oil (olive) per day
> Water: 2 quarts per day
>
> Sources: www.mypyramid.gov; http://fnic.nal.usda.gov;
> http://www.realage.com/eat-smart/food-and-nutrition/

Mr. Q must be proactive about his fluid intake, as evidenced by his dry skin condition. Examination of his urine in the temporary external collection device reveals an amber color. He states he does self-catheterization approximately 3 times per day and has had few bladder infections. With adequate hydration, he should be doing self-catheterization every 6 hours. He states he has moderately soft bowel movements stimulated, of course, with a daily suppository. This isn't always the case, the nurse remembers; so he notes that bowel management will need to be monitored.

Developmental considerations of the client/patient:

- College graduate, divorced father, businessman
- Question of unresolved adaptation to physical state; neglects physical needs; takes risks
- Has good support from and camaraderie with friends
- Lacks long-term intimate relationship of a caring companion
- Is teachable, but has a short social attention span
- Has a difficult time sitting still for long in a quiet mode and feels he has to be on the go most of the time

Mr. Q described the following goals:

- To reach a state where the infection is arrested so that he can welcome his son back into his home and spend time in activities with him. (Mr. Q's first wife was pregnant with their son at the time of the accident. She insisted on marrying him during his rehabilitation; but they divorced amicably when the son was 4-years-old. She is now remarried and has shared custody of the child.)
- To minimize time-consuming procedures that rob him of time to do his work and visit with friends
- To get stronger, feel better, and improve his appetite
- To gain more independence (He admits that this is wishful thinking, given his disability.)
- To avoid future hospitalizations

The nurse and the student consider the following factors:

- The patient must be educated and supervised in self-administration of IV Vancomycin 1230 mg every 12 hours.
- The patient will need twice daily oral temperature.

- The PICC line for the IV antibiotic must be monitored and maintained.
- Wound protocol that began in the hospital must be continued and consist of continuous wound evacuation by negative pressure equipment and intermittent Mepilex dressing when off the machine. A consult with a wound care specialist would be helpful.
- The nurse will need to examine and monitor other at-risk sites for tissue breakdown and teach methods to prevent same.
- The nurse should monitor nutritional status and educate the patient about healthy meals that he can prepare at home; he can supplement with Ensure until he reaches normal weight.
- The nurse should monitor the patient's self-catheterization and bowel evacuation technique and monitor hygiene practices.
- The nurse should provide wound culture, when ordered.
- The nurse should obtain albumin levels, when ordered.
- The nurse should request physical and occupational therapy assessment and instruction in self-care activities and self-care management in the home to accommodate his work and mobility needs.
- The nurse should support and affirm the patient's positive health behaviors and offer sensitive, caring instruction or resources for improvements. The nurse should facilitate development of self-esteem in the spirit of better self-management and reduction in health care costs.

The nurse, assisted by the student nurse, continues education as they assist Mr. Q and his mother in setting up the wound vacuum equipment. They strategize about the best configuration of furniture for access to items Mr. Q will need for work and for self-care while using the machine. It is suggested that they obtain a drinking water dispensing bottle and a small refrigerator on a cabinet that could be positioned within reach of his treatment station so that he can take in the increased fluids he needs and select healthy snacks periodically through the day without interrupting wound suctioning.

The patient and his mother have already figured out how he could work at his computer while propped on his side or lying prone. They configured his bed in the living room near his office setting and placed the wheelchair, comfort chair, refrigerator, water bottle space, and bureau around his bed. His entertainment center is nearby and can be operated remotely. The hardest job will be for Mr. Q to remain in that confinement for long periods of time in spite of the conveniences.

The home visit is planned for a time near the time of the next dose of IV antibiotic, so toward the end of the visit, the home health team demonstrates a "dry run" for Mr. Q and his mother to review them on the procedure, then observes their performance. They are satisfied with the technique. Obviously, they had been through something like this before.

Neal Theory Implications

Stage 3: The professional in this stage collaborates with other disciplines both within and outside of home care and is autonomous with the clinical aspects of the case and the logistical aspects of working with the agency.

Stage 2: The professional in this stage may not feel comfortable collaborating with the physician regarding orders for other disciplines, case managing, or working within the patient's environment to manage care.

Stage 1: The clinician in this stage will assess the patient and recognize the need for assistance with the case but may be unsure as to how to proceed in the home setting.

? CRITICAL THINKING

1. **How intensive should the nursing visits be?**
Answer:
   a. Professional nurse home visits 3 days per week for 2 weeks; then, if progress is noted, reduce to twice weekly until IV antibiotic is discontinued.
   b. The visiting nurse is to incorporate all items documented above under Orders.
   c. Because of the complex characteristics of this case, employ a holistic approach to care that particularly identifies mental health status concerns, such as signs of depression.

2. **Who else should join the care team and why?**
   a. Obtain a physician's order for physical therapy (PT) to assess for strength-building needs and physical adaptations not already adopted.
   b. Obtain a physician's order for occupational therapy (OT) to assess for adaptation needs in self-care management in the context of his neurologic deficit.
   c. Obtain an order for the wound care specialist on staff to assess the wound and evaluate the protocol being used in the home setting

Rehabilitation Needs

Physical therapy
Occupational therapy

3. What should be the educational components of each home visit?
Answer: At each visit, continue education regarding disease transmission prevention techniques, nutritional needs and meal planning, hydration, and skin care. Now that the student nurse is familiar with Mr. Q's needs, she has offered to prepare a healthy meals demonstration event for him for her next visit.

4. What other nursing considerations should be addressed?
Answer: Other areas of body at risk for pressure sores—Braden's Scale; sexual concerns and emotional attachments; pain sensation.

Interdisciplinary Care Plan

Problem	Goal/Plan	Intervention	Evaluation
Knowledge deficit regarding disease, its communicability, and the healing process	At each visit, identify opportunities to teach hygiene, bacterial transfer precautions, observation skills for changes in wound status.	Provide Internet sources of descriptive and illustrative information. Observe for interest and preventative behaviors. Take daily oral temperature and record it.	Patient and caregiver will reach satisfactory understanding of this disease and its prevention and need to maintain integrity of body tissues. He will report twice daily normal temperatures.
Attitude weakness toward disability, risk-taking, self-esteem, self-preservation	Patient will express through verbal and nonverbal cues of openness to discussion about attitudes toward his disability and adaptation to life as he can live it safely.	Allow time for reflective conversation at each visit. Support and affirm his positive health behaviors; offer sensitive, caring instruction or resources for improvements. Facilitate development of self-esteem in the spirit of better self-management and reduction in health care costs.	Patient will assume responsible and cautious concern for safe mobility, health maintenance, and hopeful attitude.

(Continued)

Problem	Goal/Plan	Intervention	Evaluation
Knowledge deficit and behavior toward nutritional needs	Patient will establish a regular, nutritious meal plan that he follows.	Nurse will instruct in a healthy diet and in foods necessary for wound healing and necessary weight gain and strength-building, providing Internet resources for learning.	Patient will demonstrate regular pattern of nutritious meals and interest in personal health.
Altered mobility: changes in self-care management of ADL	Patient will learn new safe methods of self-care and mobility in the home and in motorized vehicles by 1 month.	Examine and monitor other at-risk sites for tissue breakdown; teach methods to prevent same. PT will assess and improve patient's strength and mobility assets and provide guidance in appropriate exercises and equipment OT will assess patient's ability to conduct ADL and instruct in improved adaptations for meal preparation, housekeeping, and office work. Nurse will monitor bowel and bladder maintenance care procedures and care of equipment.	Patient will adopt safe mobility practices and demonstrate improved strength and more efficient methods of performing ADL.

Problem	Goal/Plan	Intervention	Evaluation
Wound treatment complexities	Patient and his caregivers will follow protocols as ordered for wound care.	Instruct in and monitor performance of vacuum wound suction pump according to intermittent schedule per physician and wound specialist orders. Obtain wound cultures and albumin levels when ordered.	Patient's decubitus wound will reach proliferation phase of integrity with remodeling beginning.
Knowledge and skill deficit in IV therapy	Patient and caregiver will perform antibiotic administration satisfactorily in technique and scheduling.	Nurse to educate and supervise patient in self-administration of IV Vancomycin 1230 mg every 12 hours and in precautionary care of PICC line site. Nurse will attend to IV site care and line integrity.	There will be no secondary insults to vascular integrity at IV site. Medication will be delivered as ordered. MRSA will be eliminated and no colonization (nares) will be noted in 2 months.
Social isolation	Patient will adhere to prescribed restriction to home and utilize available telephonic devices to socialize with friends. Family visitation will be restricted to caregivers until wound cultures negative.	Through visits of team, provide social stimulation and emphasize patient goals.	Patient, friends, and family will adhere to isolation protocol.

REFERENCES & RESOURCES

[1] Agency for Health Research and Quality (AHRQ). http://www.ahrq.gov/clinic/ta/negpresswtd/npwtd02.htm

[2] Aldabagh B, Tomecki K. What's new in MRSA infections? *Dermatology Nursing*, 22(2):2, http://proquest.umi.com March–April, 2010.

[3] Cuzzell J. Wound healing: Translating theory into clinical practice. *Dermatology Nursing*, 14(4): p. 405, http://proquest.umi.com January, 2002.

[4] Institute for Clinical Systems Improvement. Health care protocol: pressure ulcer prevention and treatment protocol, April, 2006.

[5] Mepilex. SMTL Dressings Datacard. http://www.dressings.org/Dressings/mepilex.html

[6] Miller S, Ortegon M, Serena T. Negative pressure wound therapy: An option for hard-to-heal wounds. *Nursing Homes*, January, 2006. Retrieved on 8/8/10 from http://www.thefreelibrary.com/Negative+pressure+wound+therapy:+an+option+for+hard-to-heal+wounds-a0141755736

[7] Noble D. Patient education on MRSA management: The nurse's role. *MedSurg Nursing*, 18(6):375–378, 2009.

[8] Sussman C, Bates-Jensen B. *Wound Care*. Aspen Publishers, 2001.

[9] Wound Ostomy and Continence Nurses Society. Position statement: pressure ulcer staging. October, 2007.

[10] YouTube Wound Pump Demonstration Videos (8/10): Negative Pressure Wound Therapy from Smith and Nephew. http://www.youtube.com/watch?v=-wxyKEStuDQ and Wound Vac Therapy http://www.youtube.com/watch?v=5onM4RzFJFE&feature=related

Section 9

Neurological

Case 9.1 Brain Stem Infarct

By Shelia Spurlock-White, MSN, RN

This case study illustrates how the home health nurse coordinates care for a very complex case, in which a sudden illness presents significant changes to a patient's life. The patient is a 45-year-old female who suffered a brain stem infarct from taking birth control pills. She had a previous history of hypertension that was controlled by medication. She was diagnosed with hemiplegia as a result of the stroke, acute respiratory distress syndrome (ARDS), *Clostridium difficile* (C-Diff) and hypertension. She was transferred from acute care hospitalization to acute care rehabilitation, and now to home. The patient lives with a paid caregiver and has one brother, who is her executor and power of attorney. He is very anxious and overwhelmed about having to care for her; he feels he has his own family to care for. Her brother believes it would be better to have her go to a nursing home to receive care. The patient does not want to go to a nursing home and believes she is able to remain in her home. Coordinating supportive care and providing rehabilitation services to improve the patient's ability to remain safe in her home are the primary foci of the home health team.

 ORDERS FOR HOME CARE

Patient: 45-year-old female
Diagnoses: Status post brain stem infarct, hemiplegia, obesity, hypertension

---

Clinical Case Studies in Home Health Care, First Edition. Edited by Leslie Neal-Boylan.
© 2011 John Wiley & Sons, Inc. Published 2011 by John Wiley & Sons, Inc.

Current medications:
- Plavix 75 mg by mouth once a day
- Lipitor 40 mg by mouth each p.m.
- Norvasc 10 mg by mouth once a day
- Lisinopril 20 mg by mouth once a day
- Flagyl 500 mg by mouth twice a day × 10 days
- Tylenol 650 mg by mouth every 6 hours as needed for pain

Relevant past medical history: Hypertension
RN: Assess, evaluate, and develop a plan of care.
PT: Assess and evaluate.

Reimbursement Considerations

The patient has private insurance coverage for 25 visits. She is too young to be eligible for Medicare, but she can petition for a Medicaid waiver for a home health aide. The medical social worker will explore options.

THE HOME VISIT

The nurse called to schedule a visit to see the patient, and the caregiver who answered the phone advised her to contact the patient's brother. The nurse contacts the patient's brother to set up a time when he can be present to assess the patient's needs and discuss a plan of care. He states that he is very busy and does not have a lot of time for this, but he reluctantly agrees to meet on a specified date and time.

The patient lives in a ground floor apartment with easy access to the parking area. The building is in need of some cosmetic repairs but appears to be structurally sound. As the nurse enters the patient's home, she sees that living areas are in disarray. There is too much furniture, including a large china cabinet. A side table and desk are pushed up against one wall in the living room, which does not leave adequate walking space. The carpet is worn, the walls are dirty, and there are clothes in bags on the floor. In the bathroom, she sees stool smeared over the toilet seat, used toilet tissue on the floor, and litter boxes in the corner. The nurse notes that there are no grab bars or any other adaptive equipment in the bathroom.

The patient, Ms. B, enters the living room area, trying to navigate herself to a chair for the meeting. She is wearing knee-high TED hose and a brace on her left leg. Neither the brother nor the caregiver move to assist her to a chair, and she almost falls trying to sit down. The nurse asks the brother and Ms. B if it is okay for the caregiver to remain in the room while they discuss the home care services that are available and the plan of care possibilities. Since the caregiver lives in Monday to Friday, they consent to the caregiver being included in the conversation. Ms. B tries to answer most of the questions, but her brother often provides an answer before she can complete her sentences. This action frustrates Ms. B who tries to get up quickly, as though she will leave the room. She forgets her quad cane and almost falls. Her brother states, "She keeps on falling because she forgets to take her cane with her." Her caregiver, Ms. Jones, shouts, "Watch where you're going before you fall again!" The nurse asks Ms. B to stay and allow her to do a brief exam. She moves closer to the patient and begins a general assessment.

Ms. B is cooperative with the nurse and allows her to continue the assessment. Her speech is slightly slurred, but understandable; pupils are sluggish, equal, and react to light. She appears to pool saliva in her mouth, frequently drooling. Her brother hands her a napkin from across the table, but she has difficulty grasping it because she cannot clearly see it. She states that her vision is very blurred, even with her glasses. She states she has not been eating well, finding it difficult to swallow, and feeling like she will choke with certain foods. Her abdomen is soft, nondistended with hyperactive bowel sounds; last bowel movement was today and remains loose and watery. She is urinating within normal limits. The nurse finds Ms. B's BP to be elevated 160/90. Her lungs are clear, heart rate reveals regular rate and rhythm, and she denies pain. Ms. B states her left arm and leg feel numb and heavy "like they are asleep" and at times she feels like she will lose her balance. Her skin is intact, but there are several ecchymotic areas on her forearms and lower leg. When asked about her recent falls, Ms. B states that she didn't hurt herself and cannot recall the number of times she's fallen.

The caregiver is asked to provide the medicine that she administers to the patient daily. Ms. Jones obtains the medication from the other room and reviews the pills and the time of day she gives them to the patient. Ms. Jones is correct on the frequency and times of administration, but does not know what each drug is taken for. The nurse provides a quick review of the medications to the three, with a detailed medication management session to follow.

When the exam is completed, the nurse explains to the patient, her brother, and the caregiver the services that are available, the frequency of her visits each week, and what to expect from each member of the care team. They discuss the goals to be reached and the approximate time it will take to reach those goals. The current goals for Ms. B are to:

- Maintain a safe environment—fall precautions.
- Manage medication and administration.
- Prevent aspiration.

- Encourage effective communication among patient, brother, and caregiver.
- Incorporate community resources to assist in regaining the maximum independence possible for the patient.
- Practice infection control and the need to prevent spread of C-diff.

Relevant Community Resources
Notification of the fire department and police department that she is disabled Transportation for shopping and socialization Respite care Housekeeping services Church outreach groups

Based on the data collected from the history and physical, and the patient assessment, the nurse discovers the following data:

- Ms. B has difficulty swallowing food; she is at great risk for aspiration.
- Ms. B is forgetful and impulsive and has impaired decision making ability. She was observed getting up quickly and making attempts to walk without the use of her quad cane, making her a high risk for falls.
- Ms. B has evidence of falls, exhibited by the bruising on her skin; she is also on Plavix which can cause bruising.
- Ms. B has a caregiver who requires further instruction on medication administration.
- Ms. B has difficulty seeing, in spite of having new glasses, placing her at risk for falls.
- Ms. B continues with loose stool as evidenced by the smearing of BM in the bathroom.
- The brother and caregiver must hire someone to clean the home or clean the patient's home themselves to eliminate clutter, remove cat litter boxes from the bathroom, and improve sanitation as needed to keep patient safe at home.
- Ms. B has elevated BP today. The caregiver should take BP daily and keep a log of the readings so that the doctor will have data to support a possible change in medication, if needed.
- The brother should contact the rental office and make arrangements for having grab bars installed throughout the apartment to assist in prevention of falls
- The caregiver requires nutritional education to make low calorie, low sodium foods for Ms. B to assist in weight loss and hypertension control

- Both the brother and the patient will meet with the medical social worker to learn of available community resources and support groups which may help in adapting to the change in the patient as a result of her illness

Neal Theory Implications

Stage 3: The RN in this case has several years of experience as a home health nurse. She is operating autonomously as she is able to assess the needs of Ms. B and her brother at the initial visit, and she formulates a plan of care that includes a multidisciplinary team. The nurse is able to foresee the possible financial impact of this sudden illness on the patient and her family and includes all essential team members, so that both current and future needs are addressed. She explains to the family the limitation of payment under the terms of Ms. B's health insurance policy and offers information about alternative forms of payment that she may be eligible for in the future, such as charity visits and benefits provided by the Medicaid waiver program. She speaks with the physician at the initial visit to alert him of the abnormal BP reading and obtains an order to cover the treatment team she knows is necessary for the rehabilitation of this patient. From the onset of the opening of this case, the nurse's primary foci included coordinating supportive care and providing rehabilitation services to improve the patient's ability to remain safe in her home.

Stage 2: The nurse at this stage will assess the patient's needs during the initial visit. She will tell the family of the plan of care for the patient, but would rely more on physical therapy, occupational therapy, and speech therapy to lead the care of this patient since many of her needs require physical rehabilitation. A nurse at this stage may go into the home and develop a plan of care that meets the immediate needs of the patient, such as medication management and patient teaching in a few visits, and discharge the patient from nursing services, leaving the rehabilitation team members to manage the remainder of her care. The nurse may not focus on the social or long term needs of this patient, which will continue to exist after home care services have ended.

Stage 1: The nurse at Stage 1 will assess the patient's needs and open the case including the rehabilitation team members and social services. She may have difficulty addressing some of the family needs, primarily focusing on the immediate needs of the patient. For example, the nurse clearly sees the clutter that creates an

(Continued)

environment that places the patient at an increased risk for fall, but may not feel comfortable directly stating to the patient's brother and caregiver the need for the clutter to be removed from the home. The patient's brother appears angry that his sister's illness will affect his life and would rather have her placed in a nursing home. The nurse at this stage may not be able to relieve the brother's concerns due to a lack of knowledge of potential resources which may assist the family with keeping the patient at home, where the patient would like to remain. It is essential that both patient and family have their needs met and that they believe the team will assist them in the patient's care. At stage 1, this can be a great challenge to the nurse, as a result her inexperience. She may and should solicit help from her clinical supervisor to properly navigate the care this patient requires.

The nurse explains to Ms. B and her brother that although Ms. B may not recover 100%, she can improve with further rehabilitation services. The rehabilitation team that includes the nurse, physical therapist (PT), occupational therapist (OT), speech therapist (ST), dietician, and medical social worker (MSW), will collaborate and provide an interdisciplinary approach to Ms. B's care to enhance her quality of life. These services will include teaching, medication management, muscle strengthening, and gait training. The team will also provide adaptive equipment that will aid in the accommodations necessary to promote independence and to enhance the quality of life for Ms. B.

Rehabilitation Needs

Physical therapy
Occupational therapy
Vocational rehab
Speech therapy
Dietician

? CRITICAL THINKING

1. How will the members of the interdisciplinary team communicate with one another?
Answer: Team members will communicate by phone and computerized charting which allows for all to view the assessment and treatment provided. There is also a monthly case conference meeting where they

will all meet by phone with the patient and her brother to assess progress, and what, if any, issues remain.

2. What is the priority for care for Ms. B?
Answer: Safety is the priority. Ms. B has many safety issues. The team will make recommendations regarding clearing the clutter in the home, removing the cat litter from the bathroom area, the installation of grab bars, and any other necessary equipment to accommodate the needs of the patient.

3. What will the speech therapist do at the visit?
Answer: Ms. B has symptoms of altered smell and taste, decreased gag and swallowing reflexes, and weakness in her tongue as a result of the stroke. She also exhibits signs of impaired judgment and decision making, which are signs that her cognitive ability has been compromised. The speech therapist can assess and determine a plan of treatment which may lessen those deficits.

4. What will the physical therapist do at the visit?
Answer: Ms. B has balance problems and left-sided weakness which increase her chances for falling. Physical therapy will perform various exercises with her to improve her balance and coordination, as well as to improve her strength. Some of the exercises will be prescribed for her to do when the therapist is not present, so the caretaker will be instructed on how to make certain Ms. B is doing the exercises correctly. Physical therapy will also make recommendations as to alternate equipment that may enhance safety in the home, such as a higher toilet, grab bars, and a shower seat.

5. What will the occupational therapist do at the visit?
Answer: The occupational therapist will assess and prescribe exercises and adaptive equipment which will aid in Ms. B's ability to assist in her own care. The occupational therapist will teach her how to wash and dress herself and possibly teach her other activities of daily living that she may be able to perform.

 BACK TO THE CASE

Cultural Competence

Ms. B is a single African American woman, who relies solely on the support of her brother. Her brother is overwhelmed by the possibility of having to care for her, as well as his own family, and feels that she would be better off in a nursing home where other people

(Continued)

can take care of her. He believes the nursing home can do a better job than he can, because he cannot imagine having to provide personal care for his sister. It is essential that the team communicates with him to acknowledge his feelings, that they assure him they will work to help get her community resources to help with her care, and that they communicate that there is a possibility that some of her current level of functioning will improve with rehab.

The nurse addresses the financial expenses that can accompany the recovery of this illness. She explains that the medical social worker will address costs not covered by insurance and will help to locate alternate funding sources available to assist in her care. The brother seems to relax slightly when hearing that there may be sources to help him financially with the care of his sister, as well as services that may continue after the home care team has discharged the patient. The nurse explains that her anticipated length of treatment would be about 4 weeks, unless a skilled need continues to exist. She also explains that the physical, speech, and occupational therapists; the dietition; and the medical social worker will assess and provide him with each of their schedules and anticipated lengths of treatment. The physician is called to confirm the orders, is provided with the elevated BP value today, and is alerted to the start of care.

? CRITICAL THINKING

1. How does the team achieve its outcomes within the financial constraints of the family?
Answer: The patient currently has a commercial insurance policy from her previous employer, which has limited benefits for home care services. She is allowed 25 home care visits per calendar year. The team needs to be aware of the limited number of visits, and make certain visits do not exceed that number. The team will try to provide the maximum interventions during a visit, as well as provide the patient and caregiver with home exercises to practice on days that the therapist cannot visit. The dietician and medical social worker services are covered for 1 visit by each profession. It is very difficult to do all of the assessment and teaching in one session. Additional sessions may be approved by requesting authorization through the insurance carrier. It may also be possible to assess charitable funds from the

organization to pay for additional services not covered by the insurance carrier.

The patient is paying the caregiver out of her income because personal care services are not covered under her insurance plan. She currently receives income from her short term disability at 65% of her salary; after 90 days, her long term disability policy should continue to provide her with income for an additional 180 days. The medical social worker will work with the patient to find alternative funds for medical care needed once her benefits have been exhausted. She may possibly qualify for Medicaid at that time, which would provide personal care assistance for a specified number of hours.

Interdisciplinary Care Plan

Problem	Goal/Plan	Intervention	Evaluation
Knowledge deficit regarding disease process	Patient and family will verbalize an understanding of the disease process and potential for rehab within 4 weeks.	Teach patient about symptoms resulting from the disease. Teach patient and caregiver about meds. Teach patient and caregiver about signs and symptoms to report to MD.	Patient and family verbalize understanding and caregiver is able to show log with vital signs. Caregiver can provide a brief description of medication actions.
Altered mobility related to left side hemiplegia	Patient will have increased mobility and improved recognition of left side in 6 weeks.	PT and OT provide strengthening and gait training exercises. ST provides cognitive training.	Patient is able to walk with improved steady gait. Patient recalls to use quad cane when ambulating.
Risk for aspiration related to weakness in tongue and decreased gag and swallowing reflexes	Patient will have improved tongue control and stronger gag reflex in 6 weeks.	ST will provide exercises to improve motor control of tongue and swallowing.	Patient is able to swallow without gagging. Patient has proper food consistency, allowing her to chew and eat without gagging.

(Continued)

Problem	Goal/Plan	Intervention	Evaluation
Risk for falls related to impaired vision and balance	Patient will have improved balance within 6 weeks.	PT/OT will provide strength training exercises to improve balance. Patient will have eyes examined and a change in lens within 4 weeks. Remove clutter to allow for safe ambulation.	Patient will have improved vision with aid of new glasses. Patient will have fewer falls than in prior 6 weeks.
Ineffective coping of family system	Patient's brother will assist as he can and exhibit improved coping skills as it relates to care of his sister.	Community resources and support will be provided. Patient and brother will attend a support group.	Patient and family will use the resources provided.
Inability to perform ADL/IADL independently	Patient will manage ADL's with minimum assistance in 90 days.	OT will assess and provide necessary equipment to aid in the independence of the patient.	Patient continues to reside in her home with the assistance of caregiver.
Potential for social isolation	Patient will verbalize satisfaction with attending adult day care in 90 days.	PT/OT will provide patient with exercise to increase strength and mobility and with adaptive devices as needed to enhance independence.	Patient has improved strength and mobility and is able to be more independent with her care. Patient is enjoying the adult day care center 2 days a week.

REFERENCE & RESOURCE

[1] National Stroke Association, http://www.stroke.org

Case 9.2 Multiple Sclerosis

By Leslie Neal-Boylan, PhD, RN, CRRN, APRN-BC, FNP

This case study illustrates how the home health nurse works with the patient and family to reach mutually agreeable goals. The patient has had relapsing-remitting multiple sclerosis for 6 years and had been living independently. She recently had an exacerbation of her symptoms, and she has not regained her former abilities or her energy level. The patient's entire life has been changed by the exacerbation of symptoms. She had been a successful, independent, single professional woman and is now confronted with the limitations of her disease and its symptoms as well as by her parents' desire to manage her care. The use of the interdisciplinary team and excellent communication among its members are keys to the management of this case.

 ORDERS FOR HOME CARE

Patient: 34-year-old African American
Diagnosis: Multiple sclerosis
Current medications:
- Lisinopril 10 mg once a day
- Betaseron 250 mcg 4 times once a day every other day
- Copaxone 20 mg SC once a day

Relevant past medical history: Hypertension controlled with medication.
RN: Assess and evaluate.
PT: Assess and evaluate.

Clinical Case Studies in Home Health Care, First Edition. Edited by Leslie Neal-Boylan.
© 2011 John Wiley & Sons, Inc. Published 2011 by John Wiley & Sons, Inc.

Cultural Competence

Ms. S is African American. Her parents clearly feel strongly about supporting her and caring for her. The team will need to praise them for this behavior and encourage their support but teach them that maximal self-care is important for Ms. S's quality of life.

 ## THE HOME VISIT

The nurse is the first to enter the home, which is a first floor apartment. The home is clean, uncluttered, and well organized. An older woman whom the nurse presumes is not the patient greets the nurse warmly. A man of about the same age as this woman is standing by the door and says hello to the nurse. The nurse presumes that these are the patient's parents. After introductions are shared, the nurse asks to see the patient. The patient's parents inform the nurse that Ms. S is in the bedroom in bed. As it is 2 o'clock in the afternoon, the nurse is dismayed to find Ms. S in bed. The nurse introduces herself to the patient, pulls up a chair alongside the bed, and begins to do the admission assessment.

Ms. S is pleasant and cooperative during the lengthy history taking and discussion. As the nurse asks the necessary questions, she notes that the patient's wheelchair is sitting in the far corner of the room. The bed is a standard double bed, and the dresser is at the far corner opposite the corner in which the wheelchair is sitting. Additionally, both parents are in the room during the history portion of the assessment and frequently answer questions for the patient.

The nurse looks in the bathroom and the kitchen, including the cabinets and the refrigerator, to assess safety and the accessibility to the toilet and tub/shower and to nutritious food in the kitchen. No accommodations have been made to increase accessibility in any part of the apartment. The nurse asks whether the patient is aware of the adaptations that are available and whether she has considered them. Ms. S's mother answers: "No. We were waiting until you came." There is nutritious food in the refrigerator and in the cupboards; and on seeing the nurse examine these areas, the patient's mother reveals, "We arrived last week and we have been doing all of the shopping and taking care of her and the apartment."

Relevant Community Resources

Housekeeping services
Notification of the fire department and police department that she is disabled

---

The nurse continues to gather data and discovers that the patient is knowledgeable about her medications and that her mother prepares them and administers them to Ms. S. Also, Ms. S's mother and father prepare her meals and bring them to her in bed or in the wheelchair.

When the nurse has finished gathering the data, she asks the parents to leave the room so she can examine Ms. S. Once the parents have left, the nurse asks Ms. S what her goals are for her care. She mentions the following goals:

- To live independently again
- To have her parents move out of her house
- To resume her work in some form
- To be able to meet her friends at the shopping mall for a day out

---

Rehabilitation Needs

Physical therapy
Occupational therapy
Potential for needing speech therapy in the future

Based on the history and physical examination, the nurse discovers the following data:

- Ms. S has profound fatigue, but is able to get 5–6 hours of uninterrupted sleep most nights.
- Ms. S has dysesthetic pain in the lower extremities.
- Ms. S has mild upper extremity weakness.
- Ms. S has profound lower extremity weakness.
- Ms. S does not know how to transfer to the wheelchair by herself.
- Ms. S has been receiving assistance with all of her activities of daily living (ADL).
- Ms. S has neurogenic bladder dysfunction.
- Ms. S is continent of bowel.
- Ms. S cannot ambulate.
- Ms. S has no current infection or spasticity.
- Ms. S has no difficulties with speech or swallowing.
- Ms. S is not currently sexually active.
- Ms. S has no history of depression but is saddened by her current situation.

Neal Theory Implications

Stage 3: The professional in this stage collaborates with other disciplines both within and outside of home care and is autonomous with the clinical aspects of the case and the logistical aspects of working with the agency.

(Continued)

Stage 2: The professional in this stage may not feel comfortable collaborating with the physician regarding orders for other disciplines, case managing, or working within the patient's environment to manage care.

Stage 1: The clinician in this stage will assess the patient and recognize the need for assistance with the case but may be unsure as to how to proceed in the home setting.

? CRITICAL THINKING

1. What is the priority for care for Ms. S?
Answer: The priority of care must always be safety. The nurse and the physical therapist will make recommendations regarding keeping the home uncluttered, installing grab bars in the shower, installing smoke and carbon monoxide detectors, and ensuring that the patient can reach the phone and the light switches in each room.

2. What will the physical therapist (PT) do when he arrives at the home?
Answer: The PT will do a PT assessment to determine Ms. S's needs and goals for therapy. The PT will also assess the home environment for safety and accessibility. Additionally, the PT will begin to teach Ms. S exercises to help strengthen her upper and lower extremities. Both the nurse and the PT will work on teaching the patient to transfer to and from the wheelchair properly. The PT will recommend adaptations to the environment to promote safety and accessibility and will examine the wheelchair for its appropriateness to Ms. S. The PT may recommend a particular wheelchair or a type of wheelchair cushion and a change to a hospital bed to prevent pressure ulcers and to allow Ms. S more control. Both the nurse and the PT will explain that an elevated toilet seat or a 3-in-1 commode can assist Ms. S to toilet herself.

3. Is there anyone else who should be called into this case?
Answer: Yes. The nurse should call the physician for orders for an occupational therapist (OT), a home health aide (HHA), and a medical social worker (MSW).

4. What will each of these disciplines do?
Answer: The OT will reinforce the teaching and interventions of the nurse and the PT as they will for the OT's recommendations. Additionally, the OT will teach Ms. S upper extremity strengthening exercises and work with her to regain her independence. The OT will introduce assistive devices such as adaptive eating utensils, a reacher,

and a long-handled shoe horn to enable Ms. S to be more independent with ADL. Along with the other health disciplines in the case, the OT will teach Ms. S how to cook her own meals and adapt her home to suit her needs. The OT will work with Ms. S toward her goal of resuming her work which was in an office in a nearby city. The OT might help Ms. S see if she could work from home or only part time in the office and may be able to obtain computer adaptations that will help Ms. S do her work.

Initially, the HHA will visit Ms. S daily to help her bathe, dress, and get into her wheelchair. The HHA will also prepare one quick meal and put one load of laundry in the washing machine. The HHA will make Ms. S's bed for her and tidy her apartment. However, the HHA will not do comprehensive house cleaning or meal preparation.

The MSW will work with Ms. S to find community resources to help her so that her parents do not have to live with her. The MSW will work with the patient to find resources that fit her ability to pay and will also work with the OT to help Ms. S return to work.

BACK TO THE CASE

The nurse explains to Ms. S that she can be independent of her parents with some outside help. The patient is thrilled and motivated to work toward her goals. When the nurse informs the patient's parents of this and that they will not be needed as live-ins in the home much longer, the parents are unexpectedly angry. The nurse is taken aback by their response. She assures them that the home care team will assist Ms. S to learn what she needs to learn to manage independently and that she will have resources from the community to supplement what she does herself. The nurse also explains that while the parents remain in the home, they can best help Ms. S by allowing her to perform as much of her own care as she can. The patient reassures her parents that she still loves and need them but that she wants to live like an adult again.

The nurse calls the primary care provider (PCP) and requests medication to assist with the bladder dysfunction, dysesthetic pain, and

Reimbursement Considerations

The patient is too young to be eligible for Medicare and has had too much income to qualify for Medicaid. However, she may eventually qualify for Medicaid. Her private insurance will cover a certain number of visits and some equipment. The nurse, as case manager on this case, will need to negotiate with the insurance case manager for visits beyond those originally allowed.

fatigue. The nurse also requests an order for intermittent self-catheterization and explains that she plans to teach the patient self-care. The physician agrees to the plan and orders Ditropan, Phenytoin, and Prozac.

? CRITICAL THINKING

1. How will the members of the interdisciplinary team communicate with one another?
Answer: Team members will communicate by phone and arrange to hold a monthly case conference that includes the patient by phone or in person.

2. What will happen after each discipline makes its initial visit?
Answer: Each team member will reinforce what the other members are teaching the patient and family. Each will work from a discipline-specific care plan and also from the interdisciplinary care plan.

Interdisciplinary Care Plan

Problem	Goal/Plan	Intervention	Evaluation
Knowledge deficit regarding disease process	Patient and family will verbalize understanding of recent changes in patient's condition within 1 week. Patient and family will demonstrate understanding of disease process within 3 weeks.	Teach patient and parents about remissions and relapses of MS. Teach patient about new medications. Teach patient and parents the importance of self-care management.	Patient will participate more fully in self-care management. Parents will only assist patient when she needs help from another person.
Pain in lower extremities	Patient will have reduced pain in lower extremities within 2 weeks.	Contact PCP regarding a prescription. Teach alternative pain management strategies.	Patient states pain is a 2–3/10.
Weakness in upper and lower extremities	Patient will have increased strength in all extremities within 2 months.	Contact PCP regarding prescription for SSRI. Teach patient strengthening exercises.	Patient is able to participate more in self-care related to increased strength.

Problem	Goal/Plan	Intervention	Evaluation
Fatigue	Patient will have strategies to manage fatigue within 1 month.	Teach patient about sleep hygiene. Teach patient to alternate rest with activity.	Patient is sleeping better and fatigue is interfering less with quality of life.
Neurogenic incontinence	Patient will have control of bladder management within 1 month.	Contact PCP and recommend evaluation of bladder dysfunction and request prescription for antispasmodic. Teach patient to self-catheterize. Teach patient timed voiding.	Patient is able to perform self-catherization as needed and has no urinary tract infections.
Ineffective coping of family system	Patient and family are able to cope with sequelae of disease process within 3 months.	Provide information about community resources, support groups, and services. MSW to provide counseling for patient and family.	Patient and family have resources for emotional support and use them effectively.
Altered mobility	Patient will have increased mobility of upper and lower extremities within 3 months.	Physical and occupational therapy for strengthening and mobility.	Patient is able to transfer properly, has no pressure ulcers, and is able to manage ADL independently.
Inability to perform ADL/IADL independently	Patient will manage ADL independently in 3 months. Patient will have help with IADL as needed in 1 month.	Team members teach patient adaptive techniques for performing activities. Obtain assistive devices and adaptive equipment for patient.	Patient is able to remain in her home with some support of outside assistance.

(Continued)

Problem	Goal/Plan	Intervention	Evaluation
Social isolation	Patient will verbalize satisfaction with social relationships within 3 months.	Improve patient's strength and mobility. Obtain adaptive devices and equipment that will enable patient to participate in activities outside of the home.	Patient has returned to work. Patient is able to meet friends at the shopping mall.

REFERENCES & RESOURCES

[1] Consortium of Multiple Sclerosis Centers, www.mscare.org/cmsc.

[2] K. Costello, J. Halper and C. Harris (eds.), *Nursing Practice in Multiple Sclerosis: A Core Curriculum*, Demos, 2003.

[3] "International Organization of Multiple Sclerosis Nurses: International journal of MS care, www.iomsn.org.

[4] "National Multiple Sclerosis Society," http://www.nmss.org.

[5] "Paralyzed Veterans of America: Multiple Sclerosis Council for Clinical Practice Guidelines."

Section 10

Maternal Health

Case 10.1 Antepartum Care

By Ruth Smillie, RN, MSN

This case study demonstrates the ongoing coordination of the many health care needs of the pregnant woman with hyperemesis gravidarum. Ms. F is a 26-year-old woman experiencing her first pregnancy. She is 12 weeks pregnant and was discharged yesterday from the hospital. She has been diagnosed with hyperemesis gravidarum. During her hospital stay, she received antiemetics, fluids, and a peripherally inserted central catheter (PICC) line for continued intravenous fluids at home. The visiting nurse will be vital in helping Ms. F through the difficult weeks ahead.

Cultural Competence

Mr. and Ms. F's family is originally from India. They may have different cultural needs and expectations. Understanding the Indian and Hindu culture may help the nurse to be a more effective teacher. In this instance, the nurse should discuss with the family if they have any special cultural needs. Making assumptions on generalizations could be hurtful. Cultural knowledge, including that most Hindus are vegetarian, helps to direct the nurse to appropriate assessments. They may have different medical beliefs including the use of different herbs or traditional medicines that should be explored with them as well. Discussing roles and expectations on an individual basis is the best assessment for any family.

Clinical Case Studies in Home Health Care, First Edition. Edited by Leslie Neal-Boylan.
© 2011 John Wiley & Sons, Inc. Published 2011 by John Wiley & Sons, Inc.

ORDERS FOR HOME CARE

Patient: 26-year-old G1P0 woman
Diagnosis: 12 weeks pregnant with hyperemesis
Current medications:
- Ondansetron 4 mg IVP every 6 hours as needed
- Lactated Ringer's with multivitamins with thiamine added 1 liter per day by PICC. Infuse each morning over 4 hours.

Relevant past medical history: Ms. F has had nausea and vomiting for the last 8 weeks and has been hospitalized 2 times for dehydration. She states that she vomits approximately 15 times a day and can no longer work as a bank manager. Prior to this pregnancy, Ms. F's medical history was unremarkable.

RN: Assess hydration and nutrition. Assess home environment. Assist with infusion; teach patient self-infusion and PICC care. Evaluate PICC site and dressing. Change dressing weekly. Evaluate mood. The patient needs to record daily weights and test urine for ketones daily.

THE HOME VISIT

The nurse climbs the metal stairs to the top floor where Ms. F's apartment is. She notes the increasing warmth as she moves upward. Ms. F's husband, dressed in a pressed white shirt and slacks, greets the nurse at the door. Inside the apartment it is very warm. Ms. F is lying on the couch in blue silk pajamas in the tidy living room with an industrial sized bucket next to her. She leans forward to greet the nurse and finds herself retching instead. She is visibly pregnant. Ms. F and her husband are from India. He is an engineer, and she is a bank manager. They speak excellent English with slight accents.

The infusion company dropped off the PICC supplies yesterday afternoon after Ms. F's discharge from the hospital. The nurse begins her assessment of Ms. F by asking her some questions. Ms. F explains to the nurse that she has not been able to work for nearly 3 months now because of the constant vomiting. She has been hospitalized twice with dehydration and is hoping this PICC line and treatment will help her feel better. Ms. F's husband wants to know what he can do to help, stating that he feels helpless and responsible since they planned this pregnancy together. Ms. F relates that the loss of her income has stressed them both. She states they will be able to manage the rent but living expenses will be very difficult to finance without her income. They have many questions regarding the health of the mother and baby. Ms. F is unable to maintain the home and has a special aversion to any cooking or food smells. Mr. and Ms. F are practicing Hindus. Mr. F. works daily and helps Ms. F with bathing and caring for the home. She sometimes feels sad and frustrated but feels confident that she will manage.

Reimbursement Considerations

Reimbursement for this visit would be covered by the patient's private insurance. In the event that the patient meets the low-income guidelines, Medicaid would provide this service.

The nurse assesses Ms. F and notes the following data:

- Ms. F is oriented and alert.
- Left antecubital double lumen PICC line is clean with clear dressing intact. Site is without redness, warmth, or drainage.
- Physical assessment is unremarkable except for the following:
    ○ Gravid uterus
    ○ Dry lips and skin
    ○ Retching and occasionally spitting saliva into bucket
- Ms. F states she has had retching 4 times today and has taken in only small amounts of liquid and some rice.
- Orthostatic vital signs show little change from lying to sitting to standing.
- Ms. F has voided 3 times today in good amounts, and the urine is light yellow in color and negative for ketones.
- Ms. F's weight is unchanged from her discharge weight.
- The nurse finds no indication of clinical depression after using a depression scale to assess Ms. F's mood.

After assessing Ms. F, the nurse asks to view the home. Ms. F and her husband live together in a small 2-bedroom apartment. The living area and the kitchen are one large room. There is a single bathroom. The apartment is much warmer than outside; there are no fans. The windows are screened and open. The apartment is tidy, clean, and sparsely furnished. The extra bedroom is an office with a laptop computer, but plans are being made to make it the nursery.

Neal Theory Implications

Stage 3: The professional nurse at this stage would be able to assess the family with confidence and access resources for them. The professional would know what community resources were available for assistance with ADL or home care. The professional may be able

(Continued)

to locate women who have had a similar experience who may want to provide emotional support to the family. This professional would clarify the essential goals for this family and help them meet those goals. The professional would assess and recognize when the patient was not progressing as expected and would act decisively to correct the situation.

Stage 2: The professional at stage 2 may be able to assess the patient and home environment but need assistance to identify resources in the community or from other disciplines. This professional would recognize changes in the patient's status, but may need assistance in what actions are appropriate to take. This professional may not be aware of community groups or support that is available. This professional would be able to effectively teach the patient aseptic technique.

Stage 1: The professional at stage 1 may feel overwhelmed and uncomfortable in the home environment. The professional may be able to accurately assess the patient, but be unsure how to proceed after identifying patient needs. This person may have difficulty communicating effectively with the family.

The nurse and Mr. and Ms. F discuss their plan for this pregnancy. They develop the following goals together:

- Ms. F will find foods and fluids that she can tolerate and that are healthful for the growing fetus.
- Ms. F will not lose weight.
- Mr. and Ms. F will access appropriate information regarding hyperemesis gravidarum.
- Mr. and Ms. F will recognize the signs of increasing depression and report them.
- Ms. F will access the PICC and do daily infusion of fluids (spike bag, prime tubing, set pump, and start infusion aseptically)
- Ms. F will be able to add vitamins to fluid bag.
- Ms. F will be able to infuse intravenous medications and recognize serious side effects of medications.
- Mr. and Ms. F will recognize signs of dehydration and infection.
- Ms. F will receive disability compensation from her work.
- The overheated apartment will be cooled.
- Mr. and Ms. F will begin to prepare for the eventual birth.

| ? | **CRITICAL THINKING** |

1. Are there any referrals that are appropriate for Ms. F?
Answer: Yes, a dietician. Ms. F would benefit from discussing foods that she can tolerate and that will provide her with the calories and nutrition she needs for pregnancy. The dietician can help her develop an eating plan that minimizes her nausea and vomiting and is considerate of her cultural and pregnancy dietary needs. The dietician can discuss timing of eating and fluid intake that may also influence the nausea and vomiting. A medical social worker (MSW) could assist Ms. F with applying for disability from her work. An MSW may be able to help her find resources to get fans or air conditioning for the apartment. They may also look into helping her find nursery items she may need. Physical therapy (PT) may be helpful to maintain muscle strength with decreased activity levels.

2. Discuss how the nurse could incorporate respect for this couple's culture into her teaching.
Answer: The effectiveness of the nurse and the teaching provided by the nurse are influenced by the perception of the learners. A nurse does not have to have the same beliefs or values, but must show respect and openness to others' cultural beliefs. Understanding the Indian and Hindu cultures may help the nurse to be a more effective teacher. In this instance the nurse should discuss with the family if they have any special cultural needs. Making assumptions or generalizations could be hurtful. Cultural knowledge including that most Hindus are vegetarians helps to direct the nurse to appropriate assessments. The nurse should not assume that Mr. and Ms. F are strict vegetarians just because they are of the Hindu faith; she should instead ask of what their diet consists. While paternalism is a part of some Indian families, this American couple may have different values. Recognizing and discussing cultural influences that affect the care of the patient is important and individualized. Understanding an individual's culture begins with an open mind, not a stereotype. Therefore, the best way to incorporate respect for their culture is to discuss it openly without preconceived judgments.

3. What are the three greatest concerns in caring for Ms. F? Explain why and prioritize them?
Answer (in prioritized order): Note that nutrition is not first. While it is important, Ms. F and the fetus can live without good nutrition for a period of time; but without hydration, both will fail quickly. Ms. F is also at higher risk for infection and the sequelae of infection (sepsis, fetal loss. etc.), which makes teaching aseptic technique a higher priority in this instance.

Dehydration in pregnancy can cause preterm labor and harm to the fetus and the mother. Maintaining hydration is extremely important and should be the priority goal for Ms. F. Therefore, teaching her to infuse the fluids, manage the vomiting, and decrease the high indoor temperatures becomes a priority.

Infection from the PICC line is also a top priority. Infection can also be extremely detrimental to Ms. F and the fetus. Therefore, teaching Ms. F to use aseptic technique when priming and attaching tubing or adding medications to the bag or to the line should be a priority as well.

Nutrition is important. Proper nutrition is vital for fetal growth and development as well as good immune function in Ms. F. Nutrition education for Ms. F will help her develop a plan to improve nutrition.

4. Ms. F is unable to leave the apartment because of her nausea, retching, and vomiting. What sources of support would you recommend for Ms. F?

Answer: The visiting nurse may find that Ms. F needs assistance with self- and home care needs. She may need assistance with her activities of daily living (ADL), shopping, and housework; right now, Mr. F. is assuming these responsibilities. In the future, if he is unable to do them, the nurse may need to help the family find someone to assist them. A home health aide may need to be involved, or a willing family or community member may be able to help. The access to the Internet may help Ms. F to connect with women who can help her through this difficult time. The website http://hyperemesis.org has information and links to support groups that may be helpful for Ms. F and her husband. Social networking on the computer may be helpful for Ms. F. She may find that this is a good way to keep in touch with friends and family and will provide support.

Seeking support within the extended family or the community to help this family prepare for the eventual birth would be helpful. Often, extended family or community members can find the resources to assist the family with their present needs and prepare the home for the eventual birth.

Relevant Community Resources

Other women who have had hyperemesis with a positive outcome
Internet support through: http://hyperemesis.org
Local charity or community group for assistance with house cleaning or nursery equipment.

5. Mr. and Ms. F are concerned about the health of the baby. What information would the nurse tell them about the baby's health?
Answer: The growing baby's well-being depends on the severity of the condition. Maternal weight loss seems to be an indicator of increasing fetal complications. With careful monitoring and treatment, Ms. F should be able to have a healthy baby.

Interdisciplinary Care Plan

Problem	Goal/Plan	Intervention	Evaluation
Fluid volume deficit related to frequent emesis	Patient and caregivers will immediately report changes in patient, especially: decreased daily weight, dizziness on rising, decreased urination or concentrated urine, ketones in urine, increased volume and/or frequency of emesis, confusion, or other change in mental status.	Teach patient and caregivers to recognize symptoms of worsening dehydration and report them to the physician or call emergency medical services (EMS). Teach patient to test urine for ketones daily. The nurse will continue to evaluate patient for dehydration on scheduled weekly visits.	Patient and husband verbalize understanding of reporting changes in health status to physician and when to call EMS. Patient continues to have nausea and some vomiting but shows no signs of dehydration. Urine is pale yellow, negative for ketones and she describes adequate urine output. Patient will continue to monitor daily. The nurse will continue to monitor on a weekly basis.
Risk for infection related to PICC line and intravenous fluid therapy	Patient will remain infection free. Patient and family will recognize signs of infection (temperature over 100.5, redness, purulent drainage or swelling at insertion site) and call the physician or EMS if they occur.	Teach patient and husband to recognize symptoms of infection and call physician or EMS if necessary. Nurse will continue to evaluate for infection on scheduled weekly visits.	Patient is free of infection after first week; continue to monitor. Patient and husband verbalize good understanding of signs of infection and when to call physician or EMS. Patient will continue to monitor daily. The nurse will continue to monitor on a weekly basis.

(Continued)

Problem	Goal/Plan	Intervention	Evaluation
Nutrition: Altered, less than body requirements related to hyperemesis	Patient will not lose weight. Patient will be able to tolerate some food and fluids.	If nausea diminishes, refer patient to dietician to help with balanced diet. Teach patient accepted dietary changes that may help her maintain nutrition such as: • Small frequent meals. • Eat solid foods separately from liquids. • Take in fluids between meals. • Eat simple carbohydrates that are easier to digest like rice, crackers, toast, pasta. • Eat dry toast or crackers before rising in the morning. • Eat proteins that are lower in fat like beans or chicken.	Patient continues with nausea; vomiting diminishing but still present. Patient maintains weight and makes small increases weekly.
Social isolation related to being homebound	Patient will state isolation has improved within next 2 days.	Discuss appropriate activities to decrease boredom. Patient may prefer movies or computer games as she may feel too nauseated for anything involving	Patient states she prefers to watch movies and is keeping a list of movies she would like to see. She signed up with a low cost movie provider. Patient has joined online hyperemesis support group and states that she feels

Problem	Goal/Plan	Intervention	Evaluation
		increased movement. Help patient use computer to access support groups for hyperemesis. Discuss patient's willingness to meet other women in the community who have had pregnancies with hyperemesis.	like she can get through this pregnancy. Patient states she will consider meeting other women who have had hyperemesis.
Knowledge deficit related to care of PICC and intravenous fluid and medication therapy	Patient and husband will demonstrate proper techniques for assembling intravenous equipment, giving medications and fluids, and PICC dressing changes.	Teach patient to assemble IV equipment and infuse fluids and medications. Teach patient and husband to use aseptic technique: • When giving intravenous medications and fluids. • When changing or reinforcing PICC dressing.	Patient and husband demonstrate excellent aseptic technique with IV medications, fluids, and dressing changes.
Potential for injury related to side effects from intravenous fluids and medications	Patient and husband will verbalize understanding of proper medication administration and potential life-threatening side effects.	Teach patient and husband proper medication administration. Teach patient and husband to recognize potential life-threatening side effects.	Patient shows no signs of side effects to medications and fluids. Patient and husband verbalize understanding of proper medication administration and potential life-threatening side effects.

(Continued)

Problem	Goal/Plan	Intervention	Evaluation
Potential for impaired home maintenance management related to husband's potential inability to maintain home	Home will remain maintained as evidenced by safe living conditions. Husband will have resources to help him maintain the home if he should find it overwhelming.	Discuss with husband to identify if home maintenance is overwhelming. Assess home safety with weekly visits. Identify any community persons or groups that may be interested in helping. Contact local charity to find resources for a fan or air conditioner.	Husband continues to maintain the home in a safe manner. A local charitable organization provided an air conditioner to the family. The nurse will continue to evaluate weekly.
Knowledge deficit related to disability compensation	Patient will receive disability benefits and compensation.	Social service referral called.	Social service able to assist patient to attain disability compensation.
Potential for ineffective individual coping related to isolation and continued illness	Patient and husband will recognize signs of ineffective coping and identify them to the nurse or call PCP as needed.	Discuss signs of ineffective coping and depression as found on the National Institute of Mental Health website [6]. Print a copy for the patient and husband to refer to as needed.	Patient and husband verbalize understanding of signs of ineffective coping and feel she is coping well. Patient and husband will continue to monitor daily. The nurse will monitor on a weekly basis.

REFERENCES & RESOURCES

[1] M. Fejzo et al., "Symptoms and pregnancy outcomes associated with extreme weight loss among women with hyperemesis gravidarum," *Journal of Women's Health*, 18(12): pp. 1981–1987, 2009. doi:10.1089/jwh.2009.1431.

[2] Hyperemesis Education and Research (HER) Foundation, (n.d.) Retrieved from: http://www.hyperemesis.org

[3] A. Jennings-Sanders, "A case study approach to hyperemesis gravidarum home care implications (Electronic version)," *Home Healthcare Nurse*, 27(6):347–351, 2009.

[4] A. Lamondy, "Managing hyperemesis gravidarum (Electronic version)," *Nursing*, 37(2):66–68, 2007.

[5] S. Munch and M. Schmitz, "The hyperemesis beliefs scale (HBS): A new instrument for assessing beliefs about severe nausea and vomiting in pregnancy," *Journal of Psychosomatic Obstetrics & Gynecology*, 28(4):219–229, 2007. doi:10.1080/01674820701262036.

[6] National Institute of Mental Health, (n.d.) "What Are the Signs and Symptoms of Depression?" Retrieved from: http://www.nimh.nih.gov/health/publications/depression/what-are-the-signs-and-symptoms-of-depression.shtml

[7] B. Poursharif, L. Korst, M. Fejzo, K. MacGibbon, R. Romero and T. Goodwin, "The psychosocial burden of hyperemesis gravidarum (Electronic version)," *Journal of Perinatology*, 28:176–181, 2008.

[8] V. Rhodes, "Rhodes Index of Nausea, Vomiting and Retching," Retrieved from: http://www.hyperemesis.org/downloads/rhodes-index.pdf, 1996.

[9] P. Sheehan, "Hyperemesis gravidarum assessment and management (Electronic version)," *Australian Family Physician*, 30(9):698–701, 2007.

[10] P. Tan, R. Jacob, K. Quek and S. Omar, "Pregnancy outcome in hyperemesis gravidarum and the effect of laboratory clinical indicators of hyperemesis severity," *Journal of Obstetrics and Gynecology Research*, 33(4):457–464, 2007. doi:10.1111/j.1447-0756.2007.00552.x.

[11] S.L. Ward and S.M. Hisley, *Maternal-Child Nursing Care*, F.A. Davis Company, 2009.

Case 10.2 Postpartum Care following Uncomplicated Delivery

By Ruth Smillie, RN, MSN

This case study describes how the nurse develops a plan with the family during a brief exposure with minimal intervention. The patient is a 17-year-old gravida 1, para 1 woman who delivered a healthy infant girl vaginally at a local hospital. She had an uncomplicated delivery with a second-degree perineal tear. She is breast-feeding the infant. The option for a nurse to visit in the first days postpartum was offered to the woman and agreed to during her hospital stay. The patient desired continued support with breast-feeding and general support with her new role as a parent. The new mother's desire to successfully parent will guide the nurse's assessment and interventions in this case study.

Cultural Competence

Ms. N is 17; she is a teenager. The developmental needs of the teen differ from the more mature mother. She will need support and encouragement to parent effectively and to develop adequate self-care. She is at higher risk for poor parenting, abuse, and rapid subsequent births. The professionals caring for Ms. N should evaluate the special needs of the adolescent when planning care.

Clinical Case Studies in Home Health Care, First Edition. Edited by Leslie Neal-Boylan.
© 2011 John Wiley & Sons, Inc. Published 2011 by John Wiley & Sons, Inc.

ORDERS FOR HOME CARE

Patient: 17-year-old postpartum female
Diagnosis: G1P1; 3400 gm, 5-day-old infant girl born at 39 weeks gestation; breast-feeding
Current medications:
- Prenatal vitamins, once a day
- Docusate 100 mg twice a day
- Ibuprofen 600 mg every 6 hours as needed for pain
- Acetaminophen 1–3 regular strength tablets every 4 hours as needed for pain

Relevant past medical history: Uncomplicated prenatal course, no missed visits. Blood type A+. Rubella immune, Group B Strep negative, no sexually transmitted infections. The mother had the influenza and H1N1 vaccines during pregnancy. The infant is average for gestational age and passed her hearing screen. The bilirubin at discharge was at the low risk level. Breast-feeding was well established at discharge with the infant voiding and stooling normally. The first physical exam on the infant was within normal limits.
RN: Assess breast-feeding and perineal repair; provide parenting support. Assess infant weight, vital signs, and voiding and stooling patterns.

Reimbursement Considerations

Reimbursement for this visit would be covered under Medicaid. Many areas of the country provide these services without cost through grant monies. The infant assessment and the maternal visit need to take place on the same date and in the residence of the parent.

THE HOME VISIT

The nurse arrives at the neat 3-bedroom cape in a tidy residential neighborhood on a paved, tree-lined street. Greeting her at the door is a woman in her 40s, who warmly ushers her in. The home smells of freshly baked cookies and is clean and well kept. The woman introduces herself as Grandma and calls out to Ms. N, the mother of the infant, to come and greet the nurse. Ms. N arrives holding the infant; both are dressed appropriately. Ms. N smiles at the nurse shyly and introduces the baby as Liddy, gently making her wave at the nurse.

Grandma brings cookies and ice tea to the living room where the nurse and the new mother have begun to discuss the visit. Grandma excuses herself and retires to the kitchen, offering to help if needed. Ms. N explains that her own family was not supportive of her pregnancy and that she has been living with the father of the baby and his parents for the last 6 months. She feels at home here.

The nurse assesses the infant, explaining to Ms. N each step as she progresses. The infant is dressed in a clean, one-piece pink outfit with a matching hat and booties. She is alert and active. Vital signs (HR: 133, RR: 44, Axillary, T: 36.9C) and assessment are normal. The nurse is able to answer many of Ms. N's questions concerning normal skin irregularities, like the milia on the baby's nose, as well as pointing out normal reflexes that infants have. Ms. N explains that she thinks that the infant is afraid of her, as she often seems to jump when she picks her up. She is relieved to know that that was the Moro reflex and that it is normal. Ms. N tells the nurse that the baby feeds about 10 times a day. The nurse watches as Ms. N breast-feeds the baby; she notes a good latch and frequent swallowing. Next, the nurse weighs the infant, noting only a 4 percent weight loss from birth. The nurse finishes by changing the diaper, discussing normal voiding and stooling patterns for infants, and finding that the baby is voiding at least 6 times a day and often has several yellow stools.

Ms. N has many questions for the nurse concerning infant care. She is worried about breast-feeding and about whether the baby is getting enough to eat. She wants to know when the baby will start sleeping though the night, how she can get the father of the baby more involved in infant care, and when the baby will learn to smile and talk. She said she enjoys the baby but sometimes feels very alone and isolated. She states that the grandmother is very supportive and helps her care for the infant sometimes. She is happy with her new family and wants to be a good mother to this baby. Her boyfriend works construction, and she is planning to finish her last year of high school in the fall.

After assessing the infant, the nurse asks to view the home. She notes a working carbon monoxide detector and fire alarm. The home is tidy; the infant sleeps in a crib next to the parent's double bed. The crib is filled with stuffed animals and has a bumper around the mattress and several blankets in it. There is a mobile hanging above the crib. The family cat is sleeping in the crib. Safety covers are already in place over the outlets and doorknobs. The baby has a new car seat and stroller. In the living room, there is an old, wide, mesh-sided playpen with several rips in the mesh and one side broken in the down position. In the bathroom the nurse notes the perineal wash bottle and a sitz bath, as well as fresh feminine hygiene pads.

The nurse takes a few moments to do a physical assessment on Ms. N. She notes the following data:

- VS: BP: 122/78, HR: 74, RR: 16, T: 36.8C
- Lochia: Scant rubra, no foul odor or clots
- Fundus: Firm, 3–4 cm below umbilicus
- Perineal repair: Clean with no redness, slightly swollen
- No hemorrhoids noted.
- Breasts with everted nipples, slight redness on areola bilaterally, no breakdown
- Breasts are firm and warm; mother feels "stretched."
- There are no problems with voiding.
- The mother is stooling normally with return to normal once-a-day pattern.
- Breath sounds clear.
- There is some perineal discomfort and occasional cramping abdominal pain, especially with breast-feeding. Ms. N takes Ibuprofen once or twice daily, with relief.
- Ms. N is using the perineal wash bottle appropriately.

The nurse helps Ms. N to focus on what needs and goals she has now that she is a new parent. Ms. N informs the nurse of the following goals:

- To be a good parent
- To meet other teens like herself
- To breast-feed without pain
- To be able to go to a movie without the baby
- To get the father more involved in caring for the baby

Neal Theory Implications

Stage 3: The professional nurse at this stage would be able to assess the mother and infant with confidence and access resources for the new parent. The professional would know what community resources were available. The professional would be able to find parenting groups or classes that would be appropriate for this teen mother and utilize other disciplines as needed. The professional could identify where to find low cost or free infant equipment if needed. This professional would identify safety issues immediately and effectively resolve them.

Stage 2: The professional at stage 2 may be able to assess the patient and home environment, but need assistance to identify resources in the community or from other disciplines. This professional would identify safety issues, but may need assistance communicating or resolving them. This professional may not be aware of community groups or support that is available. This professional would be able to effectively teach the patient self-care.

Stage 1: The professional at stage 1 may feel overwhelmed and uncomfortable in the home environment. This professional may be able to accurately assess the patients, but be unsure how to proceed after identifying patient needs. This person may have difficulty communicating safety issues to the patient.

? CRITICAL THINKING

1. Identify 2 areas of concern for the mother and the infant.
Answer:
Mother:

- Pain related to engorgement of breasts
- Pain related to perineal swelling
- Abdominal pain and cramping with breast-feeding
- Skin breakdown and potential interruption of breast-feeding
- Social isolation related to infant care

Baby:

- Risk for bodily injury related to old playpen
- Risk for suffocation related to crib with bumpers, stuffed toys, and cat

2. Using the voice of the nurse, discuss each of these concerns with the mother of the baby. Include suggestions and treatments if needed.

Instruct the new mother about breast engorgement.
Answer: "Your breasts are a little swollen as a result of your milk coming in. Inside your breasts are a series of little sacs that fill with milk, like bunches of grapes. These all connect with tiny ducts to the nipples of the breasts and empty when the baby feeds. As your milk increases, the blood vessels around the sacs swell; and sometimes there is some fluid around the sacs as well. This is all very normal; and as long as the baby continues to feed well, it will decrease in the next few days. Until then, the best way to lessen the discomfort is to feed the baby often and take the ibuprofen and acetaminophen that is prescribed for you. If you find that you are having trouble getting your baby to latch because the breast is firm and swollen, you should express some milk manually or with a pump to "soften" the breast and then put the baby to the breast. Using warm compresses before feeding will help to soften the breast. Cold compresses on the breast for a few minutes after the feeding may help to lessen swelling. If the baby isn't emptying the breasts with feeding, using a breast pump after she feeds will help."

Instruct the new mother about perineal swelling.
Answer: "You have a little swelling around the area where the baby came out and where you have some stitches. This is normal and should get better over the next few days. To keep the area clean, keep using the perineal wash bottle that you have here in the bathroom after you pee or poop. You can also use the sitz bath filled with warm water for 20 minutes, 3 or 4 times a day. This will help the swelling go down and may lessen the pain. It also will help to keep the area clean. Wash your hands before and after taking care of this area. Taking ibuprofen or acetaminophen as ordered will help to lessen the pain. Remember to change your perineal pad several times a day and to avoid tampons, douching, and sex until you see your provider next month."

Instruct the new mother about the care of her breasts.
Answer: "You are doing a great job breast-feeding, but there is some redness around your nipples that we want to make sure gets better so you can keep feeding comfortably. You got the baby on the breast well. Did you notice how most of the brown part of the breast around the nipple, called the areola, was in the baby's mouth? That is really important; it is part of a good latch or attachment to the breast that will keep the breast from getting sore. You need to wash the nipples with warm water only, because soaps can dry out the nipple. You should squeeze out a little breast milk after you feed, spreading it on your nipple and areola; let that dry. Then you can use a small amount of lanolin cream to help prevent soreness."

Instruct the mother regarding the risk of social isolation.
Answer: "Taking care of a baby sure does change your social life. You are not alone; in our community, there are many women your age who have infants. There are several teen-parenting groups that meet locally. Let's see which one you might be interested in. I can help you find something that fits your needs. I think we can find a breast-feeding support group just for teens. You can also become a Women, Infants and Children (WIC) participant. WIC can help you with nutritional foods and may also assist you to rent a breast pump. That may make it possible for you to get out for a few hours."

Relevant Community Resources

Teen parenting education groups
Breast-feeding group
Local charity or community group for assistance with infant equipment
Local Women, Infants and Children (WIC) Program: Breast pump rental and food assistance
School-based parenting education

Instruct the new mother about infant safety.
Answer: "I see that you have an older playpen here in the living room. These older playpens are dangerous. The baby could suffocate and die in this side that won't go up. The holes in the mesh also may be a strangulation problem as the baby gets older. I can help you take it down and get rid of it, and then we can call and see if the local thrift shop has a safe one. I see that you have many blankets, stuffed animals, and the family cat here in the baby's crib. While I know these things seem fun and harmless, they can actually hurt your baby. Studies have shown that bumpers, blankets, stuffed animals, and other loose objects in the crib can cause the baby to suffocate. Sudden Infant Death Syndrome (or SIDS) can occur when a baby sleeps with bumpers, loose blankets, or stuffed animals. Let me help you take these things out of the crib. The best way to keep the baby warm is to dress her in a warm sleeper and keep the room at a temperature that is comfortable for you and the baby. Keep the baby warm, but do not overheat her. Remember to always put her on her back to sleep, never on her side or tummy.

Pets should be kept out of the crib as they can make the baby sick. The baby doesn't have a strong system to fight off germs and diseases like you and I do, so it is best to limit her contact with the kitty until she is older."

3. Which concern has the highest priority?
Answer: Safety is the highest priority. The crib and playpen are unsafe and should be addressed immediately.

4. Is jaundice a concern? Which infant assessments are important with regard to jaundice?
Answer: Assessment of risk for jaundice is important in all infants. Sixty percent of full-term newborns will show some signs of jaundice; most require no intervention. Very high levels of unconjugated bilirubin can cause illness in the newborn and will need treatment. The visiting nurse has an important role in evaluating jaundice in the newborn. In the home setting, evaluating feeding and elimination patterns are vital to establishing the risk for complications from jaundice. The infant who feeds well and voids and stools frequently will be eliminating bilirubin and lowering the risk of jaundice. The best evaluation of feeding effectiveness is steady weight gain. Weighing the infant and comparing the weight to the infant's birth weight provide important information about how the baby is feeding. A loss of more than 7 percent of the birth weight is concerning and should be reported to the health care provider.

5. What resources should the nurse recommend for this family?
Answer: A breast-feeding group or individual consultation with a board-certified lactation consultant (IBCLC), parenting classes for teens, and infant care classes.

Interdisciplinary Care Plan

Problem	Goal/Plan	Intervention	Evaluation
Risk for injury to infant related to out-of-date playpen in use in home	Patient and family will discard it immediately.	Teach parents and grandmother about hazards of old baby equipment. Assist them in discarding it. Discuss local thrift shops where they can obtain safe equipment for infants.	Parents and family discard playpen. Local charity donated new portable crib to family.
Risk for suffocation related to stuffed animals, cat, and bumpers in crib	Patient and family will remove bumpers and stuffed animals from crib immediately. Cat will never be allowed in crib.	Teach patient and family the risks of SIDS related to stuffed animals, pets, and crib bumpers. Assist them to remove these items from the crib and sleeping areas of the infant during visit.	Crib is free from extra plush items that can cause suffocation. Cat is no longer allowed in bedroom where crib is kept.
Risk for altered parenting related to maturity and age of parents	Parents will provide safe and effective care for their infant in 1 month.	Encourage parents to seek information and educational opportunities to enhance parenting. Recommend local teen parenting classes.	Parents enrolled in local teen parenting class. Mother will be attending school-based parenting class in fall.
Risk for infection and interrupted breast-feeding related to dry, cracked nipples	Patient will continue to breast-feed. Nipples will be healed within 2 weeks. Breasts will have no sign of infection (redness, swelling, fever, etc.).	Contact lactation consultant to teach patient breast care. Suggest breast-feeding teen group for ongoing support.	Patient still breast-feeding exclusively at 2 months. Nipples are well healed; breasts are without infection.
Risk for infection related to perineal tear	Patient shows no signs of infection in 6 weeks (fever; foul-smelling lochia; increased pain, redness, or drainage).	Reinforce use of perineal wash bottle and proper hygiene. Teach patient signs of infection.	Patient remains free of infection at 6 week physician visit.

Problem	Goal/Plan	Intervention	Evaluation
Pain related to perineal injury and swelling	Patient will express pain has improved within 1 week.	Reinforce anti-inflammatory medication use. Discuss use of sitz bath.	Swelling is diminished, and patient is pain free.
Pain related to engorgement	Patient will have reduced pain within 1 week.	Discuss treatment options and consult IBCLC if this becomes an ongoing issue.	Swelling is diminished, and patient is pain free.
Loss of social interaction related to isolation	Patient will verbalize decreased isolation within 1 month.	Identify local teen parenting groups. Access WIC for breast pump rental or purchase so patient may have some time without infant and still breast-feed.	Patient pumping breast milk, is able to go to the movies with boyfriend, and is meeting other teen parents at classes.

REFERENCES & RESOURCES

[1] B. Barnet, J. Liu, M. DeVoe, K. Alporovitz-Bichell and A.K. Duggan, "Home visiting for adolescent mothers: Effects on parenting, maternal life course and primary care linkage," *Annals of Family Medicine*, 5(3):224–232, 2007. doi:10.1370/afm.629.

[2] B. Barnet, J. Liu, M. DeVoe, A.K. Duggan, M.A. Gold and E. Pecukonis, "Motivational intervention to reduce rapid subsequent births to adolescent mothers: A community-based randomized trial," *Annals of Family Medicine*, 7(5):436–445, 2009. doi:10.1370/afm.1014.

[3] Consumer Product Safety Commission, "Deaths Associated with Playpens," Retrieved from: http://www.cpsc.gov/library/playpen.pdf, 2001.

[4] D. Keister, K.T. Roberts and S.L. Werner, "Strategies for breast-feeding success," *American Family Physician.*, 78(2):225–231, 2008.

[5] A.J. Macarthur and C. Macarthur, "Incidence, severity, and determinants of perineal pain after vaginal delivery: A prospective cohort study," *American Journal of Obstetrics and Gynecology*, 191:1191–1204, 2004.

[6] S. Mass, "Breast pain: Engorgement, nipple pain and mastitis," *Clinical Obstetrics and Gynecology*, 47(3):676–682, 2004.

[7] National Institute of Child Health and Human Development, "What Does a Safe Sleep Environment Look Like [Brochure]," NIH Pub no. 06-5759. Retrieved from: http://www.nichd.nih.gov/publications/pubs/upload/BTS_safe_environment.pdf, 2006.

[8] L.A. Savio Beers and R.E. Hollo, "Approaching the adolescent-headed family: A review of teen parenting," *Current Problems in Pediatric and Adolescent Health Care*, 39:216–233, 2009. doi:10.1016/jcppeds.2009.09.001.

[9] E. Sebesta, (ND) "American Academy of Pediatrics Breast-Feeding Residency Curriculum: Management of Breast-Feeding Situations," [PowerPoint slides]. Retrieved from: http://www.aap.org/breast-feeding/curriculum/tools.html#preparedPresentations

[10] A.S. Stiles, "Parenting needs, goals, and strategies of adolescent mothers," *The American Journal of Maternal/Child Nursing*, 30(5):327–333. 2005.

[11] U.S. Department of Health and Human Services, Centers for Disease Control and Prevention, (ND) "Infants and Young Children, Animal Safety Tips," Retrieved from: http://www.cdc.gov/healthypets/child.htm

[12] S.L. Ward and S.M. Hisley, *Maternal-Child Nursing Care*, F.A. Davis Company, 2009.

[13] L. Wenner, "Care of the breast-feeding mother in medical-surgical areas," *MEDSURG Nursing*, 16(2):101–104, 2007.

[14] Woman, Infants, and Children, "WIC Fact Sheet—English," Retrieved from: http://www.fns.usda.gov/wic/WIC-Fact-Sheet.pdf

Case 10.3 Postpartum Care following Complicated Delivery

By Ruth Smillie, RN, MSN

This case study describes how the nurse coordinates care and uses community resources to support a woman suffering with postpartum depression (PPD). The patient is a 28-year-old, first-time mother. She delivered a baby girl vaginally 4 weeks ago without complications. Working throughout her pregnancy as a dental hygienist, she planned to be a stay-at-home mother after the birth. Postpartum depression was an unexpected development that has saddened and confused this family. Community and family resources are vital to the success of this family.

ORDERS FOR HOME CARE

Patient: 28-year-old; gravida 1, para 1; first-time mother. She is an Italian-American woman with a 4-week-old infant.
Diagnosis: Postpartum depression
Medications:
  • Prenatal vitamins once a day while breast-feeding
  • Sertraline 50 mg once a day
Relevant past medical history: She has no significant past medical history. She was discharged from the hospital 2 days after an uncomplicated birth. Her husband called her health care provider last week to discuss his wife's inability to care for herself and to discuss her extreme fatigue. She was seen and started on sertraline. The patient

Clinical Case Studies in Home Health Care, First Edition. Edited by Leslie Neal-Boylan.
© 2011 John Wiley & Sons, Inc. Published 2011 by John Wiley & Sons, Inc.

is breast-feeding, and the infant is gaining weight appropriately and generally doing well.

RN: Follow up for recent identification of depression and medication evaluation. Evaluate infant care, weigh infant, and assess breast-feeding and maternal attachment.

Cultural Competence

Ms. A and Mr. A are Italian-American and live in a large city. Extended family may play an important role in their lives. It would be important for the nurse to explore their cultural expectations and needs. Resources should be assessed on an individual basis. The community they live in may be part of a large city, yet it may offer support and charitable organizations specifically focused on this smaller geographic area.

 ## THE HOME VISIT

Small local markets filled with hanging cheeses and smoked meats dotted the street where the nurse would visit her patient today. It is late afternoon when the subway stops only a block from the brownstone where Ms. A lives with her husband and new baby girl. The nurse presses the bell and identifies herself, and the door clicks open. The nurse enters, and walks up the stairs to the second-floor flat. Ms. A's husband greets her warmly, holding a dark-haired baby dressed in a tiny, white-eyelet dress with a bow in her hair. He puts the baby down and explains that Ms. A is in bed. The nurse moves to the bedroom. Ms. A is lying awake. She smells of perspiration, and her hair is knotted and disheveled around her face. She is in a stained and torn nightgown. She sits up, moving very slowly, greets the nurse while staring at the floor, and cries softly.

Ms. A explains to the nurse in a monotone voice how excited she was for this pregnancy and baby, and how guilty and sad she feels because she is failing as a mother. Ms. A wonders out loud if she will ever be able to be a good enough parent, stating she feels useless. Ms. A's husband reassures her that she is going to be a wonderful mother as soon as she feels better. The bedroom is cluttered with clothes strewn around the floor and draped over furniture. The nurse assesses Ms. A and discusses her feelings and goals while Ms. A's husband attends to the baby in the living room.

Relevant Community Resources

Postpartum depression groups
Breast-feeding group
Baby basics classes for basic infant care
Local charity or community group for assistance in the home
Other women who have had postpartum depression with a positive outcome
Local family members who are willing to help with infant and home care

The nurse notes the following after assessing Ms. A:

- The patient completes the Edinburgh Postnatal Depression Scale with a score over 13 (indicating depressive illness).
- She is breast-feeding about every 3 hours 8–10 times a day; good latch is noted.
- VS: T 36.8C, HR 77, RR 18, BP 116/72.
- She complains of some nipple pain; dry. chapped-appearing nipples are noted by the nurse.
- Lochia is described as just some whitish flow, no odor.
- The patient doesn't sleep well and is tired all day.

The nurse assesses the infant and finds the following:

- There has been adequate weight gain since delivery.
- The infant is voiding and wets diapers 6 times a day; the infant is stooling 3 to 4 times a day.
- Vital signs and examination are within normal limits.
- The infant is clean and appropriately dressed.
- The crib is safe, and the baby is positioned appropriately.

Reimbursement Considerations

Reimbursement for this visit would be covered by the patient's private insurance. In the event that the patient meets the low-income guidelines, Medicaid could provide this service. The MSW may need to get involved to help the patient find resources to pay for treatments and therapies that may not be covered by insurance or Medicaid.

After speaking with Ms. A, the nurse evaluates the rest of the home. The living area is tidy, but the kitchen sink is filled with dirty dishes. The table is covered with mail and newspapers. The bathroom is unkempt with towels on the floor and dirty diapers filling the trash. Ms. A tells the nurse that she feels like a failure as a mother and wife. She is embarrassed about the state of her home, telling the nurse she kept a cleaner house when she worked full time. She really thought she would have lots of time to keep up with housework and cooking but is finding it all overwhelming. She is breast-feeding the baby and states, "This baby seems to need to eat all the time. I'm so tired; I barely have a minute of rest or time for myself." Except for breast-feeding, Mr. A and his mother have been caring for the infant. Mr. A explains that his mother is staying with them while on vacation and must return to work.

The nurse discusses goals with Ms. A but finds that Ms. A has trouble focusing and identifying any particular needs.

Neal Theory Implications

Stage 3: The professional nurse at this stage would recognize immediately that Ms. A needs support in her role as mother. The professional would know what community resources were available for assistance with ADL or home care. The professional would know where local support groups are and how to contact them. This professional would arrange immediate interventions to insure the safety of the mother and infant in this situation. The professional would assess and recognize when the patient was not making improvement in her depression, and would coordinate with other providers to effect change.

Stage 2: The professional would know which community resources were available for assistance with ADL or home care. The professional may be able to locate women who have had a similar experience and may want to provide emotional support to Ms. A or the family. This professional would clarify the essential goals for this family and help them meet them. The professional would assess and recognize when the patient was not progressing as expected and would act decisively to correct the situation.

Stage 1: The professional at stage 1 may feel overwhelmed by the emotions and the needs of this family. The professional may be able to accurately assess the patient but may underestimate the seriousness of the situation. This person may have difficulty discussing the situation therapeutically with the family.

?	CRITICAL THINKING

1. From the description of Ms. A, what indicators indicate that she is suffering from postpartum depression?

Answer: Ms. A exhibits the following signs of depression:

- Disheveled appearance
- Sleeping in the middle of the day
- Not getting dressed
- Poor hygiene
- Fatigue
- Poor sleeping at night
- Not making eye contact with the nurse
- Lethargic movement
- Crying
- Monotone voice
- Feelings of worthlessness
- Inability to focus

Her score on the depression scale simply reinforces what the nurse would have deduced through her assessment of Ms. A. It also provides a baseline assessment to evaluate progress in the future [1].

2. How does postpartum depression affect the mother-baby relationship? Identify the clues that Ms. A and her infant may have an attachment problem.

Answer: Postpartum depression can interfere with the maternal-infant attachment process. This can cause long-lasting problems for the infant. Infant learning, social development, and emotional maturity are gained through interactions with people who care for them. A mother with postpartum depression may not be able to respond to the infant's needs, and that may have a negative impact on development. The nurse should assess the maternal-infant attachment by looking for how the mother interacts and cares for the infant. The following observations may indicate that there is an attachment problem for Ms. A and the infant.

- Ms. A is not caring for the infant except to breast-feed her.
- Ms. A describes herself as a poor mother.
- Ms. A is not caring for herself.
- Ms. A does not handle the infant during the visit.

3. In Ms. A's case, what safety concerns should take priority?

Answer: The nurse would be most concerned that Ms. A not do harm to herself or the baby. Postpartum depression can lead to suicide or infanticide.

4. What resources would the nurse recommend for Ms. A?

Answer: Ms. A is unable to care for herself or the infant appropriately at this time and will need a great deal of support until she can assume these responsibilities. The nurse should work with Mr. and Ms. A to look into who can assist her. Perhaps during the day, a family member or a home health aide can assist Ms. A in self-, infant-, and home care. If they can afford to hire someone as a caregiver, that would be appropriate as well. It would be inappropriate to leave Ms. A alone at this time. The nurse can also advise the following:

- Individual and group counseling for treatment of postpartum depression. The nurse will be able to recommend to Ms. A where she can get the help she needs to begin to get treatment.
- Crisis phone numbers that Ms. A can call for support or if she feels like she is going to harm herself or the infant.
- A medical social worker (MSW) evaluation can assist with finding resources to help care for the infant while Ms. A recovers. Social work may also be involved to find resources to pay for therapies and treatments that are not covered under insurance or Medicaid.
- Local charitable organizations may be able to assist in caring for the home and helping with grocery shopping, cooking, and errands if needed.
- A lactation consultant who may be able to assist Ms. A to better care for her breasts, to be sure that the baby continues to latch well and to decrease the nipple pain.

Interdisciplinary Care Plan

Problem	Goal/Plan	Intervention	Evaluation
Risk for violence directed at self or infant	Patient and infant will remain safe. Family will recognize behaviors that may indicate worsening depressive illness. Patient will get support for her postpartum depression.	Inform family members of risk for suicide and assist them to recognize behaviors that may indicate worsening depressive illness. Identify and help patient get to support groups and individual therapy for postpartum depression (MSW may assist here). Monitor effectiveness of medication and contact provider with follow-up information so medications may be adjusted as needed.	Patient attending weekly postpartum depression group and twice weekly individual therapy with MSW. Family can identify behaviors to watch for that may indicate worsening illness or impending suicide. Patient and infant remain safe.

Problem	Goal/Plan	Intervention	Evaluation
Altered health maintenance related to postpartum depression	Home support will assist patient with ADL until she can manage them herself. Patient will manage ADL within 1 month.	Provide information about support groups. Notify physician for medication followup. MSW to assist with locating charitable organization or family that can assist with ADL now.	Home health aide assisting with ADL during the day. Sisters of patient take turns assisting patient each evening with ADL. Patient manages own ADL after 4 weeks.
Altered parenting related to postpartum depression	Parenting assistance until patient able to manage infant care independently. Patient will manage infant care independently within 1 month. Infant will be safe in care of mother.	Provide information about support groups. Assess support systems of family and community to help with infant care. Assist with finding baby care classes.	Home health aide assigned to family immediately. Patient attending infant care classes and slowly assuming more and more care of the infant after 1 month.
Impaired home maintenance related to postpartum depression	Home care assistance will be provided until patient can maintain safe home environment independently.	Provide information regarding community support. Assess support systems of family and community to assist with home maintenance.	Home health aide assists with home care. At 1 month, patient beginning to assume more care of the home. Safety maintained.
Pain related to nipple condition.	Patient will experience no further pain with breast-feeding in next 2 weeks.	Provide information on breast care. Refer patient to a lactation consultant. Refer patient to breast-feeding support group.	Breasts and nipples without redness or chafing. Patient feeding without pain at 2 weeks.

REFERENCES & RESOURCES

[1] J. Cox, J. Holden and R. Sagovsky, "Detection of postnatal depression: Development of the 10-item Edinburgh postnatal depression scale," *British Journal of Psychiatry*, 150:782–786, 1987.

[2] S. Dimidjian and S. Goodman, "Nonpharmacologic intervention and prevention strategies for depression during pregnancy and the postpartum," *Clinical Obstetrics and Gynecology*, 52(3):498–514, 2009. Retrieved from http://www.clinicalobgyn.com

[3] J. Horowitz, C. Murphy, K. Gregory and J. Wojcik, "Community-based postpartum depression screening: Results from the CARE study," *Psychiatric Services*, 60(11):1432–1434, 2009. Retrieved from http://www.psychiatryonline.com

[4] J. Kim, L. La Porte, M. Corcoran, S. Magasi, J. Batza and R. Silver, "Barriers to mental health treatment among obstetric patients at risk for depression," *American Journal of Obstetrics and Gynecology*, 202:312e1–312e5, 2010.

[5] T. Lanza Di Scalea and K. Wisner, "Antidepressant medication use during breast-feeding," *Clinical Obstetrics and Gynecology*, 52(3):483–497, 2009. Retrieved from http://www.clinicalobgyn.com

[6] L. Mayberry, J. Horowitz and E. Declercq, "Depression symptom prevalence and demographic risk factors among U.S. women during the first 2 years postpartum," *Journal of Gynecologic and Neonatal Nursing*, 36:542–549, 2007. doi:10.1111/J.1552-6909. 007.00191.x.

[7] J. Payne and S. Meltzer-Brody, "Antidepressant use during pregnancy: Current controversies and treatment strategies," *Clinical Obstetrics and Gynecology*, 52(3):469–481, 2009. Retrieved from http://www.clinicalobgyn.com

[8] D. Sit and K. Wisner, "Identification of postpartum depression," *Clinical Obstetrics and Gynecology*, 52(3):456–468, 2009. Retrieved from http://www.clinicalobgyn.com

[9] S.L. Ward and S.M. Hisley, *Maternal-Child Nursing Care*, F.A. Davis Company, 2009.

[10] K. Wisner, B. Parry and C. Piontek, "Postpartum depression," *New England Journal of Medicine*, 347(3):194–199, 2002.

[11] C.R. Zauderer, "A case study of postpartum depression and altered maternal newborn attachment," *The American Journal of Maternal/Child Nursing*, 33(3):173–178, 2008.

[12] J.J. Kim, L.M. La Porte, M. Corcoran, S. Magasi, J. Batza and R.K. Silver, "Barriers to mental health treatment among obstetric patients at risk for depression." *American Journal of Obstetrics & Gynecology*, Mar 2010, 202(3): 312.e1–312.e5, 0p; DOI: 10.1016/j.ajog.2010.01.004.

Section 11

Pediatrics

Case 11.1 Premature Infant with Apnea and Reflux

By Teresa LaMonica, PhD, MSN, RN, CPNP

This case study illustrates some of the more common concerns of a family with a premature infant and how the home health nurse guides the family in the infant's care and family adjustment. Angela, a 34-week-gestational infant was discharged after a 2-week stay in the neonatal intensive care unit (NICU) at a large community hospital. There were problems during the antepartum period. The infant required resuscitation at birth, with Apgar scores of 1/2 initially. Later concerns were apnea, bradycardia, and gastrointestinal reflux. She was discharged home on an apnea monitor with reflux, feeding problems, colic, and some hypotonia. The patient's mother was found to have a bacterial infection while in the hospital (*Clostridium difficle*) and had hypertension. These may have been in place before birth and may have contributed to early delivery. The mother was at risk for postpartum depression and needed guidance with nursing/pumping.

The home care nurse meets with the family shortly after the infant's discharge from the hospital, then weekly for the first 2 weeks at home, at 2 months of age, and again at 4 months of age. The nurse has the following concerns regarding the infant and family: Prematurity, apnea, gastrointestinal reflux and feeding, insufficient communication and parent teaching in the postpartum period and parenting adjustment.

This is the first baby for this professional couple: Mother 34 (gravida 1, para 1) and father 36. Prenatal care was regular at a health maintenance organization (HMO), with no problems until the last trimester at 32 weeks, when the obstetrician noticed that the mother's weight was not increasing enough and a sonogram showed the baby's weight

---

Clinical Case Studies in Home Health Care, First Edition. Edited by Leslie Neal-Boylan.
© 2011 John Wiley & Sons, Inc. Published 2011 by John Wiley & Sons, Inc.

slightly below what should be expected for growth. The obstetrician advised followup in 2 weeks for another sonogram, at which time the mother did not feel fetal movement and was rushed into the HMO. A challenge test was done, and the mother was admitted to the hospital with a diagnosis of intrauterine growth retardation and decreased fetal movement. After close monitoring and a trial of intravenous Pitocin to stimulate labor, dangerous dips in the fetal heartbeat followed (decelerations); and an emergency Cesarean section was warranted.

The infant had to be resuscitated at birth, with Apgar scores of 1/2. Weight was 4 pounds 2 ounces. The infant was admitted to the NICU on a respirator with apnea monitors. The infant did well in the NICU and was extubated on the second day, eventually taking nasogastric breast-feeds in small amounts, but having frequent apnea and bradycardia periods. Cranial bleeds were ruled out (sometimes seen with this age of prematurity); but the infant had significant reflux.

The mother had further hypertensive episodes postpartum and had to stay in the hospital for several days. Unfortunately, there was poor communication between the postpartum floor and the NICU. The mother received little assistance with pumping, and she was not kept informed on the baby's progress, nor encouraged to visit those first few days. On day 3 of her pumping, despite the nurses on the floor saying that they would get the milk down to the nursery, the mother found out that it had never been delivered and that the baby was receiving formula instead.

Once home, the parents visited at intervals during day and evening; sometimes with paternal grandparents. The maternal grandmother lived in Bolivia and arrived the second week. The father had to return to work a few days after the birth, and the mother often had difficulty getting to the hospital unless she had a ride. The father had not held the baby yet, saying "She is too small; I might hurt her." The mother had held the baby but was not encouraged to nurse until the second week. The mother continued to pump every day but found it increasingly difficult, and she said she was very sad without her baby at home.

The hospital had not set up a lactation consultation until 2 weeks postpartum, when the request was made by a family member who was a health professional. By then the mother's milk supply was diminished, and she was tired and beginning to feel depressed. It was discovered at this time that she had *Clostridium difficle* and antibiotics were started by the HMO doctor, who told her she could not breast-feed for 2 weeks but could keep pumping. At the mother's request, he did not consult with the pediatrician to try to find another antibiotic that would allow her to continue to breast-feed.

The baby continued to grow well, and by 2 weeks (now 36 weeks gestational age) was discharged on an apnea monitor (after the parents were given an infant CPR class) with medication for reflux and on formula. (The mom was told to continue to "try to breast-feed but to also supplement with formula.") The baby was beginning to be more alert but still had some hypotonia. Discharge planning included a home health nurse along with the apnea monitoring technician to come in the first week and at regular intervals during the first month.

Cultural Competence

The mother is from another country, and her mother often provides advice that is different from that of her pediatrician or nurse. Both parents have good family support, but the maternal grandmother is clearly the dominant caregiver. The team should view this as a strength, but remind them to try to maximize their relationship as a couple and as parents.

ORDERS FOR HOME CARE

Patient: 34-week-old premature infant
Diagnoses: Prematurity, apnea, gastrointestinal reflux, hypotonia
Current medications: Prevacid
Relevant past medical history:
- 34 weeks gestation
- Intrauterine growth retardation (IGR)
- Mother's preeclampsia
- Resuscitation at birth
- NICU x2 weeks
RN: Assess and evaluate.
Lactation consult: Assess and evaluate.

THE HOME VISIT

The nurse makes the first home visit that week at 2 o'clock in the afternoon to a 2-bedroom apartment in a suburban area. The home is clean but the living room is cluttered with baby equipment—rocker, stroller, and infant seat. The maternal grandmother greets the nurse; the infant is lying on the sofa in the living room on a pillow with the apnea monitor on. The grandmother shows the nurse into the back bedroom where the mother is in bed. There is a portable crib and diaper area set up in the mother's room, but the grandmother explains that the infant usually stays in the living room with her so as not to disturb the mother. The nurse introduces herself to the mother and asks her if she can come into the living room so the nurse can do the admission assessment on the infant and can ask the mother some questions.

The mother is pleasant and cooperative but seems tired; she looks to the grandmother to answer most of questions, saying that the grandmother takes care of the baby during the night. She says that the father of the baby comes home each day at lunch to check on the baby and does most of the getting up with the baby at night. The mother does not try to feed the baby at night due to fatigue. The grandmother reaches for the baby whenever the baby cries or needs changing.

Reimbursement Considerations

This patient is not eligible for WIC due to the parents' income, nor is the family eligible for Medicaid. They are in an HMO; and though they are not satisfied with the care they get for themselves or the baby (they always see someone different and it feels hurried), they at least have regular medical care. The state they live in has a good intervention program, and they have revisited looking into this. The HMO will cover child care visits, visits to the pulmonologist for apnea evaluation, and most of the apnea equipment. The nurse, as case manager on this case, will need to negotiate with the insurance case manager for specialists, such as a developmental pediatrician, lactation consultant, or additional home care visits beyond those typically allowed.

The nurse observes the 2 bedrooms in the apartment. The grandmother is presently staying in the room that was to be the nursery. She has recently arrived from Bolivia to help "as long as they need me." The nursery has not been finished and has boxes everywhere, no decorations, and no crib yet because "the baby was born early." The grandmother sleeps on a sofa bed. The baby sleeps in the parents' room in a portable crib at night. The bathrooms and kitchen are clean, with a formula preparation area in the kitchen where the grandmother makes up the formula daily and fixes all of the meals for the family. There is a cat in the home and a litter box in bathroom.

The nurse continues to gather data about the prenatal, birth, and neonatal histories. She discovers that the mother is a good historian but blames herself for the early birth, saying "I tried to eat right; I gave up all caffeine and alcohol and sugar and ate well. Maybe I should have quit work early." She is frustrated about being left out in the hospital regarding the baby's care and not being able to visit much. Also, she is frustrated at not being able to breast-feed due to the antibiotic she is on and says that pumping makes her more tired.

The mother is knowledgeable about the infant's medication; she shows the nurse how much she gives in the dropper. They discuss the baby's feeding, elimination, and sleep patterns.

After the nurse gets the history, she examines the baby, explaining about infant states and involuntary reflexes. Based on the history and physical examination, the nurse derives the following data:

Infant:
- Growth: The infant is now 4 pounds 12 ounces (5th percentile) and is 18 inches long. HC is within normal limits.
- Infant has normal variable states.
- Infant shows hypotonia consistent with prematurity.
- Still having reflux
- Still having occasional apnea alarms

Rehabilitation Needs

Early infant intervention for premature infant with developmental delay

Family:
- The mother has fatigue, seems depressed, and is critical of her own parenting abilities.
- Both parents are overly anxious about the baby and do not want to leave the baby alone, even with grandmother.

The nurse identifies the following goals:
- An order for an antibiotic that will allow the mother to breast-feed, if possible
- In the meantime, help with pumping, making sure that the mother is getting enough fluids, rest, and proper nutrition
- Good hygiene in the bathroom (to prevent spread of *C. difficle*)
- The cat is kept away from the baby. The litter box is kept in a separate area of the apartment.
- The baby is awakened during the day if he has gone 4 hours without a feeding.
- The infant has at least 6–8 wet diapers daily and 1–2 stools per day.
- The father is involved in diapering and holding the baby during the night, helping the mother to breast-feed.
- The grandmother supports her daughter in her attempts at mothering skills but does not do everything.
- Once the mother is feeling stronger, the mother and father get out of the house together during the week, even for a short time.

- The baby is taken for walks in the neighborhood perhaps with the father or grandmother.
- The mother understands the need to stay in a routine.
- The family understands the signs and symptoms of postpartum depression and when to call for help.

Neal Theory Implications

Stage 3: The professional in this stage collaborates with the pediatrician, the pulmonologist, and the lactation consultant to provide comprehensive care to mother and baby.

Stage 2: The professional in this stage may not feel comfortable collaborating with other disciplines, case managing, or working within the patient's environment to manage care.

Stage 1: The clinician in this stage will assess the patient and recognize the need for assistance with the case but may be unsure as to how to proceed in the home setting.

?   **CRITICAL THINKING**

1. What is the priority for care for the parents in caring for a premature infant?
Answer: The priority of care for this baby is support as the baby grows. The nurse, in conjunction with the pediatrician, the pulmonologist, and the lactation consultant, will make recommendations regarding the infant's care, especially with regard to feeding and reflux and aspiration precautions. Sudden infant death syndrome (SIDS) precautions, the importance of a firm mattress, and no pillows or bed-sharing should be communicated to the parents. The nurse should make sure that the parents know how to use the apnea monitor and review emergency measures with them. The nurse should be familiar with the gestational age assessment and also infant reflexes. It is important to explain the physical and developmental aspects of prematurity to the parents.

2. Assuming the mother would like to continue breast-feeding, what recommendations should the nurse, along with the lactation consultant make to facilitate this?
Answer: Both the nurse and the lactation consultant should explain the importance of hygiene and hand washing, especially since the mother

has *C. difficle*. It may be possible that the mother can be switched to another antibiotic to make breast-feeding possible. In the meantime, the mother will require support for pumping.

3. How should the nurse counsel the mother regarding the challenges unique to the premature infant?
Answer: The nurse should recommend consultation with the pediatrician or nurse practitioner for careful screening for developmental delays or failure to progress. The infant should have followup at regular intervals.

 BACK TO THE CASE

At a followup in 1 week, the nurse finds that the baby has developed colic and that the mother has stopped breast-feeding. She has changed formulas, but this did not help the colic. The baby is still taking Prevacid and had a first cold, but has had fewer apnea spells.

Relevant Community Resources

State intervention services
Premie support group/autism or other developmental support groups
Notification of the fire department and EMS that infant has an apnea monitor at home

---

During a 6-month followup (4.5 months corrected age), some of the problems have resolved. The baby is off of the apnea monitor and still has some reflux and some hypotonia and delays even for the corrected age. The nurse discusses this with the family and recommends a referral for early intervention.

At the 8-month old followup (6.5 months corrected age), the reflux has nearly resolved. The baby is taking solid foods and formula. The mother is back at work full time. The grandmother is still living in and is the primary caretaker. When she returns to her home, the baby will require daycare. The mother is very happy to be back at work, states that her depression has resolved ("I feel like a different person.") and both parents are involved in the infant's care when they are home from work at night. The baby still has hypotonia, a backward crawl, and other developmental concerns such as decreased eye contact and delayed vocalization. The nurse reiterates the need for early intervention, which the parents had not pursued previously.

Interdisciplinary Care Plan

Problem	Goal/Plan	Interventions	Evaluation
Knowledge deficit regarding parenting/ prematurity	Family will verbalize understanding of caring for newborn, premature infant upon discharge visit.	Teach parents about caring for newborn premature infant, infant states and reflexes, sleep, elimination, and feeding expectations.	Mother and father will participate more fully in caring for newborn. Grandmother will become knowledgeable about assisting in care.
Sleep—infant	Infant will have safe area for sleep—placed "back to sleep" with apnea monitor on.	Coordinate need for apnea monitoring with apnea practitioner. Review apnea monitor with parents and grandmother. Discuss SIDS risk, no pillows, second hand smoke, etc.	Infant continues monitoring as required.
Elimination— infant	Infant will have 6–8 wet diapers per day and at least 1–2 soft stools per day.	Hydration—Have parents and grandmother check diapers.	Infant will be adequately hydrated.
Feeding— infant	Infant will take either breast or bottle every 2–3 hours when awake.	Teach mother proper pumping technique and breast-feeding.	Family will verbalize understanding and show support.
Development— infant	Infant will continue to show progress based on corrected age.	Continue to screen for developmental progress. Recommend appropriate infant stimulation.	Infant will develop normally given corrected age.
Risk for postpartum depression— mother	Mother will become more involved in infant's care, holding and feeding infant during the day. Mother will get dressed in the morning and be up more during the day.	Provide information about postpartum depression. Suggest an appointment with PCP this week for evaluation and followup.	Family will provide support and mother will not develop postpartum depression.

Problem	Goal/Plan	Interventions	Evaluation
Risk for ineffective coping of family system	Mother and father will take more of an active parenting role, with grandmother assisting.	Mother will help feed, hold, and care for baby more during the day, with father taking an active part at night.	Grandmother will recognize need to help but allow parents more control over infant care.
Social isolation	Mother will get out for daily walks or activities.	Family will support mother in efforts to get out of the house temporarily for brief periods of respite.	Mother will not feel socially isolated.

REFERENCES & RESOURCES

[1] American Academy of Pediatrics, "Guidelines for Parents with a Newborn," http://www.aap.org

[2] C. Beckman et al, *Obstetrics and Gynecology*, Lippincott, 2010.

[3] C. E. Burns, A. M. Dunn, M. A. Brady, N. B. Starr, C. G. Blosser, *Pediatric Primary Care*, Saunders/Elsevier, 2009.

[4] N. Hacker and J. Gambone, *Hacker & Moore's Essentials of Obstetrics & GYN*, Saunders, 2010.

[5] M. Hall, "Early recognition of developmental delays," *Journal for Nurse Practitioners*, 5(9):690–691, 2009.

[6] M. Hoekenberry and D. Wilson, *Wong's Essentials of Pediatric Nursing*, Mosby/Elsevier, 2009.

[7] E. McKinney, S. James, S. Murray and J. Ashwill, *Maternal and Child Nursing*, Saunders/Elsevier, 2009.

[8] Mayo Clinic, "Premature Baby? Understand Your Preemie's Special Needs," http://www.mayoclinic.com/health/premature-baby/FL00108

[9] National Institutes of Health, "Premature Babies," http://www.health.nih.gov/topic/prematureBabies

[10] K. Rais-Bahrami and B. Short, *Children with Disabilities*, M. Batshaw, L. Pellegrino, and N. Rosizen (eds.), Brooks, 2007.

Case 11.2 Asthma

By Teresa LaMonica, PhD, MSN, RN, CPNP

This case study illustrates a situation with a family of a preschool-aged child (3-year-old Felicity) with significant ear, nose, throat (ENT), and respiratory problems. Felicity was born at 37 weeks gestation. Her 30-year-old mother, gravida 4, para 3 (one stillbirth), had a C-section. There was infant ABO-incompatibility and a need for jaundice bilirubin lights. Felicity was discharged by 5 days, had a normal neonatal course, and was breast-fed. Her first cold occurred at 2 months of age.

The child's father is active-duty military with long deployments. The child's mother works as a nurse part-time in a geriatric setting. They live on a military base and have no family in the area. The family has military benefits and insurance.

The mother noticed that the child was snoring and wheezing at night and had long pauses when she didn't breathe. When the child woke up, she looked pale and coughed a great deal. The rescue EMS was called, and the child was admitted for seizures and aspiration. A sleep study and bronchoscopy were done. Following these, the child was diagnosed with sleep obstructive apnea (SOA) and adenoidal and tonsillar hypertrophy. Pulmonary function tests showed asthma. Albuterol nebulization and steroids helped resolve the asthma. Other tests: electro-brain wave (EEG) and upper gastrointestinal (UGI) tests were normal.

Clinical Case Studies in Home Health Care, First Edition. Edited by Leslie Neal-Boylan.
© 2011 John Wiley & Sons, Inc. Published 2011 by John Wiley & Sons, Inc.

Cultural Competence

The mother is a part of a military culture which includes unique needs of spouse/family, especially while the father is away in a war.

 ORDERS FOR HOME CARE

Patient: 3-year-old girl
Diagnoses: SOA, new onset asthma, mild gastrointestinal reflux, parent anxiety
Current medications:
- Albuterol nebulizers
- Flovent
- Prednisone (Prelone)
- Cephalex
- Prevacid

Relevant past medical history:
- 37-weeks gestation
- Jaundice
- ABO incompatibility
- Eye surgery for probing at 12 months
- Frequent conjunctivitis
- Dacryostenosis as an infant
- Episodes of otitis media, bronchiolitis, mild conductive hearing loss with speech delay

Surgeries:
- Eye–tear duct probing at age 12 months for Dacryostenosis,
- Ear tubes (x2) at age 3 years for chronic otitis media

Relevant family history:
- Paternal grandmother: asthma, hypertension
- Maternal grandfather: hypertension
- Father: Age 32 with allergies
- Mother: Clinical depression following still birth of first child (8 years ago, at age 22)
- Two older siblings (brother, age 7, with mild asthma; sister, age 5, with chronic otitis media [COM], allergies).

RN: Assess and evaluate

Reimbursement Considerations

This patient is eligible for military benefits, due to her husband's active military status. She is not eligible for Medicaid due to income and insurance. Most of the hospital bill should be covered by military insurance. The military insurance should cover upcoming specialty visits to the ENT and pulmonologist, and eventually the allergist. The nurse will need to make sure that the patient can be seen in a timely manner and that previous test results are sent to each provider. As the mother is often in the car with her children, the nurse can help the family explore insurance coverage for a battery-operated portable nebulizer. The nurse, as case manager on this case, will need to negotiate with the insurance case manager for specialty services in this case.

 ## THE HOME VISIT

The nurse makes the first home visit the afternoon of discharge to reinforce hospital teaching, use of the nebulizer, and to review medications. It was decided in the hospital that there was no need for apnea monitoring in the home and that oral steroids would decrease the tonsillar hypertrophy enough until surgery could be scheduled.

The townhome is fairly clean and neat but" well lived in"; the family room has toys scattered about; and there are dishes in the kitchen sink. Pets include a large dog (golden retriever) and a gerbil. There are no cats or other animals in the home. The child is on the sofa in the family room watching TV and looks pale and tired. Older children pay in the kitchen and family room. There are 3 bedrooms.

The mother is pleasant and cooperative but is often distracted with the other children's needs. She looks harried and tired. She comments that she has had no sleep, as she is always up all night with a sick child. The mother is anxious and worried about caring for Felicia alone at night if she stops breathing again or has another asthma attack. A neighbor has been helping with the other children while the youngest was in the hospital. She says she doesn't know many people, as this has been a recent move and her family is on the West Coast. The mother is anxious about the child's medication; the nurse reviews these with her and shows her how to use the nebulizer.

The nurse continues to gather data about the prenatal, birth history, and neonatal history and gathers the following additional data:

- Mrs. L is tired and anxious over the recent hospitalization and upcoming surgery.
- The siblings, ages 5 and 7, are playful and alert.

The nurse identifies the following goals:

- To have the child's asthma under control
- To not have any apnea episodes
- To have no signs respiratory distress

- To explore triggers for asthma events, such as upper respiratory infections (URI), allergies to dust, pets, or outside allergies, such as pollen and grass
- The mother will feel comfortable with the nebulizer and know the signs of respiratory distress.
- The mother understands what reflux is and the possible role it plays in asthma.
- There is a plan for help with child care now and for the upcoming surgery.

Neal Theory Implications

Stage 3: The home care nurse in this stage collaborates with other disciplines: Pediatrician, ENT, and pulmonary doctors, as well as the home care team. He/she is autonomous with the clinical aspects of the case, as well as the assessment and teaching roles.

Stage 2: The home care nurse in this stage is beginning to develop a working relationship with the ENT staff and is learning to collaborate with the physician regarding home care.

Stage 1: The home care nurse in this stage will assess the patient and recognizes the need for assistance with the case but may be unsure as to how to proceed in the home setting, especially with regard to what military resources may be available to the mother.

? CRITICAL THINKING

1. What is the priority for care for this child? Her mother?
Answer: The priority of care must always be safety. The nurse, in conjunction with the pediatrician and pulmonologist, need to make sure that the mother knows how to monitor for respiratory distress, how to use the nebulizer, and is aware of emergency measures.

2. Explain sleep obstructive apnea (SOA) and why this is considered a true or absolute indication for an adenoidectomy/tonsillectomy.
Answer: Apnea is defined as pauses in breathing for at least 15 seconds [4]. Absolute indications for adenoidectomy/tonsillectomy include airway obstruction secondary to hypertrophy of adenoids and/or tonsils [3]. Symptoms of SOA in this age group include mouth breathing, snoring, and apnea, especially with colds or upper respiratory infections [2, 5].

3. Discuss asthma goals and the use of a stepwise approach for management of asthma in this age group.
Answer: The nurse should be familiar with the National Institutes of Health (NIH) [6] asthma classification and guidelines, as they represent the gold standard in asthma management. It is important to assess asthma triggers, which may or may not be allergic in nature. Goals for treatment include being symptom free during both daytime and night time and the ability to do daily activities, including play and school [2] (www.nih.gov). Having a written asthma plan is important, in a stepwise approach to management that is clear for the parent to follow. Use of the peak flowmeter will help the parent to provide more information to the pediatrician, as well as to provide a more objective measure of respiratory distress. Preschoolers are able to use peak flow but it will take more effort to teach them; often stickers on the numbers help as an incentive to blow harder.

4. What are other goals of home care management at this time?
Answer: To have the mother determine the child's asthma triggers, both allergic and nonallergic, and to work toward reducing these. To become comfortable with asthma management, recognizing respiratory distress and the need for intervention. Knowledge decreases anxiety and empowers parents in the care of their children's illnesses.

5. What are important interventions for additional family support?
Answer: While the father is deployed in a war zone, the mother's anxiety is bound to be increased, especially with a sick child. Her previous history of losing a child at birth may make her feel more vulnerable at this time, especially given the emergent nature of the last emergency room visit. Finding support in the community, especially within the military, is helpful at this time. Keeping the father informed of his child's condition is also important. The nurse will help Mrs. T to find community resources, especially through military services, and other resources within her financial means.

Relevant Community Resources

Child-care services/respite care, if needed.
Counseling for the mother, as needed during this difficult time
Notification of the fire department and EMS that a child requires a nebulizer at home

---

 BACK TO THE CASE

The nurse explains to the mother the use of the nebulizer and peak flowmeter. She also explains what each medication is used for. She reviews signs of respiratory distress and the asthma management plan. The hope is that the apnea will be controlled through the use of oral steroids at this time. Once the child has her scheduled tonsillectomy and adenoidectomy surgery this problem should be resolved. The nurse helps coordinate care and also assesses the child for any distress. The nurse also encourages the mother to get some help from her neighbors or have a family member come in anticipation of the surgery.

? CRITICAL THINKING

1. How will the members of the interdisciplinary team communicate with one another?
Answer: Team members will communicate by phone and arrange appointments, tests, and preoperative scheduling within 1 week.

2. What is the role of the nurse in the coordination of these services?
Answer: The nurse should reinforce the ENT and pulmonary discharge orders. It is especially important to help coordinate information from the previous hospital and ensure that appointments are made so that the surgery can be done in a timely manner. Each will work from a discipline-specific care plan and also from the interdisciplinary care plan.

Interdisciplinary Care Plan

Problem	Goal/Plan	Intervention	Evaluation
Knowledge deficit of parent regarding asthma	Mother will verbalize basic understanding of asthma, its presentation, and treatment steps, at discharge and reinforced at 1 week.	Teach parent basic recognition of asthma symptoms. Use written asthma care plan (use of step-wise approach) to show treatment and when to call for help. Teach peak flow use and nebulizer use and show use of other mediations.	Parent will be able to list symptoms of worsening asthma/ respiratory distress and state what she would do in each instance. Parent will give a demonstration of peak flowmeter, nebulizer use and drawing up medications.
Respiratory distress	Child will remain free of respiratory distress.	Teach parent proper medication administration, including oral steroids and rescue drugs/nebulizer.	Child will exhibit clear breath sounds and show no signs of respiratory distress.

Problem	Goal/Plan	Intervention	Evaluation
		Parent will be able to recognize signs of worsening distress.	Parent will verbalize medication schedule and step-wise asthma plan. Parent will verbalize signs of respiratory distress/worsening asthma or apnea.
Apnea	Child will have no apnea episodes. Parent will recognize apneic episodes and need for intervention.	Contact EMS if child has color changes or prolonged distress associated with apnea. Reassure parent that regular medication should reduce apnea.	Child is apnea free. Parent is able to verbalize what to do in case of an emergency. Parent understands the need for upcoming surgery.
Parenting fatigue	Child's asthma will be under control and have no apnea episodes. Parent and child will have been able to sleep through the night.	Keep child on a good sleep/bedtime schedule. Keep child on a regular nap/rest schedule during the day.	Both child and parent are sleeping better. Parent's fatigue is interfering less with quality of life.
Preparation for upcoming tonsillectomy and adenoidectomy surgery	Child will have age- appropriate understanding of upcoming surgery. Parent will understand need for surgery and for preoperative instructions.	Coordinate with ENT surgeon and nurse, as well as hospital for preoperative tour and for preoperative instructions to mother.	Child is able to verbalize need for surgery in her own words. Parent is able to verbalize preoperative instructions, as well as medications up until surgery.
Ineffective coping of family system	Parents and siblings are able to cope with new diagnosis and upcoming surgery and postoperative course.	Provide information about community resources, support groups, and services, especially through the military hospital.	Parents and siblings have resources for emotional support and use them effectively.
Social isolation for parent	Parent will verbalize satisfaction with social support within next few weeks.	Obtain support information for parent. Support parent who is away at war through military resources, leave of absence if needed.	Parent has social support via extended family and military support group/other military friends. Parent at war has counseling and leave of absence (LOA) if needed.

REFERENCES & RESOURCES

[1] A. Alario and J. Birnkrant, *Practical Guide to the Pediatric Patient*, Mosby, 2008.

[2] C. Burns et al., *Pediatric Primary Care*, Lippincott/Elsevier, 2009.

[3] M. Hoekenberry and D. Wilson, *Wong's Essentials of Pediatric Nursing*, Mosby/Elsevier, 2009.

[4] R. Kliegman, K. Marcdante, H. Jensen and R. Behrman, *Nelson's Essentials of Pediatrics*, Saunders/Elsevier, 2006.

[5] E. McKinney, S. James, S. Murray and J. Ashwill, *Maternal and Child Nursing*, Saunders/Elsevier, 2009.

[6] National Institutes of Health, "Guidelines for Asthma Management," http://www.nih.org/asthma guidelines, 2007.

Case 11.3 Adolescent with Neurodevelopmental Disability

By Teresa LaMonica, PhD, MSN, RN, CPNP

This case study illustrates some of the more common concerns of a family of a child with neurodevelopmental disabilities and illustrates the role of the home health nurse in coordinating complex care for an adolescent with severe disability, guiding both child and family in optimal care, and assisting in transition toward adulthood.

This 17-year-old adolescent boy, Freddy, was diagnosed soon after birth with brain damage secondary to meconium aspiration and severe hypoxia at birth, with resulting cerebral palsy (CP) and severe mental retardation. Freddy was born at 42 weeks at a small community hospital to a 30-year-old mother (gravida 1, para 1). The mother had received regular prenatal care; and other than going past her due date, she had no foreseeable problems. Although she was post term, the obstetrician (OB) felt no need to induce labor. Once labor started, the primary OB was unavailable; and a "backup" doctor ended up delivering the baby at a different hospital. (They had originally planned to have the baby at a large medical center where they had taken their tour and childbirth classes.)

Once the mother's membranes were broken in the labor room, the nurse noticed meconium and immediately alerted the doctor who performed a Cesarean (C-section) soon after. The baby was not breathing at birth and required cardiopulmonary resuscitation (CPR) and vigorous suctioning in attempts to remove meconium from the airway and lungs. Although the parents were both in the delivery room, they were not allowed to see or hold baby at this time, due to the emergency measures. Later, they were advised that the baby was in the neonatal

Clinical Case Studies in Home Health Care, First Edition. Edited by Leslie Neal-Boylan.
© 2011 John Wiley & Sons, Inc. Published 2011 by John Wiley & Sons, Inc.

intensive care unit (NICU) on a respirator but "probably would not survive more than a few hours."

Later in the afternoon, the mother was wheeled down to the NICU window accompanied by the postpartum nurse and her husband to see her son, "who was full of tubes." The baby ended up "surprising everyone" by steadily improving while in the NICU, requiring ventilator support, nasogastric (NG) feeds, and constant monitoring. The doctors cautioned that he would most likely be very brain damaged due to the long interval without oxygen and the amount of meconium that had been in his lungs. At this time, Freddy developed seizures that were controlled by medication.

The NICU stay ended up being 6 weeks. The parents visited, and the mother continued to pump her breast milk for NG feedings. Despite the best efforts by the speech pathologist, the baby was not able to suck. The baby was discharged to the parents by 6 weeks, after the parents had learned CPR and how to care for a baby with an NG tube and apnea monitor.

At first, home care nursing was instituted at 3 days a week and gradually diminished to once per month. Although devastated, the parents were happy that the baby had at least survived. They had good family support: The maternal grandmother had come from another state but remained for the first 2 months, and the paternal grandparents who lived nearby would visit frequently. Neighbors were also supportive to the family, often bringing over meals. Weeks turned into months and the first 2 years were full of learning to care for a baby with special needs. The home health nurse reinforced how to perform NG feedings. It was the nurse who suggested that the colic that Freddy had been diagnosed with at 2 months (he was crying continually and not sleeping) was really severe gastroesophageal (GE) reflux.

The nurse referred him to a developmental pediatrician who was much more tuned into his special needs. After a trial of medication and thickened feeds, a Nissen Fundoplication surgery was done at Children's Hospital; and a gastrostomy tube (G-tube) was inserted at this time. The parents were never quite comfortable with having to put in the NG tube every few days. In addition, the G-tube decreased the risk of aspiration.

Developmentally, Freddy did not progress much beyond early infancy, similar to a 3-month level in areas of language (babbling, giggling), social (smile, receptive to voice and songs), gross motor (unable to roll over or sit up on his own), and fine motor abilities (had no pincer grasp but was able to hold hands and move his fingers well). He has always been very receptive to family members, friends, and caretakers that he knows. Some other concerns have been partial seizures, hip dysplasia, severe scoliosis, skin and respiratory infections.

Freddy's parents have remained very engaged in his daily care, and 3 years later they had another son (Jon, born at term without difficulty).

The mother has stayed home since Freddy's birth while the father has remained at his accountant job, maintaining the family's insurance. His work has been flexible during Freddy's numerous hospitalizations and illnesses. The younger brother, Jon, is now 14 and beginning high school. Grandparents on both sides have remained active in Freddy's care and in supporting Jon's activities.

Cultural Competence

The parents often work with different caretakers from other countries with language barriers and often different cultural practices. The home care team can help provide them with resources for communicating with these providers.

Freddie has been in a special-needs program from 5 years of age until the present, which has been a main source of support for the family, providing in-services on topics such as community resources, financial assistance, trusts, and wills. The school and the primary care provider have been an anchor for Freddy and his family. The pediatrician continues to coordinate care with specialists, such as neurology (seizures); orthopedics (contractures, scoliosis); plastic surgeon (pressure sores); nutrition (NG, G-tube feeds, nutritional needs); pulmonary (reactive airway disease, admissions for pneumonia, bronchiolitis); physical, occupational, and speech therapies (PT, OT, ST); and home care nursing.

Since infancy, Freddy has required braces and splints, an apnea monitor, occasional oxygen, NG feeds and later a G-tube (Kangaroo Joey pump), nebulizer, bulb syringe, and suction machine. Freddy has ongoing problems such as severe developmental delay; mental retardation; contractures; severe scoliosis; frequent respiratory infections; skin issues; orthodontic problems; gum hyperplasia; feeding and bowel problems; incontinence; some spasticity; and hypotonic, muscle atrophy.

A home care nurse known to the family arrives at the house the day after Freddy has been discharged from the hospital after a recent admission due to pneumonia. This nurse is part of a team that has been following Freddy since birth on a monthly basis. The mother explains that this admission was particularly difficult due to the emergency nature as he had to be taken by ambulance to the nearest hospital and the staff did not know him. Instead of being on a pediatric unit, he was in an adult ICU. A variety of doctors cared for him there.

Current concerns that were identified included neurodevelopmental, orthopedic, speech, educational, respiratory, feeding, and incontinence issues. Caretaker fatigue and the need for emotional support for

Freddy's parents as Freddy moves toward adulthood are other concerns. Freddy's sibling also needs support as he and Freddy grow older.

> ### Relevant Community Resources
>
> State intervention services
> Neurodevelopmental support group, respite care, other developmental support groups, transitional support as Freddy moves toward adulthood
> Notification of the fire department and EMS of home O^2 use and monitoring if this has not been done
> Support for sibling

 ## ORDERS FOR HOME CARE

Patient: 17-year-old adolescent with severe cerebral palsy, recovering from pneumonia

Diagnoses: Cerebral palsy, severe mental retardation, seizures, hypotonia, spasticity, and respiratory problems.

Current medications:
- Depakane (Valporic Elixir) 18 mL twice a day
- Lorazepam (Ativan) 1 mg mixed with water every p.m.
- Chloral hydrate 12 mL elixir at bedtime
- Dulcolax suppository every other day
- Pulmocort nebulizer twice a day
- Albuterol nebulizer every 4–6 hours, as needed
- Cephalex IV antibiotic twice a day

Relevant past medical history
- Cerebral palsy
- Severe mental retardation
- Seizures
- Spasticity
- Contractures
- Hypotonia
- Severe scoliosis
- Frequent respiratory and skin infections
- Pressure sores
- Cellulitis
- Orthodontic problems
- Gum hyperplasia
- Feeding and bowel problems
- Incontinence
- Severe gastroesophageal reflux

Previous hospitalizations: NICU, aspiration pneumonia, severe GE reflux, pressure sores, contractures, cellulitis, scoliosis and hip repairs, recurrent pneumonia (at ages 4, 8, 15 years and last admission at age 17 years).

Surgeries: Nissen Fundoplication, G-tube, hip dysplasia, scoliosis repair, contracture repair.

Interdisciplinary team: OT, PT, ST, special education teachers, social worker, dietician, developmental specialist, neurologist, pulmonologist, orthopedic surgeon, nurses, and developmental pediatrician (primary care provider).

Reimbursement Considerations

This patient has private insurance. Although insurance pays for a large portion of medicines, it may still be a struggle to pay for the remainder. The nurse, as case manager on this case, will need to negotiate with the insurance case manager for possible respite care and additional visits after this hospitalization.

THE HOME VISIT

The nurse makes the home visit at 10:00 a.m. to a moderate-sized home, where she finds the mother, caretaker, and Freddy. The home is clean and organized with Freddy in his own room off of the main hall. A daybed is in the room; the mother sleeps there during the week. There is a large family room off of the kitchen where equipment is also kept. There is a ramp off of this room to a deck and another ramp at the side of the house to enter a carport. There is an accessible bathroom with a shower stall (with roll-in access and a shower chair) and sink that accommodates a wheelchair.

Freddy is in bed and appears alert and smiling, making sounds in "greeting." The nurse observes that the home is pleasant and cheerful, surrounded by pictures of family with a "lived in" but clean appearance; items needed for Freddy are apparent in the kitchen, family room, and Freddy's room. There are pictures of the Jon with Freddy and Jon's sports awards in the room.

The nurse asks about other interval history and new medications. The mother is an excellent historian and keeps a notebook with a time line of recent events with medication and lab results. She is very knowledgeable about Freddy's medications and care. She voices her frustration about the recent admission and lack of coordination of care.

After the nurse collects the interval history, she examines Freddy. She gathers the following data:

- General: Alert, smiling, and vocalizing, no apparent distress at this time.
- Skin: Pale, no cyanosis. No areas of redness noted.

- Head/neck: Scalp clear, no lesions, brown hair brushed and clean. No lymphadenopathy.
- Eyes/ENT: Eyes, clear. Ears, no discharge. Nose, yellow secretions, nasal prongs in place. Mouth, teeth protruding, crooked, no lesions. Throat, no lesions, no redness.
- Respiratory: Respiratory rate (RR)—22; breath sounds (BS) coarse bilaterally; no wheezing, no rales. There is an occasional moist productive cough with yellow secretions.
- Cardiac: Heart rate (HR) 62 and regular, no murmurs. Brachial and femoral pulses are strong.
- Neurodevelopmental: Severe developmental delays; at 3 month level for gross motor and speech.
- Orthopedic/spine and extremities: Severe curvature of the spine (scoliosis); contractures of wrists, legs, and feet. Splints not on at this time.
- Abdomen: Abdomen distended but soft, G-tube is in place, slight redness around site, no discharge, diaper on, and bed pad on.

Rehabilitation Needs

Educational needs and socialization needs for the child with severe developmental delay continue as before, through school.
Use of physical, occupational, and speech therapy

After consulting with the pediatrician and pulmonologist, the nurse identifies the following goals:

- Respiratory: Improvement in pneumonia.
- Abdomen: The G-tube remains patent; prevent aspiration risk.
- Skin: There are no pressure sores and the IV is patent.
- Neurological: Level of consciousness remains the same as baseline; patient remains seizure free.
- Developmental: Patient's developmental and emotional needs are met through participation in family, neighborhood, and school activities.
- Educational: Potential for development and socialization are maximized through school activities.
- Family: The parents are able to take advantage of respite care and take time to participate in the sibling's school and sporting events and activities. Caretaker fatigue is lessened through nursing support and respite care. Freddy's parents feel supported in their need to express their fears of loss/death and feel comfortable seeking counseling.

Neal Theory Implications

Stage 3: This professional understands the complexities of this case and knows how to address them. The nurse in this stage will be aware of community resources and will have efficient and success-ful interdisciplinary communication. The nurse will proactively work to help the family transition to adult care.

Stage 2: The professional in this stage may not feel comfortable collaborating with the physician regarding orders for other disci-plines, case management, and working within the patient's envi-ronment to manage care. This nurse may be aware of some resources but may not be as adept at coordinating all aspects of care or working toward Freddy's future.

Stage 1: The clinician in this stage will assess the patient and rec-ognize the need for assistance with the case but may be unsure as to how to proceed in the home setting. This nurse will need a lot of support, as this is a challenging case. This care may not be suit-able for a stage 1 nurse.

? CRITICAL THINKING

1. Discuss CP, its etiology, and its manifestations.
Answer: CP, once thought of as stemming mainly from birth hypoxia, actually is associated with many factors of prenatal, perinatal, and postnatal causes [4]. Prenatally, besides anoxia or birth trauma, other causes are maternal infections, Rh or blood type incompatibility, and genetic or congenital abnormalities [4]. Problems during birth include asphyxia and factors related to prematurity and low birth weight [4]. Other factors happen after birth, such as injuries to the infant's devel-oping brain in the form of infection (bacterial meningitis), trauma (shaken baby syndrome, falls), or poisoning [3, 4].

Symptoms of CP include the infant not meeting developmental mile-stones, such as not being able to sit up without support or not walking, and persistence of involuntary reflexes, such as Moro and crossed extensor reflex [3, 4].

2. What is the incidence of CP following asphyxia at birth?
Answer: The incidence of CP due to birth asphyxia is actually quite low [6].

3. What is the priority of care for an infant or child who is diagnosed with CP?

Answer: Treatment goals include: 1) early recognition, usually through developmental and neurologic assessments, 2) early intervention to promote optimal development, and 3) ongoing multidisciplinary team involvement with the overall goal of living as normally as possible [3].

Care of the infant or child with CP should use a multidisciplinary team approach. Home care nurses will coordinate care with the primary care doctor and neurologist, with other specialists, including the OT, dietician, and social worker or case manager. The home care nurse will help guide the parents in day-to-day care of their child, such as medication administration, feeding (which may include NG or G-tube feedings) skin care, mobility issues, safety concerns, and emotional support [3].

4. What is the priority of care for Freddy at this time?

Answer: The priority of care at this time is to support respiratory improvement. Management of pneumonia in a child who is immobilized and has immunity risks is critical. Regular use of oxygen, suctioning, and monitoring of respiratory status is important. Assessment of level of consciousness (LOC) as an indicator of sepsis is also important. The nurse, in conjunction with the pediatrician and pulmonologist, needs to make sure that IV antibiotics and fluids are being administered properly and that aspiration precautions are in place.

5. What safety measures should be put in place?

Answer: Safety measures in the home should include working fire alarms, an evacuation plan if there is a fire or emergency, and EMS notification that oxygen, suctioning, and monitors are in use. There need to be extra precautions for lifting, managing wheelchair transfers to and from bed, shower, and car. There should also be precautions for reducing aspiration risk.

6. Regarding going back to school, what does the nurse need to review with teachers and the school nurse?

Answer: The nurse should review with the school nurse and teacher the need for any new medication while at school and assessment parameters for respiratory distress.

7. How can the home care nurse help foster a smoother transition toward adult care? What are family priorities at this time?

Answer: The nurse needs to provide support as well as referrals at this time.

8. How will the home health team help the family during the transition from primary care and children's services to those of adulthood?

Answer: Each team member will reinforce Freddy's care and goals and respect the family's wishes and needs. Each will work from a discipline-specific care plan and also from the interdisciplinary care plan.

Interdisciplinary Care Plan

Problem	Goal/Plan	Interventions	Evaluation
Ineffective breathing/ risk of infection	Parents and caretaker will verbalize understanding of patient's worsening respiratory status. Parents and caretaker will continue to use oxygen as indicated, suction airway as needed, and use chest physical therapy (CPT via vest or manually).	Review with parents and caretaker respiratory assessment and use of pulse oximeter. Review with parents and caretaker about oxygen use, suctioning, and CPT.	Patient will maintain adequate gas exchange and show effective breathing through pulse oximeter parameters, with no signs of respiratory distress. Parents and caretaker will verbalize respiratory assessment parameters and signs of respiratory distress. Parents and caretaker will demonstrate proper suctioning and CPT.
Risk for nutritional impairment	Patient will have adequate nutrients and fluids through consistent G-tube feedings and G-tube site will remain infection-free.	Continue to support parents and caretaker to give proper nourishment through G-tube feeds and assess abdomen for signs of distention and G-tube for signs of infection.	Parents and caretaker will state G-tube feeding schedule and state signs of G-tube infection.
Caretaker fatigue	Parents will have strategies to get more rest and have respite care for child.	Help parents to get proper rest and allow for times for relaxation.	Parents are sleeping better and fatigue is interfering less with quality of life. Parents are able to have regular relaxation times.
Neurogenic incontinence/ potential for infection and skin breakdown	Patient will have needs met for bladder and bowel incontinence through hygiene measures.	Regular diaper changes Keep track of wet diapers and stool. Use antispasmodic medication as prescribed.	Patient is kept clean and dry, without skin breakdown or urinary tract infections.

(Continued)

Problem	Goal/Plan	Interventions	Evaluation
Risk for ineffective coping of family system	Patient has emotional and developmental needs met. Family members are able to maintain a sense of normalcy and contentment as a family unit.	Provide information about community resources, support groups, and services. Individual or family counseling as needed.	Patient and family have resources for emotional support and use them effectively.
Social isolation	Patient will be up and dressed during the day. Patient will continue school. Family will begin to explore other avenues for transition to adulthood once school program ends.	Parents and caregivers will dress patient daily and take patient outdoors regularly. Home health team will assist family to find resources to explore transitional options.	Patient has returned to school. Family has a plan for transitional care.

The author would like to thank the parents of this patient for their contribution to this case.

REFERENCES & RESOURCES

[1] C. Beckman et al., *Obstetrics and Gynecology*, Lippincott/Williams & Wilkins, 2010.

[2] N. Hacker and J. Moore, *Hacker & Moore's Essentials of Obstetrics and Gynecology*, Saunders/Elsevier, 2010.

[3] M. Hockenberry and D. Wilson, *Wong's Essentials of Pediatric Nursing*, Mosby/Elsevier, 2009.

[4] E. McKinney, S. James, S. Murray and J. Ashwill, *Maternal and Child Nursing*, Saunders/Elsevier, 2009.

[5] National Multiple Sclerosis Society, http://www.nmss.org.

[6] L. Pellegrino and M. Batshaw, *Children with Disabilities*, Brooks, 2008.

Section 12

Pediatric Intensive Care

Caring for the Chronically Ill Pediatric Patient in the Home

Caring for a chronically ill child in the home requires expertise in pediatrics, specialized training, compassion, empathy, competence, and confidence. A pediatric home health nurse must be alert and know how to immediately respond to life-threatening situations, since the home setting does not readily offer a cardiac arrest/code blue team. The home health nurse must rely upon his/her individual skill set and best practices to guide the pediatric patient through any given situation and to prevent emergency room admissions and hospitalizations.

Of equal importance are techniques to manage and cope with stress because caring for ailing children and their families can be overwhelming and laden with anxiety. Hence, pediatric nurses new to pediatric intensive care in the home should complete a thorough orientation. The ability to perform a comprehensive assessment is necessary to be able to formulate a plan for the continuum of care in order to reach optimal clinical outcomes and to ensure patient satisfaction, safety, and comfort.

Before the Assessment: 5 Musts

1. Delve into the patient's diagnosis through evidenced-based research from credible sources and institutions to become familiar with common symptoms, treatment options, medication regimens, and prognoses. Understanding the pathophysiology will help to adjust and align expectations for care protocols.
2. Consider the patient's discharge summary a valuable tool. Discharge plans are often underutilized, yet they provide detailed insight and/or recommendations from physicians to be incorporated in the patient's care plan and future protocols.
3. If the home health agency permits, set up a brief, informal visit with the patient and his/her parents and caregivers prior to the initial assessment to begin building a relationship and, hopefully, to alleviate some of the anxiety associated with caring for a child with complex medical needs in the home. A candid conversation may be able to place all involved parties at ease and promote a more free-flowing exchange of pressing concerns and questions. Although the visit may require additional time and effort, the nurse will gain a greater understanding of family dynamics that can only help during the formal assessment process.
4. Reviewing the home health agency's policies and procedures specific to the patient's condition(s) can serve to remind the nurse of the best practices associated with a condition/disease. Review of the agency's pediatric medication administration policy is vital as pediatric medication errors are 3 times more likely than with adults. Copy the policies and refer to them often.

5. Prior to the patient's discharge, the patient's local EMS and fire departments should be contacted with the home's address to inform them that a chronically ill patient resides at the address. If a call is placed from the address, the EMS or the fire department will be immediately dispatched, which could prevent a delay in treatment when seconds count!

A note about the cases in this section: One of the cases concerns a 28-year-old patient. This patient has the mental capacity of a child, has been cared for by pediatric nurses since childhood, and continues to receive this type of care. Therefore, his case is included in this section.

Case 12.1 Alpha-Thalassemia X-Linked Mental Retardation Syndrome

By Lannette Johnston, RN, BSN, MS, CPST

This case illustrates how the private duty pediatric home health nurse works with the patients, patients' parents/caregivers, and health care team to care for a patient with mental retardation. The two patients presented in this case study are Caucasian males who are biological brothers. Alex, who is 10 years old, and Patrick, who is 6 years old, have inherited the Alpha X-Linked chromosome and are diagnosed with Alpha-Thalassemia X-Linked Mental Retardation Syndrome (ATRX syndrome).

ATRX syndrome is an X-linked mental retardation syndrome which is a rare, inherited condition characterized by severe mental retardation, characteristic facial features, and mild anemia. Due to the inheritance pattern of this disorder, only males are affected [2].

Alex has the mental ability of a 16–20-month-old and is more advanced than his brother Patrick, who has the mental ability of a 9–12-month-old. The boys are in the infant stage of growth and development and continue to have the oral/tactile fixation. (Figure 12.1.1)

 ORDERS FOR HOME CARE

Patients: 10- and 6-year-old Caucasian males
Diagnosis: Alpha-Thalassemia X-Linked Mental Retardation Syndrome
 (ATRX syndrome)

Clinical Case Studies in Home Health Care, First Edition. Edited by Leslie Neal-Boylan.
© 2011 John Wiley & Sons, Inc. Published 2011 by John Wiley & Sons, Inc.

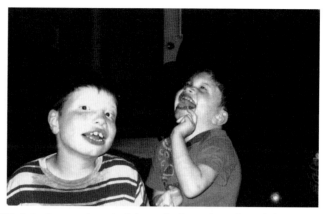

Figure 12.1.1. Despite their disabilities, the boys show their ability to have fun and express joy, happiness, and love for family.

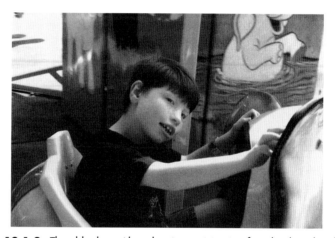

Figure 12.1.2. The older boy, Alex, showing anticipation for what lies ahead on the great elephant ride.

Current Medications:
Alex:
- Prevacid 30 mg by mouth once a day
- Fluoride 1 mL by mouth at bedtime
- Tylenol infant drops (1.8 mL) 3 droppers by mouth every 4 hours as needed
- Gas drops 1.6 mL by mouth as needed
- Metoclopramide (5 mg/5 mL) 2 mL by mouth four times a day
- Acyclovir cream topical as needed for cold sores
- MiraLAX 1½ tsp by mouth once a day
- Bethanacol 2.5 mg by mouth four times a day
- Maalox ½–1 tsp by mouth four times a day as needed
- Melatonin 3 mg at bedtime as needed (Figure 12.1.2)

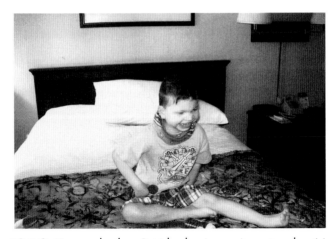

Figure 12.1.3. Younger brother, Patrick, showing excitement and anticipation for summer vacation.

Patrick:
- Zantac syrup 37.5 mg (2.5 cc) by mouth once a day
- Milk of Magnesia ¼ tsp by mouth nightly as needed
- Maalox 1 tsp by mouth as needed
- Gas drops 0.8 mL by mouth as needed
- Benadryl 3.12 mg by mouth as needed
- Tylenol infant drops (80 mg/0.8 mL)
- Prevacid 15 mg by mouth twice a day
- MiraLAX ½ tsp by mouth once a day
- Triamcinolone Cream 0.1% topical as needed for facial rash
- Nystatin Cream topical as needed facial rash
- Melatonin 3 mg at bedtime as needed
- Vaseline to cover the topical creams twice a day as needed (Figure 12.1.3)

Alex's relevant past medical history:
- Multiple hospitalizations for pneumonia (PNX) and respiratory syncytial virus (RSV)
- Hypoxia
- Short periods of apnea
- Orchiopexy surgery (surgical transposition of an undescended testicle from the abdomen and permanently placing it in the scrotum)
- Severe gastroesophageal reflux disease (GERD)
- Poor oral motor skills

Patrick's relevant past medical history:
- A traumatic birth related to hypoxia and cardiac dysthymia supraventricular tachycardia (SVT) that led to intubation and transport to a level one trauma center for a 6-week hospitalization.
- He currently suffers from:

- GERD
- Poor oral motor skills
- Hypoxic episodes
- Will need orchiopexy surgery in the future

RN: Assessment and evaluation.

PT/OT: Assessment and evaluation.

 ## THE HOME VISIT

The nurse enters the ranch-style home and introduces herself to the mother, Ms. U. The home is clean, well maintained, uncluttered, organized, and thoroughly childproofed. The mother greets the nurse warmly and introduces the nurse to her sons. The boys are safely playing on the floor at the mother's side. The mother gives a detailed explanation of the children's medical conditions to the nurse. The nurse asks the mother questions related to the ATRX syndrome and takes notes during their discussion. She tells the nurse that the condition is genetically passed from mother to son and becomes tearful saying that she is the carrier for the gene that is passed down to males. However, the mother also comments that if she had had a daughter, her daughter would have been a carrier, but would not have the disease.

Ms. U was told that the chance of having another child with Alex's symptoms was highly unlikely. So she and her husband decided to have another child. During her second pregnancy (with Patrick), an accurate diagnosis was made of Alex's condition—ATRX syndrome. She and her husband were told that if the gender of the second fetus was male, he would also have ATRX syndrome. Despite the prognosis, the parents decide to continue the pregnancy.

Ms. U explained that having children with disabilities is accompanied by a myriad of complex emotions. There are instances when she and her husband experience bouts of sadness followed by happiness. She quickly straightens her posture, smiles, and states, "I would do it all over again. We love our beautiful children."

Cultural Competence

The parents are faith-based Christians and are very religious. They attribute the children's survival thus far to God. The parents feel strongly about supporting and caring for their children forever and are adamant that institutionalization is not an option. The team will need to praise them for this behavior and encourage their continued support. The family may want to involve their church to help them obtain some respite or to help with running errands and completing household chores.

The nurse sits on the floor to assess the boys and begins interacting with them. She observes their developmental age, behaviors, and cognitive abilities. The boys are very pleasant. They are unable to speak, but make cooing noises. The nurse observes that Alex has greater mobility than Patrick. The boys are unable to walk or complete simple tasks performed by most children their age such as playing with toy trucks and cars, coloring pictures for their parents, writing a special birthday card, playing ball in the yard, or singing a song. Ms. U is not discouraged and is very upbeat. Although her boys cannot perform age-appropriate milestones, they have mastered individual milestones that have taken their parents' breath away.

Rehabilitation Needs

Physical therapy
Occupational therapy
Potential for speech therapy in the future
Neurodevelopmental therapy

The nurse asks to view the children's bedroom. Their bedroom is clean and well organized. For safety, they sleep in twin beds placed on the floor. Ms. U explains all of the aspects of the bedtime routine, which consists of the parents assisting the boys with personal care such as brushing their teeth and bathing. After bedtime rituals are complete, the parents enjoy reading a story and kissing them good night. The mother explains that her sleep is disturbed and can be difficult if the boys deviate from their sleep routine between 7:30 p.m. and 5:30 a.m. The nurse checks the room for any safety concerns. All outlets are covered and a smoke detector is placed just outside of the room.

Ms. U reviews the boys' medication regimens and daily routines with the nurse. The mother is a seasoned intensive care unit (ICU) nurse who is very knowledgeable about her children's disease process, prognosis, dietary needs, and treatment options. The father is a carpenter; however, mom thoroughly updates him on all of the above.

The nurse and mom review expectations and goals for the pediatric private home care plan for the children:

- To prevent choking and aspiration
- To ensure constant supervision
- To prevent injury
- To provide complete care of the children's activities of daily living (ADL)
- To act quickly to react to any distress the children may experience including choking and seizures

> ### Reimbursement Considerations
>
> The primary insurance for the boys is Medical Assistance (MA) with a secondary insurance through the mother. MA will cover in-home skilled nursing services of 33 hours per week to be shared for the boys while parents work. One nurse will deliver the care for both boys. The home health nurses will need to thoroughly complete nursing documentation for each child and have the mother or father sign the visit tickets. The paperwork and visit tickets must be submitted to the home health office within 48 hours of services. The supervisor on the case will need to complete recertification assessments and complete required MA paperwork: Letter of Medical Necessity (LOMN), Parent Work Letters/Schedules, Care Plan for each child, Physician Orders, and copies of the nursing documentation. All paperwork must be submitted to MA by the required time line to ensure adequate reimbursement of services.

Based on the history and physical examination, the nurse discovers the following data:

- The boys continue to be in the oral fixation phase; they place everything in their mouths.
- The boys require 10–12 hours of sleep at night for their developmental age. Melatonin is used as a sleep aid when necessary.
- They experience severe global developmental delays.
- They are incontinent of bladder and bowel elimination.
- They cannot ambulate and require total assistance of transfer.
- They have visual and speech limitations.
- They have muscle rigidity, spasticity, and limited range of motion of the extremities.
- They have difficulty swallowing and poor oral motor function.
- They currently have no infections.
- They require total assistance of all ADL.
- They require administration of all medications.

> ### Neal Theory Implications
>
> Stage 3: This nurse has experience in pediatric intensive home care. This nurse feels capable of handling the many facets of a complicated case that involves 2 patients as well as the parents.
>
> Stage 2: The professional in this stage may have experience providing intermittent home care but not intensive care over a shift. This

nurse will need a lot of support from the other disciplines that are involved. He/she will need to adjust to the complexity of the care and may want to defer to a more experienced home health nurse to manage this case.

Stage 1: The clinician in this stage may have pediatric experience but may not know how to adapt that experience to the home setting. This nurse should probably not be assigned to this case but might be able to make observational visits in order to learn how to manage such a complex case.

? CRITICAL THINKING

1. What are the priorities for Alex and Patrick's care?
Answer: The priorities are to prevent choking, aspiration, and seizures. The nurse recognizes that the oral fixation phase and swallowing disability place the brothers at high risk for choking and aspiration. In addition, the nurse acknowledges the high risk for seizures related to their disease process and the importance of feeding the children pureed foods slowly followed by constant vigilance to prevent aspiration. The children should be fed separately (never together). The nurse will obtain orders for supplemental oxygen and pulse oximetry in the home.

2. What are the roles and objectives of the physical therapist (PT)?
Answer: The PT will complete a PT assessment to determine the boys' needs and goals for therapy and evaluate the home environment for safety and accessibility. Additionally, the PT will teach the mother and nurse exercises to help strengthen the boys' upper and lower extremities. The PT will recommend adaptations to the environment to promote safety and accessibility and examine the wheelchairs and strollers for appropriateness. The PT may recommend a particular wheelchair/stroller for an easier transfer. The nurse and PT will recognize the parents' involvement in neurodevelopmental therapy for the boys.

The approach of neurodevelopmental therapy uses no medication or any invasive medical interventions. It is effective in treating many conditions ranging from learning disabilities to stroke recovery. The process involves using primitive reflexes present in automatic responses set off by the nervous system. (See: [3])

The children's neurologist highly recommends the therapy and believes that it has significantly helped the children.

3. Are there any other health care professionals who should be contacted?
Answer: Yes. The nurse should call the physician for orders for a medical social worker (MSW).

4. What is the role of MSW?
Answer: The MSW will work with the parents to find community resources to help them with respite hours, financial assistance for medical equipment not covered by insurance, and transportation expenses as well as information on support groups for parents of children with disabilities.

BACK TO THE CASE

The nurse can help the boys reach the mother's intended goals. The nurse also explains how the home health agency can assist parents with respite hours provided by a licensed nurse. The mother is very pleased and describes the difficulty she and her husband have finding leisure time due to demands of the children's medical conditions.

Relevant Community Resources

Housekeeping services
Notification of the fire department and police department that the home has two critical pediatric patients
Support groups for parents of chronically ill children

The nurse and Ms. U discuss the need to have supplemental oxygen and pulse oximetry in the home since the children have occasional hypoxic events. Once a physician order is obtained for oxygen and the pulse oximeter, the nurse will have the family's preferred durable medical equipment (DME) supplier deliver the equipment.

CRITICAL THINKING

1. How will the members of the interdisciplinary team communicate with one another?
Answer: The children's home health nurses will communicate with parents and the nursing supervisor for the children's needs and health issues. The supervisor will effectively communicate with the children's primary care physician (PCP) regarding all health concerns and orders.

The supervisor will have monthly clinical meetings with the home health nurses to ensure that the care plans and medication regimens are followed accurately and to discuss any concerns. The PT and Occupational Therapist (OT) will communicate and educate the home health care nurses regarding exercises for the boys.

2. What will happen after each discipline makes the initial visit?
Answer: Each team member will reinforce what the other members are teaching the patient and family. Each will work from a discipline-specific care plan and also from the interdisciplinary care plan.

Interdisciplinary Care Plan

Problem	Goal/Plan	Intervention	Evaluation
Risk for aspiration and choking	Patients will be free of aspiration and choking. Family will verbalize understanding of keeping all small objects away from patients and the importance of feeding the patients slowly pureed food by day 1.	Teach family about signs and symptoms of choking and aspiration. Teach family the importance of attending a cardiopulmonary resuscitation (CPR) class.	Family will verbalize the signs and symptoms of choking and aspiration. Family will be CPR certified.
Risk for injury	Patients will continue to be free of injuries. Family will continue to closely supervise patients and protect patients from injury. Family will closely monitor home environment for possible causes of potential injuries.	Teach family safety precautions.	Patients will be free of injuries. Family will continue to supervise patients at all times.
Risk for impaired skin integrity	Patients will not have impaired skin integrity. Family will verbalize importance of changing soiled diapers' and keeping perineal area dry. Parents will verbalize the importance of changing the patients' positions every 2 hours.	Teach parents the signs and symptoms of impaired skin integrity.	Patients will have intact skin integrity.

(Continued)

Problem	Goal/Plan	Intervention	Evaluation
Ineffective coping of family system	Patients and family are able to cope with sequelae of disease process within 3 months.	Provide information about community resources, support groups, and services. MSW to provide counseling for family.	Patients and family have resources for emotional support and use them effectively.

REFERENCES & RESOURCES

[1] American Academy of Pediatrics, *Guidelines for Pediatric Home Health Care*, Author, 2009.

[2] Healthline, "Alpha-Thalassemia X-Linked Mental Retardation Syndrome," http://www.healthline.com/galecontent/alpha-thalassemia-x-linked-mental-retardation-syndrome 6/6/10

[3] Methods of Healing, "Neurodevelopmental Therapy," http://www.methodsofhealing.com/Types_of_Healing/neurodevelopmental-therapy

Case 12.2 Anoxic Brain Damage/Achondroplasia

By Lannette Johnston, RN, BSN, MS, CPST

This case study illustrates how the home health nurse works with the patient, patient's parents/caregivers, and health care team to reach mutual goals. The patient, Brooke, is a 6-year-old Caucasian female with the diagnosis of anoxic brain damage/achondroplasia. The patient has the mental level of a 3-month-old baby. The patient was born at 34 weeks' gestation. Anoxic brain damage happens when the brain receives inadequate oxygen for several minutes or longer. Brain cells begin to die after approximately 4 minutes without oxygen. Brooke receives 16 hours per day of skilled nursing care, 7 days a week. Her mother has a diagnosis of achondroplasia, but the patient's father is of normal stature. Achondroplasia is a genetic condition of dwarfism.

> "Achondroplasia is a form of short-limbed dwarfism. The word achondroplasia literally means 'without cartilage formation.' However, the problem is not in forming cartilage but in converting it to bone (a process called ossification), particularly in the long bones of the arms and legs.
>
> All people with achondroplasia have short stature. The average height of an adult male with achondroplasia is 131 centimeters (4 feet, 4 inches), and the average height for adult females is 124 centimeters (4 feet, 1 inch). Characteristic features of achondroplasia include an average-size trunk, short arms and legs with particularly short upper arms and thighs, limited range of motion at the elbows, and an enlarged head (macrocephaly) with a prominent forehead. Fingers are typically short and the ring finger and middle finger may diverge, giving the hand a three-pronged

Clinical Case Studies in Home Health Care, First Edition. Edited by Leslie Neal-Boylan.
© 2011 John Wiley & Sons, Inc. Published 2011 by John Wiley & Sons, Inc.

(trident) appearance. People with achondroplasia are generally of normal intelligence.

Health problems commonly associated with achondroplasia include episodes in which breathing slows or stops for short periods (apnea), obesity, and recurrent ear infections. In adulthood, individuals with the condition usually develop a pronounced and permanent sway of the lower back (lordosis) and bowed legs. Older individuals often have back pain, which can cause difficulty with walking." [3]

The patient has had pediatric private duty home health nurses since the age of 2 years.

The use of the interdisciplinary team and excellent communication among its members are keys to the management of this case and optimal patient outcome.

 ORDERS FOR HOME CARE

Patient: 6-year-old Caucasian female named Brooke
Diagnosis: Anoxic brain damage/achondroplasia
Current medications:
- Nystatin Cream 1 unit dose topical as needed for yeast rash
- Calmoseptine 1 unit dose topical as needed for erythema
- Sween cream 1 unit topical as needed to affected areas
- Hydrocortisone 1% cream 1 dose topical as needed to affected area
- Nystop powder 1 unit dose topical twice a day as needed to red areas of skin folds and perineum
- Bactroban 1 unit dose topical twice a day as needed open skin
- Destin or A& D Cream apply a thick layer every diaper change
- Glycerin suppositories 1 unit dose per rectum as needed
- Lactulose 5 mL three times a day as needed
- Simethicone 0.6 mL every 3–4 hours as needed
- Prevacid 15 mg twice a day
- Zantac 30 mg every 8 hours
- Diastat 5 mg per rectum as needed for seizure > 5 minutes may repeat in 5 minutes
- Zaditor 1 drop both eyes three times a day
- Tylenol 160 mg every 4–6 hours as needed
- Motrin 100 mg every 6 hours
- Zyrtec 5 mg once a day
- Saline nasal spray 1 spray each nostril as needed
- Flintstone vitamin 1 tablet once a day
- Flouride 0.5 mg once a day

- Calcium carbonate 100 mg every 12 hours
- Ferin solution 37.5 mg once a day
- Peptamen Junior with Prebio 58 mL via G-tube at 60 cc per hour × 4 hours during the day then Peptamen Junior 400 mL via G-tube overnight
- Scopolamine patch 1 unit dose topical every 72 hours
- Robinol Liquid 0.2 mg every 6–8 hours
- Benadryl Liquid 12.5 mg/5 mL, give 6 mL as needed
- Albuterol 4 puffs inhalation with spacer via tracheostomy three times a day and every 4 hours as needed
- QVar MDI with spacer 5 puffs every 12 hours
- Oxygen 1–4 liters via trachmist collar to maintain oxygen saturation between 95% and 100%

Relevant past medical history:
- Prematurity at 34 weeks' gestation
- Skull fracture related to a fall
- Cardiac arrest resulting in anoxic brain damage
- Frequent hospitalizations
- MRSA
- Tracheostomy
- Gastrostomy tube
- Mental retardation
- Skin breakdown
- Constipation
- Pneumonia
- Seizures
- Mediport placement

RN: Assess and evaluate.
PT: Assess and evaluate.
OT: Assess and evaluate.
Speech therapist: Assess and evaluate.

 ## THE HOME VISIT

Brooke's home is two stories. The Make-a-Wish Foundation recently renovated her bedroom. The bedroom was designed to help cognitively stimulate Brooke and to accommodate her medical equipment. The room looks like it came out of Disneyland and is every little girl's dream bedroom, designed with princesses and pastel colors. (Figure 12.2.1)

Brooke lives with her parents, Mr. and Ms. P. The home is clean, uncluttered, and well organized. Brooke's room is pristine, and all of the supplies are neatly organized.

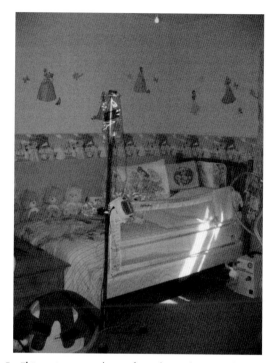

Figure 12.2.1. This patient was chosen from the Make-A-Wish Foundation to have a wish granted. Since Brooke's condition is life threatening and makes it difficult for her to travel to Disney World, her parents chose to have Disney come to Brooke's room. Make-A-Wish Foundation granted her the wish of having her bedroom transformed into a Disney Princess Room.

The pediatric nursing supervisor enters the home to interview Brooke's parents and to assess Brooke. Brooke's parents welcome the nurse into their home with open arms. Brooke's mother shares Brooke's life story. She begins her story as follows:

"When Brooke was born she was a normal little girl, other than having dwarfism. Our struggles began when we went shopping. Brooke was in her car seat in the back seat. We arrived at the store. When we were getting her out of her car seat she was limp, blue, and not breathing. My husband ran into the store and called 911. The ambulance came; and while they were transporting her to the back of the ambulance, they dropped her. My baby hit her head on the floor; that is how she got her skull fracture. This was the start of our nightmare. Our little girl was hospitalized for 3 months. The doctors told us that she would not be normal because she suffered brain damage and vocal-cord paralysis and would need a tracheostomy for breathing for the rest of

Cultural Competence

Brooke is Caucasian. Her parents are practicing Christians. Brooke's parents clearly feel strongly about supporting and caring for her. Their primary goal is to keep her at home as long as possible. Institutionalism is not an option. The team will need to praise and support them for their dedication to and care of Brooke. The parents will need education on the importance of leisure time and time alone to maintain a healthy relationship.

her life. It was awful. As bad as it was, we are thankful she is alive."

The nurse enters Brooke's room to assess her. The nurse is greeted with a big smile from Brooke. She attempts to communicate with the nurse by making some vocal noises. She can say "hi," "tickle," and "out" and is currently working with nurses and a speech therapist to say her vowels. Brooke is a pleasant little girl who thrives on interaction with others. (Figure 12.2.2)

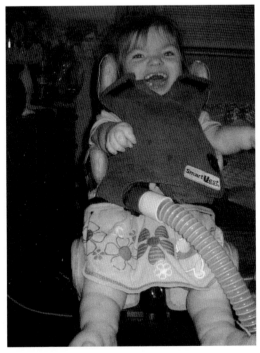

Figure 12.2.2. This high wall chest percussion (HWCP) vest provides percussion and vibration to the chest wall aiding in secretion clearance.

Brooke is alert and oriented to her name. She is able to kick her legs back and forth when she gets excited. Her tracheostomy is a number 4.0 uncuffed Bivona tracheostomy. Brooke's tracheostomy is for maintaining a patent airway. She has poor head and neck control. She receives 1.5 liters via tracheostomy collar mist at night. During the day she is on room air. She does utilize supplemental oxygen when she is sick. Her pulse oximeter reading is 99% on room air.

The nurse inspects Brooke's skin and does not notice any areas of skin breakdown. The nurse realizes that Brooke is at high risk for impaired skin integrity. Brooke's G-tube (gastrostomy tube) is healed, and no signs of infection are noted. Brooke receives tube feedings for her nutritional requirements. The tube feedings are: Peptamen Junior with Prebio 58 mL via G-tube at 60 cc per hour × 4 hours during the day, then Peptamen Junior 400 mL via G-tube overnight. The nurse recognizes that Brooke is at high risk for aspiration and the importance of administering the tube feedings in the upright position.

The nurse observes Brooke's poor head and neck control and recognizes the importance of support for Brooke's head and neck at all times to prevent injuries. (Figure 12.2.3)

The nurse looks closely at the room and observes: A high wall chest percussion (HWCP) vest, a suction machine, lab supplies, a smoke detector located in the hall outside Brooke's room, and 2 handicapped accessible fire exits close by. The home also has numerous fire extinguishers. In the event of a fire, Brooke would require complete assistance to evacuate her home. The mother reassures the nurse that the local fire, police, and emergency authorities have been notified that a chronically ill child resides in the home.

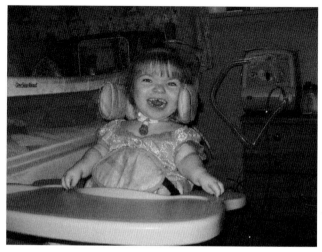

Figure 12.2.3. This customized high chair is used to keep Brooke secure and in an upright position in order to keep her airway open and assist with breathing.

Relevant Community Resources

Financial assistance with major utility bills, if needed
Notification of the fire department and police department that
   patient is disabled
Support groups for parents of chronically ill children

The nurse continues to gather data and discovers that the parents
are very knowledgeable about Brooke's medications and care plan.
Brooke receives skilled nursing services 16 hours a day, 7 days a week.
The nurse and mother review expectations and goals for the pediatric
private duty care plan for Brooke:

- To have complete safety for Brooke
- To prevent future hospitalizations
- To prevent choking and aspiration
- To prevent injury
- To provide complete care of Brooke's activities of daily living
  (ADL)
- To act quickly to resolve any distress she may experience including
  choking and aspiration

Based on the history and physical examination, the nurse discovers the
following data:

- Brooke requires 10–12 hours of sleep at night for her developmental
  age.
- Brooke experiences severe global developmental delays.
- She is incontinent of bladder and bowel elimination.
- She cannot ambulate and requires total assistance of transfer.
- She is nonverbal, but able to look to a person when her name is
  called.
- She has muscle rigidity, spasticity, and limited range of motion of
  the extremities.
- She has poor head and neck control.
- She is unable to eat by mouth and requires tube feeding.
- She is currently free of infections or skin breakdown.
- She requires total assistance of all ADL.
- She requires administration of all medications.
- She requires supplemental oxygen via tracheostomy collar to main-
  tain adequate tissue perfusion.
- She requires frequent tracheal suctioning related to copious
  secretions.

Neal Theory Implications

Stage 3: This professional considers family dynamics when planning care. The nurse has adequate resources that she can go to for answers to questions or concerns regarding the patient's disease process and medical interventions.

Stage 2: The nurse in this stage may not be able to foresee future issues related to the care of the patient and family or be aware of the need for resources and referrals.

Stage 1: The clinician in this stage may not be ready to handle such a complex case but could be mentored by a stage 3 nurse.

? CRITICAL THINKING

1. What should be the priorities for Brooke's care?
Answer: The priorities are to prevent choking, aspiration, and injury. The nurse recognizes that Brooke's condition places her at risk for choking, aspiration, skin breakdown, and infection. In addition, the nurse acknowledges the high risk for hypoxia and respiratory arrest related to the need for a tracheostomy and the need for supplemental oxygen. She realizes the importance of completing a thorough respiratory assessment and for recognizing the signs and symptoms of respiratory distress.

2. What are the roles and objectives of the physical therapist (PT) in this case?
Answer: The PT will complete a PT assessment to determine Brooke's needs and goals for therapy as well as the home environment for safety and accessibility. Additionally, the PT teaches the mother and nurse exercises to help strengthen Brooke's upper and lower extremities. The PT will recommend adaptations to the environment to promote safety and accessibility and examine the wheelchairs and Hoyer lift for appropriateness. The PT may recommend a particular wheelchair for an easier transfer. The nurse and PT will reinforce each other's involvement in Brooke's care.

3. Are there any other healthcare professionals who should be contacted?
Answer: Yes. The nurse should call the physician for orders for a medical social worker (MSW) and Pride Support Services. Brooke is also receiving occupational (OT) and speech therapy (ST).

4. What is the role of MSW?
Answer: The MSW will work with the parents to find community resources to help them with respite hours, financial assistance for medical equipment not covered by insurance, transportation expenses, electric bills, and information about support groups for parents of children with disabilities.

Pride Support Services is a mental health and mental retardation (MHMR) government support service for patients with an MHMR diagnosis. They establish a comprehensive individual support plan to help the patient and family achieve positive outcomes.

Rehabilitation Needs

Physical therapy
Occupational therapy
Speech therapy

BACK TO THE CASE

The nurse can help Brooke reach the parents' intended goals. The nurse also explains how the home health agency can assist parents with respite hours provided by a licensed nurse or financially assist with other medical needs not provided by insurance.

Reimbursement Considerations

The primary insurance for Brooke is Medical Assistance (MA). There is not a secondary insurance. MA will cover in-home skilled nursing services of 112 hours per week. The home health nurses will need to thoroughly complete nursing documentation of the child and have the mother or father sign the visit tickets. The paperwork and visit tickets must be submitted to the home health office within 48 hours of services. The supervisor on the case will need to complete recertification assessments and complete required MA paperwork: Letter of Medical Necessity (LOMN), Parent Work Letters/Schedules, Care Plan for the child, and Physician Orders, and copies of the nursing documentation. All paperwork must be submitted to MA by the required time line to ensure adequate reimbursement of services.

1. How will the members of the interdisciplinary team communicate with one another?
Answer: Brooke's home health nurses will communicate with the parents and the nursing supervisor for her needs and health issues. The supervisor will effectively communicate with the children's primary care physician (PCP) regarding all health concerns and orders. The supervisor will have monthly clinical meetings with the home health nurses to ensure that the care plans and medication regimens are followed accurately and to discuss any concerns. The PT, OT, ST, and Pride Support Service Coordinator will communicate and educate the home health care nurses on recommended exercises for Brooke.

2. What will happen after each discipline makes the initial visit?
Answer: Each team member will reinforce what the other members are teaching the family. Each will work from a discipline-specific care plan and also from the interdisciplinary care plan.

Interdisciplinary Care Plan

Problem	Goal/Plan	Intervention	Evaluation
Impaired gas exchange	Patient will have adequate oxygenation and tissue perfusion daily. Parents will verbalize signs and symptoms of respiratory distress: cyanosis, labored breathing, use of accessory muscles, low oxygen saturations <90%, asymmetrical chest rise, tracheal deviation, adventitious breath sounds, copious secretions, tachycardia, tachypnea, and anxiety by day 1. Patient will be free of infections and complications related to mechanical ventilation daily.	Teach the parents how to suction patient properly. Teach the parents the DOPE pneumonic: D—Displaced tube O—Obstruction P—Pneumothorax E—Equipment failure Have parents verbalize their emergency plan in the event patient goes into respiratory arrest.	Patient maintains adequate gas exchange. Patient maintains adequate airway clearance and effective breathing patterns. Patient will be free of infections and complications.

Problem	Goal/Plan	Intervention	Evaluation
Risk for aspiration	Patient will be free of aspiration. Family will verbalize understanding of keeping the head of the bed elevated at least 30 degrees during tube feedings by day 1.	Teach family about signs and symptoms of aspiration. Teach family the importance of attending a cardiopulmonary resuscitation (CPR) class.	Family will verbalize the signs and symptoms of choking and aspiration. Family will be CPR certified.
Risk for impaired skin integrity	Patient will not have impaired skin integrity. Family will verbalize importance of changing soiled diapers, keeping perineal area dry, and changing the patient position every 2 hours by day 1.	Teach parents the signs and symptoms of impaired skin integrity. Teach parents how to properly use the specialized air mattress and bed. Teach parents the signs of skin breakdown and to report it to the nurses immediately.	Patient will have intact skin integrity.
Risk for infection	Patient is free of infection. Patient's family will continue to practice meticulous infection control and limit ill visitors on a daily basis. Patient's primary care physician will continue to provide monthly and as-needed home visits.	Provide information about infection control practices and the importance of hand washing and cleaning equipment on a regular basis. Educate parents and nurses on the importance of reporting any signs and symptoms of infection to the physician immediately. Nursing supervisor will draw monthly blood work per physician order and report lab results to physician.	Patient will remain infection free.

(Continued)

Problem	Goal/Plan	Intervention	Evaluation
Risk for constipation	Patient will have normal elimination. Parents and nurse will continue to follow bowel regime ordered by physician daily.	Parents will verbalize the signs and symptoms of constipation: distended abdomen, hypo-/hyperactive bowel sounds, absence of daily bowel movement, abdominal discomfort, and facial grimacing. Educate parents on the importance changing the patient's position every 2 hours.	Patient will have normal elimination.

REFERENCES & RESOURCES

[1] American Academy of Pediatrics, *Guidelines for Pediatric Home Health Care*, Author, 2009.

[2] Children's Hospital of Philadelphia, http://www.chop.edu/healthinfo/head-injury.html

[3] Genetics Home Reference, "What Is Achondroplasia?" http://ghr.nlm.nih.gov/condition=achondroplasia

Case 12.3 Cerebral Palsy/ Acute Respiratory Failure

By Lannette Johnston, RN, BSN, MS, CPST

This case study illustrates how the home health nurse works with a patient requiring intensive services, the patient's parents/caregivers, and the health care team to reach mutual goals. The patient is a 28-year-old Caucasian male with the diagnosis of cerebral palsy and acute respiratory failure. The patient has the mentality level of a 2-year-old toddler and a body of a 12-year-old. Despite being an adult, the patient has had Pediatric Private Duty home health nurses since the age of 17. Prior to the initiation of services, the parents provided all of the care to the patient. All of his life, the patient has required complete assistance with all activities of daily living (ADL). He became ventilator dependent in 2004, which required the parents to ask for additional help for his care.

 ORDERS FOR HOME CARE

Patient: 28-year-old Caucasian male named Sam
Diagnoses: Cerebral palsy and acute respiratory failure
Current medications:
- Ketoconazole shampoo 1 unit dose topical as needed
- Calmoseptine Topical as needed
- Clotrimazole/Bethameth cream 1 unit topical as needed to affected areas
- Hydrocortisone 1% cream 1 dose topical as needed to affected area

Clinical Case Studies in Home Health Care, First Edition. Edited by Leslie Neal-Boylan.
© 2011 John Wiley & Sons, Inc. Published 2011 by John Wiley & Sons, Inc.

- Nystop powder 1 unit dose topical as needed to affected area
- Neosporin Plus pain ointment topical 1 dose to affected area
- Bactroban 1 unit dose topical to affected area 3 times daily as needed
- Lactulose 30 mL 4 times daily as needed
- Mylicon 2.5 cc 3 times daily
- Senna Syrup 5 mL 3 times daily
- Dulcolax suppository 1 dose as needed
- Tylenol 650 mg every 4 hours as needed
- Valium 2 mg at bedtime
- Prevacid 30 mg twice daily
- Reglan 5 mL 4 times daily
- FeSO4 1 tsp daily
- Robinul 1 mg twice daily as needed
- Oxygen 5 liters via tracheostomy (trach)/ventilator to maintain oxygen saturation between 95% and 100%
- Duoneb Inhalation 1 vial every 4 hours as needed

Relevant past medical history:

- Traumatic birth
- Frequent hospitalizations
- Halo brace
- MRSA
- Tracheostomy
- Ventilator dependent
- Gastrostomy tube
- Mental retardation
- Skin breakdown
- Constipation
- Pneumonia
- Thrombocytopenia

RN: Assess and evaluate.
PT: Assess and evaluate.
OT: Assess and evaluate.

Cultural Competence

It is important that the nurses and interdisciplinary team determine whether there are cultural factors of which they should be aware as they care for Sam. His parents clearly feel strongly about supporting/caring for him. Their primary goal is to keep him at home as long as possible. Institutionalism is not an option. The team will need to praise/support them for their dedication and care of Sam. The parents will need education on the importance leisure and time alone to maintain a healthy relationship.

THE HOME VISIT

Sam's home is a ranch-style, handicapped-accessible home that was designed with Sam's needs in mind. Sam lives with his parents, Mr. and Mrs. D, and his younger sister, Mia. The home is clean, uncluttered, and well organized. Sam's room is very meticulous and all supplies are neatly organized.

The pediatric nursing supervisor enters the home to interview Sam's parents and assess Sam. Sam's parents welcome the nurse. Sam's mother shares Sam's life story and the struggles he has encountered since birth. She begins her story:

"Sam was born at 42 weeks; He didn't want to enter this world. Now I can see why. When he was born his Apgar score was 0 at first, and then after they resuscitated him it only came up to 6. He spent the first week of his life in the neonatal intensive care unit (NICU). Once we were discharged from the hospital, I began to enjoy my sweet little bundle of joy. When Sam was 4 months old, Sam's Aunt Jean (a practicing nurse) noticed that Sam wasn't a normal baby. At 6 months he was diagnosed with cerebral palsy (CP). Sam had to be fed pureed foods by mouth because of his disease. He required constant supervision.

When he was 5-years-old, he had his first halo brace to support his head and neck. During the time of his halo brace he had to have a bone from his hip placed in his neck. He had to wear the halo for 5 months. Unfortunately, 5 years later he had to have another halo placed. We continued to love and care for our beautiful Sam. He taught us how to enjoy life to the fullest.

Over the course of his life he has had numerous hospitalizations for arm fractures, pneumothorax, pneumonia, and respiratory infections. At the age of 18, Sam had to have a tracheostomy and be on a ventilator. Now that he is 28, he continues to thrive and appreciate everything people do for him. I want people to know how it is to have a child with fragile medical conditions. It is not easy, but life isn't easy either. We love him so much." (Figure 12.3.1)

The nurse is eager to meet Sam. The nurse enters Sam's room, approaches the head of his bed and says, "Hi, Sam." Sam immediately looks at the nurse and begins to smile. He knows the nurse is there to see him. Sam's room is decorated in a vibrant, colorful jungle theme. On the ceiling above Sam's head is a mural of the blue sky and clouds. Hanging from the light fixture is a green-leaf swag draped down with colorful Christmas lights. Every wall in Sam's room has a different jungle mural. On the left side of Sam is a TV and a variety of children's movies and cartoons. (Figure 12.3.2)

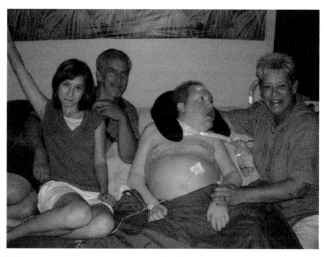

Figure 12.3.1. Sam is so happy surrounded by his loving family.

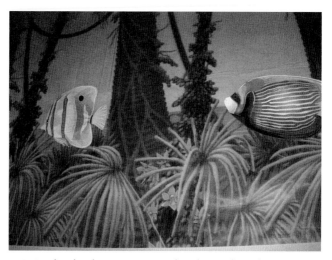

Figure 12.3.2. The detail Sam's parents placed in making their son's room vibrant and colorful to help keep him alert.

Sam is alert and oriented to his name. He is nonverbal, but smiles when spoken to. His trach is a number 6.0 shiley with an inner canula. He is being mechanically ventilated with an LP 10 ventilator. His pulse oximeter reading is 98% oxygen saturation level with a heart rate of 86. His ventilator settings are: Assist Control mode, rate of 12, tidal volume 600, PEEP (positive end expiratory pressure) of 5, humidified air 28–30 degrees, low-pressure alarm set at 8, and a high-pressure alarm rate of 45. Sam's bed is a specialized hospital bed that provides frequent

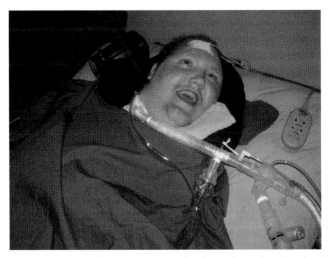

Figure 12.3.3. Assistive devices are required to keep Sam's head and neck aligned properly to maintain an open airway.

rotation and is equipped with an Airsoft mattress. The nurse inspects Sam's skin and does not notice any areas of skin breakdown. The nurse realizes that he is at high risk for impaired skin integrity.

Sam's gastrostomy tube (G-tube) is healed, and no signs of infection are noted. He is currently receiving tube feedings of Nutramen at 175 cc per hour. The nurse observes the rest of the room and notes the following: A Hoyer lift, a high wall chest percussion vest, a suction machine, lab supplies, a smoke detector located in the hall outside of Sam's room, and a handicapped-accessible fire exit close by. (Figure 12.3.3)

Relevant Community Resources
Financial assistance with major utility bills, if needed Notification of the fire department and police department that he is disabled Support groups for parents of chronically ill children

The home also has numerous fire extinguishers. In the event of a fire Sam would require complete assistance to evacuate his home. There are two means of exit in the home; both have ramps to safely accommodate Sam and all of his medical equipment.

The mother reassures the nurse that local fire, police, and emergency authorities have been notified that a chronically ill person resides in the home.

The bathroom was added to meet Sam's hygiene needs. The shower is a very large, handicapped shower. The nurse is impressed with the cleanliness and organization of Sam's room and bathroom.

The nurse continues to gather data and discovers that the parents are very knowledgeable about Sam's medications and care plan. Sam receives skilled nursing services 10 hours a day while his parents work. The nurse and mother review expectations and goals for the pediatric private duty care plan for Sam:

- To have complete safety for Sam
- To prevent future hospitalizations
- To prevent choking and aspiration
- To prevent injury
- To provide complete care for Sam's activities of daily living (ADL)
- To act quickly to respond to any distress he may experience including choking and aspiration

Rehabilitation Needs

Physical therapy
Occupational therapy

Based on the history and physical examination, the nurse discovers the following data:

- Sam requires 10–12 hours of sleep at night.
- He experiences severe global developmental delays.
- He is incontinent of bladder and bowel.
- He cannot ambulate and requires total assistance of transfer.
- He is nonverbal, but is able to look to a person when his name is called.
- He has muscle rigidity, spasticity, and limited range of motion of extremities.
- He is unable to eat by mouth and requires tube feeding.
- He is currently free of infections or skin breakdown.
- He requires total assistance of all ADL.
- He requires administration of all medications.
- He requires mechanical ventilation and supplemental oxygen to maintain oxygen saturations of 95% to 100%.

Neal Theory Implications

Stage 3: This nurse is comfortable managing all of the equipment in the home setting, is able to troubleshoot without difficulty, and is very aware of community and other resources that can help the patient and family.

Stage 2: The professional in this stage may not realize that the parents are valuable resources and can teach the nurse how best to care for Sam's individual needs. This nurse may need assistance transferring his/her knowledge of intensive care practices into the home setting.

Stage 1: The clinician in this stage will assess the patient and recognize the need for assistance with the case but may be unsure as to how to proceed in the home setting.

? CRITICAL THINKING

1. What are the priorities of Sam's care plan?
Answer: The priorities are to prevent choking, aspiration, and injury. The nurse recognizes that Sam's condition places him at risk for choking, aspiration, skin breakdown, and infection. In addition, the nurse acknowledges the high risk for hypoxia and respiratory arrest related to the need for mechanical ventilation. She realizes the importance of completing a thorough respiratory assessment and recognizing the signs and symptoms of respiratory distress.

2. What are the roles and objectives of the physical therapist (PT)?
Answer: The PT will complete a PT assessment to determine Sam's needs and goals for therapy and evaluate the home environment for safety and accessibility. Additionally, the PT will teach the mother and nurse exercises to help strengthen the patient's upper and lower extremities. The PT will recommend adaptations to the environment to promote safety and accessibility and will examine the wheelchairs and Hoyer lift for appropriateness. The PT may recommend a particular wheelchair for an easier transfer.

3. Are there any other health care professionals who should be contacted?
Answer: Yes. The nurse should call the physician for orders for a medical social worker (MSW) and North Star Support Services.

4. What is the role of the MSW?
Answer: The MSW will work with the parents to find community resources to help them with respite hours, financial assistance for medical equipment not covered by insurance, transportation expenses, electric bills, and information on support groups for parents of children with disabilities.

North Star Support Services is a mental health and mental retardation (MHMR) government support service for patients with a MHMR diagnosis. They establish a comprehensive individual support plan to help the patient and family achieve positive outcomes. They can assist the parents in obtaining skilled nursing services for Sam. This service is provided for patients over the age of 21.

BACK TO THE CASE

The nurse can help Sam reach the mother's intended goals. The nurse also explains how the home health agency can assist parents with respite hours provided by a licensed nurse or financially assist with other medical needs not provided by insurance.

Reimbursement Considerations

The primary insurance for Sam is an Independent Waiver through the Department of Public Welfare. In each fiscal year, he is awarded so many units of skilled nursing services while his parents work. One unit is equal to 15 minutes. It is important that the nursing supervisor perform monthly reviews in the Department of Public Welfare's Home and Community Services Information System (HCSIS) to determine the number of units utilized. It is important to stay within the allotted units. The home health nurses will need to thoroughly complete nursing documentation of Sam and have the mother or father sign the visit tickets. The paperwork and visit tickets must be submitted to the home health office within 48 hours of services. The supervisor on the case will need to complete recertification assessments and complete required paperwork: Sam's MHMR support coordinator submits the required documentation to the Department of Public Welfare through the HCSIS system. The coordinator also provides an in-depth Individual Support Plan to the mother and the agency for coordination of care. All documentation must be submitted to the business office by the required time line to ensure adequate reimbursement of services.

CRITICAL THINKING

1. How will the members of the interdisciplinary team communicate with one another?
Answer: Sam's home health nurses will communicate with parents and the nursing supervisor for his needs and health issues. The supervisor

will effectively communicate with the child's primary care physician (PCP) regarding all health concerns and orders. The supervisor will have monthly clinical meetings with the home health nurses to ensure that the care plans and medication regimens are followed accurately and to discuss any concerns. The PT, OT, and North Star Support Service coordinator will communicate and educate the home health care nurses on recommended exercises for the patient.

2. What will happen after each discipline makes the initial visit?
Answer: Each team member will reinforce what the other members are teaching the family. Each will work from a discipline-specific care plan and also from the interdisciplinary care plan.

Interdisciplinary Care Plan

Problem	Goal/Plan	Intervention	Evaluation
Impaired gas exchange	Patient will have adequate oxygenation and tissue perfusion daily. Parents will verbalize signs and symptoms of respiratory distress: cyanosis, labored breathing, use of accessory muscles, low oxygen saturations <90%, asymmetrical chest rise, tracheal deviation, adventitious breath sounds, copious secretions, tachycardia, tachypnea, and anxiety by day 1. Patient will be free of infections and complications related to mechanical ventilation daily.	Teach the parents how to suction patient properly. Teach the parents the DOPE pneumonic: D—Displaced tube O—Obstruction P—Pneumothorax E—Equipment failure Have parents verbalize their emergency plan in the event the patient goes into respiratory arrest.	Patient maintains adequate gas exchange. Patient maintains adequate airway clearance and effective breathing patterns. Patient will be free of infections and complications.
Risk for aspiration	Patient will be free of aspiration. Family will verbalize understanding of keeping the head of the bed elevated at least 30 degrees during tube feedings by day 1.	Teach family about signs and symptoms of aspiration. Teach family the importance of attending a cardiopulmonary resuscitation (CPR) class.	Family will verbalize the signs and symptoms of choking and aspiration. Family will be CPR certified.

(*Continued*)

Problem	Goal/Plan	Intervention	Evaluation
Risk for impaired skin integrity	Patient will not have impaired skin integrity. Family will verbalize importance of changing soiled diapers, keeping perineal area dry, and changing the patient position every 2 hours by day 1.	Teach parents the signs and symptoms of impaired skin integrity. Teach parents how to properly use the specialized air mattress and bed. Teach parents the signs of skin breakdown and to report it to the nurses immediately.	Patient will have intact skin integrity.
Risk for infection	Patient is free of infection. Patient's family will continue to practice meticulous infection control and limit ill visitors on a daily basis. Patient's primary care physician will continue to provide monthly and as-needed home visits.	Provide information about infection-control practices, the importance of hand washing, and cleaning equipment on a regular basis. Educate parents and nurses on the importance of reporting any signs and symptoms of infection to physician immediately. Nursing supervisor will draw monthly blood work per physician order and report lab results to physician.	Patient will remain infection free.

Problem	Goal/Plan	Intervention	Evaluation
Risk for constipation	Patient will have normal elimination. Parents and nurse will continue to follow bowel regime ordered by physician daily.	Parents will verbalize the signs and symptoms of constipation: distended abdomen, hypo-/hyperactive bowel sounds, absence of daily bowel movement, abdominal discomfort, and facial grimacing. Educate parents on the importance changing the patient position every 2 hours.	Patient will have normal elimination.

REFERENCES & RESOURCES

[1] American Academy of Pediatrics, *Guidelines for Pediatric Home Health Care*, 2009.

[2] http://www.halobrace.com

[3] National Institute of Neurological Disorders and Strokes, http://www.ninds.nih.gov

Section 13

Infectious Disease

Case 13.1 *Clostridium difficile*-Associated Disease (CDAD)

By Debra Riendeau, MN, APRN, BC, PMHNP-BC

This case study illustrates how the home health nurse works with a patient with several challenging conditions to collaboratively meet realistic goals. The patient, Mr. J, was paralyzed from the waist down due to a snowboarding accident 4 years ago. He receives financial support from the state in which he resides and is on permanent disability. He is wheelchair bound and independent in his home, which has been remodeled to incorporate his physical disability. Approximately 4 weeks ago, he developed a decubitus ulcer on his left buttock due to his seat cushion in his wheelchair being improperly inflated causing increased pressure and decreased circulation to the area. Despite treatment, the decubitus ulcer progressed to a stage III. He was hospitalized and a surgeon performed a skin graft using skin taken from his left bicep area. While in the hospital, he was started on a course of intravenous antibiotics. The patient's mother and sister have been trained by the hospital nursing staff to administer the patient's clindamycin by intravenous (IV) pump using his peripherally inserted central catheter (PICC) line. He is now returning home to complete his course of antibiotics and his surgical recovery process.

Reimbursement Considerations

The patient is currently receiving state disability payments due to his initial injury and is covered for his medical care.

Clinical Case Studies in Home Health Care, First Edition. Edited by Leslie Neal-Boylan.
© 2011 John Wiley & Sons, Inc. Published 2011 by John Wiley & Sons, Inc.

ORDERS FOR HOME CARE

Patient: 27-year-old Caucasian male
Diagnosis: Paraplegia, status post skin graft to left buttock and donor site left bicep
Allergies: Penicillin
Current medications:
- Clindamycin 600 mg IV every 12 hours
- Protonix 40 mg by mouth every evening at bedtime

Relevant past medical history: Snowboarding accident with subsequent lower extremity paralysis
RN: Assess and evaluate. Skilled procedure: Cover the buttock wound with a nonstick dressing, covered with gauze and secured in place with soft cloth surgical tape. Apply a hydrocolloid dressing to donor site. Perform a weekly sterile PICC line dressing change.
PT: Assess and evaluate.

Rehabilitation Needs

Physical therapy to assist the patient to return to his former level of wheelchair independence and mobility

THE HOME VISIT

The nurse opens the case and notes that the patient lives in a ranch-style home with appropriate wheelchair access. The home is clean, but it has many medical supplies in boxes scattered in various locations around the living room. There is one main hallway from the front door, which is clear of clutter and provides easy access to the kitchen and the patient's bedroom in the back of the house. There is a bathroom off the main hallway for visitors and a large wheelchair accessible bathroom that is attached to the patient's bedroom. This bathroom has no tub, but it allows for a shower chair to be wheeled directly into the stall. There are several sturdy grab bars and a personal shower present.

The nurse discovers that Mr. J is lying supine in his hospital bed. He is cooperative and social. He states, "Ask whatever you need to. I stopped being shy during rehab after the accident." He recounts several stories while the nurse gathers his history. The nurse performs a basic head-to-toe admission assessment noting that the skin on the donor site is granulating without infection. The patient has a PICC in his right antecubital fossa for his intravenous antibiotics. He willingly turns on his side in bed with the use of his overhead grab bar. The nurse notes that his graft site is covered. The nurse continues to gather data and discovers that the patient is knowledgeable about his medications. Additionally, the nurse is informed that due to his decreased independence and being bedridden, his meals are being made by his mother and his sister who live close by and take turns visiting him for each meal.

Cultural Competence

This patient is a young man who typically manages his own care and socialization. He now needs the help of his mother and his sister. While it might be tempting to confer with his mother and/or sister regarding his care, Mr. J is an adult and is capable of making his own decisions. The home care team must be certain to consult with him regarding the treatment plan.

As the assessment is being completed, the nurse asks the patient what his treatment goals are. He lists the following goals:

- To get his wounds to heal so that he can be up in his wheelchair again
- To be off of antibiotic therapy
- To regain his independence, especially in his activities of daily living (ADL)
- To be able to leave his home by using the public wheelchair van again
- To be able to meet his friends at their favorite restaurant

Relevant Community Resources

Renewal of notification of the fire department and police department that he is disabled and has returned home

Based on the history and physical examination, the nurse discovers the following data:

- Mr. J has been receiving assistance with his bathing twice a week.
- Mr. J self catheterizes every 6 hours.
- Mr. J is continent of bowel with a daily bowel routine done by his mother early every morning.
- Mr. J has an infection in the left buttock graft area.
- The PICC line has an occlusive dressing and shows no sign of infection at the site.

> ### Neal Theory Implications
>
> Stage 3: The nurse in this case demonstrated autonomy by independently making clinical and other decisions as well as seeking referrals to other health care professionals caring for the patient. The nurse is able to make arrangements to transfer the patient to a local hospital at the end of the case.
>
> Stage 2: The professional in this stage will demonstrate more comfort in dealing with health care issues (like *Clostridium difficile*) and the complexity of the home care environment. There is still a need to seek the experience of other health professionals to problem solve and negotiate the care needs of the patient in the home care setting. The nurse may need help facilitating a smooth transition from home to hospital.
>
> Stage 1: The clinician in this stage will assess the patient and recognize the need for assistance with the case but may be unsure as to how to proceed in the home setting. The nurse will need to ask questions of a more experienced nurse concerning a *Clostridium difficile* infection and require assistance in managing the patient's care and treatment plan.

? CRITICAL THINKING

1. What is the priority for nursing care for Mr. J?
Answer: Since the patient has successfully maintained his life for the last 4 years and his home has been fully adapted for his disability, the priority of care is infection control. The nurse will reinforce education with the patient and the family in regard to sterile technique. Sterile technique must be maintained in conjunction with contact and use of the PICC line and intravenous therapy. Additionally, the buttock wound must be kept clean and dry for the wound to heal and the graft to take.

2. What education should be provided by the nurse to the family on this initial visit?
Answer: The nurse will reinforce education with the patient and the family with regard to sterile technique and with regard to the use of the PICC line and intravenous antibiotic therapy. Additionally, the buttock wound must be kept clean and dry for the wound to heal and the graft to take.

3. What will the physical therapist (PT) do during the first visit to the home?
Answer: The PT will do an initial assessment to determine Mr. J's needs and goals for home therapy. The PT will also assess the home environment for safety and accessibility. Since this patient has been living with his disability for 4 years and the house has proper accommodations, the PT will focus on assessing the cushion in the wheelchair since this was the initial problem which caused the decubitus ulcer. However, the patient is bedridden for the time being. The PT will make an appointment to return later in the patient's recovery when he is able to return to wheelchair mobility.

4. Is there anyone else who should become involved in the care of this patient?
Answer: Yes. Even though the patient had been having a home health aide twice a week before the decubitus ulcer occurred, the nurse should call the physician for orders for a home health aide (HHA) who will visit Mr. J daily (initially) to help him with a bed bath, oral care, and dressing until he can return to his former activity level.

↻ BACK TO THE CASE

For the next several days, the nurse sees the patient on a daily basis to perform a general nursing assessment including vital signs and to assess both wounds for healing as well as signs and symptoms of infection. Additionally, the nurse performs wound care to the left buttock graft site and assesses the PICC line insertion site for infection and patency. The nurse determines that the patient's mother or sister continues to administer the patient's clindamycin by IV pump using his PICC line without incident.

? CRITICAL THINKING

1. With regard to side effects, what signs and symptoms should be monitored while the patient is receiving IV clindamycin?
Answer: The patient should be monitored for mild diarrhea, nausea, and vomiting. More severe side effects include rashes; hives and itching; and swelling of the mouth, face, lips, or tongue. The nurse should also monitor for difficulty breathing and tightness in the chest. Additionally, the patient may also experience severe stomach cramps with severe, persistent diarrhea that could be bloody.

ↄ **BACK TO THE CASE**

On the third visit, the patient is markedly distressed. He reports that he is feeling nauseated and is having severe, painful abdominal cramping. He states he has been awake for most of the night due to several bouts of nonbloody diarrhea with a foul odor. He had called his mother around midnight, and she has been helping him use the bedpan. He is concerned about what is happening.

? **CRITICAL THINKING**

- With this patient's current status, what is the nurse's first priority?
  Answer: Due to the fact that this patient has been on intravenous antibiotic therapy during his hospitalization, the nurse must consider the possibility that the patient is experiencing *Clostridium difficile*-associated disease (CDAD). CDAD can occur while a patient is in the hospital or at a later time after discharge. This patient is also on a proton-pump inhibitor that was started at the time of his surgical procedure to prevent stress ulcers. Proton pump inhibitors are considered a risk factor for CDAD.
- What is the nurse's best course of action in the treatment of this patient at this time?
  Answer: The nurse should make arrangements to have the patient transported to a hospital for treatment due to the severity of his symptoms. The physician for this patient should be notified of his symptoms as well as his transfer to the hospital.

ↄ **BACK TO THE CASE**

While waiting for the ambulance to transfer him back to the hospital, the patient and his mother ask what they can expect to happen now. They are concerned and are wondering if the new condition is life threatening. The nurse calmly reassures them concerning the possible expected interventions. The nurse also provides important education for the mother who has been caring for her son throughout the night.

? **CRITICAL THINKING**

1. What is the typical treatment for CDAD?
Answer: Additional diagnostic and laboratory testing will be conducted. Intravenous fluid replacement therapy will be ordered for con-

tinued hydration. A stool sample may be obtained from the patient. The current antibiotic will mostly likely be stopped. The patient may be started on metronidazole (Flagyl) intravenously.

2. What additional education should be provided to the mother concerning her health before they both leave for the hospital?
Answer: *Clostridium difficile* can be spread to others either from person to person or from contacts in the living environment of the infected patient. The most important prevention is with good hand washing techniques. Alcohol based handwashing gels are not effective in killing *Clostridium difficile* spores. It is important that the patient's mother decontaminate the environmental surfaces of his bedroom and bathroom as well as the bedpan and other items used in his care with a 1:100 dilution bleach solution. It is also important that all linens and other material items be cleaned using hot water and a dryer. The patient's mother should be educated to watch for signs and symptoms of the infection in her own health status and to seek medical care immediately should they occur.

Interdisciplinary Care Plan

Problem	Goal/Plan	Intervention	Evaluation
Potential for infection	The patient's donor site and skin graft sites will heal without infection in 3 weeks. Patient's PICC line will remain patent and without signs or symptoms of systemic infection.	Teach the patient and family the signs and symptoms of wound infection (redness, heat, tenderness and drainage). Teach the patient and family the correct procedure to access the PICC line for antibiotic therapy to maintain sterility.	Patient's donor and skin graft sites heal without infection.
Knowledge deficit: Skin graft and donor site care	Patient and family will verbalize the correct care of the skin graft and donor site in 1 visit.	Educate the patient and family to leave the skin graft and donor site dressing intact.	Patient and family did not disturb the dressings.

(Continued)

Problem	Goal/Plan	Intervention	Evaluation
Care of the PICC line	PICC line will remain patent.	Teach the patient and family the correct procedure to access and flush PICC line to maintain sterility.	Patient and family consistently demonstrated the correct procedure for PICC line use.
Correct understanding of clindamycin antibiotic therapy	Patient and family will demonstrate the proper procedure for administering antibiotics safely thru PICC line. Patient and family will verbalize the adverse reactions to clindamycin antibiotics.	Teach the patient the signs and symptoms of adverse reactions to clindamycin.	Patient and family recognized several of the adverse reactions to clindamycin administration and sought medical care.
CDAD disease process	Pt and family will verbalize the signs and symptoms, course, and treatment of CDAD. Family will verbalize the decontamination procedures for CDAD in the home.	Teach the patient and family the signs and symptoms of CDAD, the course of the disease, and the treatment of the disease. Teach the family the decontamination measures for the home in regards to CDAD.	Patient and family recognize and verbalize the signs and symptoms, the course of disease and the treatment, as well as decontamination procedures for CDAD in the home environment.
Altered comfort: pain	Patient will receive pain medications that relieve pain to the patient's acceptable level (2–3/10) in 1 hour.	Assess patient's pain every 2 hours and administer pain medications as ordered by the physician.	Patient reported pain level was managed to 2–3/10 in 1 hour.
Inability to perform ADL/IADL (instrumental activities of daily living) independently	Patient's ADL/IADL needs will be met in 1 day.	Referral to physical therapist in regards to mobility needs. Home health aide will provide bed baths daily until patient is able to shower after wounds heal without infection.	Patient reports ADL/IADL needs have been met.

Problem	Goal/Plan	Intervention	Evaluation
Social isolation	Patient will verbalize satisfaction with social relationships in 2 weeks.	Develop a plan with patient for friends to visit during his convalescence.	Patient's friends visit 1–2 times a week to watch movies and play video games.
Neurogenic bladder incontinence	Patient will self-catherize every 6 hours.	Review self-catherization technique as needed and reinforce proper procedure.	Patient resumes and continues his self-catherization routine every 6 hours around the clock.
Alteration and bowel evacuation	Patient will have a formed bowel movement every day.	Review digital stimulation and manual evacuation procedure with patient's mother.	Patient's mother continues with patient's preoperative bowel routine.

REFERENCES & RESOURCES

[1] L. Sehulster and R. Chinn, "Guidelines for environmental infection control in health-care facilities," Recommendations of CDC and the Healthcare Infection Control Practices Advisory Committee (HICPAC). 52 (RR-10) 1–42. Retrieved from http://www.cdc.gov/mmwr/preview/mmwrhtml/rr5210a1.htm, 2003.

[2] J. Snyder, H. Doyle and T. Delbridge, "Applying split-thickness skin grafts: A step-by-step clinical guide and nursing implications," *Ostomy Wound Management*, 47(11):20–26, 2001. Retrieved from http://www.o-wm.com/article/1080

[3] R. Sunenshine and L. McDonald, "Clostridium difficile-associated disease: New challenges from an established pathogen," *Cleveland Clinic Journal of Medicine*, 73(2):187–197, 2006.

Case 13.2 Community-Associated, Methicillin-Resistant *Staphylococcus aureus* (MRSA)

By Debra Riendeau, MN, APRN, BC, PMHNP-BC

This case study illustrates how the home health nurse works with the patient and family to reach mutually agreeable goals. Mrs. H is a 37-year-old female who has been diagnosed with insulin-dependent diabetes mellitus (IDDM) for the last 5 years. She attended a wedding recently and wore new shoes throughout the daytime service and the evening reception, which caused a sore area on her right fifth toe. The injury went unnoticed for over a week. At that time, she sought medical care; but despite treatment, the toe became necrotic and was amputated 4 days ago. Due to her recent toe amputation, she is temporarily off from her job as a secretary for a local school department, is unable to drive, and is homebound. She lives with her 18-year-old nephew, who is a senior in high school. He is a wide receiver on his high-school football team and is hoping to go on to college on a football scholarship. His high school football team has been dealing with an outbreak of MRSA among the football players. The school nurse sent a letter home notifying the family that the son is at risk and that the nurse has instituted a school-wide program to combat the outbreak.

Cultural Competence

Mrs. H is an African American woman who is head of her household. There are racial and ethnic considerations for this patient and her nephew. The rate of MRSA in African Americans is more than twice as high as in Caucasians [2].

Clinical Case Studies in Home Health Care, First Edition. Edited by Leslie Neal-Boylan.
© 2011 John Wiley & Sons, Inc. Published 2011 by John Wiley & Sons, Inc.

ORDERS FOR HOME CARE

Patient: Obese 37-year-old African American female

Diagnoses: Right fifth-digit foot amputation, insulin-dependent diabetes mellitus (IDDM), hypertension (HTN), community-associated MRSA

Current medications:
- Lisinopril 10 mg once a day
- Lantus insulin 35 units subcutaneous at bedtime
- Novolog insulin subcutaneous sliding scale for blood sugars 15 minutes before each meal

Relevant past medical history:
- Recent amputation of the fifth digit on her right foot
- Insulin-dependent diabetes mellitus (IDDM)

RN: Skilled assessment and evaluation. Skilled procedure: Pack wound with Iodoform gauze, cover with a 2 × 2, and wrap with a Coban wrap daily.

Rehabilitation Needs

Diabetes educator for diabetes management plan
Consider physical therapy if the patient has difficulty walking since the amputation.

THE HOME VISIT

The nurse enters the home, which is a first floor apartment, and notices that the home is clean, uncluttered, and well organized. The nurse introduces herself to the patient, pulls up a chair alongside the couch, and begins to do the admission assessment.

Mrs. H is pleasant and cooperative during the lengthy history-taking and assessment process. During the visit, the nurse looks in the bathroom to observe the accessibility to the toilet and tub/shower and to assess safety. The tub is designed for easy entry, and there is a place where the patient can rest her right foot to keep it dry during bathing. The nurse notes that the kitchen is fully stocked, and the patient says that her nephew has been going to the grocery store for the two of them. The nurse also observes that there are several candy dishes in the living room filled with chocolate candies and jelly beans. Mrs. H states, "I still have a sweet tooth, even though I have diabetes. Whenever I eat a handful throughout the day, I just take a little extra shot of insulin."

> **Relevant Community Resource**
>
> Community diabetes support groups

When the nurse has finished gathering the data, she examines Mrs. H. She notes that, in addition to the right-toe bandage, the patient has a raised reddened area with some crusting at the center on her left calf, which the patient describes as a new "spider bite."

Based on the history and physical examination, the nurse discovers the following data:

- Obese African American female
- Finger-stick blood sugars that range between 180–220 on a daily basis
- Amputation of the fifth digit of the right foot
- Raised red area with crusting on left mid calf
- Using front-wheel walker to ambulate

> **Reimbursement Considerations**
>
> The patient's care in this case is covered under her employer-provided health benefits. Her private insurance will cover the daily nursing visits, the MSW, the diabetes educator, and the durable medical equipment (the front-wheel walker).

Together, the nurse and Mrs. H set goals for treatment, as follows:

- Mrs. H states her goal is to recover from the amputation as soon as possible and return to work.
- The nurse outlines a goal for the patient to improve her control of the diabetes by learning more about food exchanges and long-term diabetes management.

> **Neal Theory Implications**
>
> Stage 3: The professional in this stage collaborates with other disciplines both within and outside of home care and is autonomous with the clinical aspects of the case and the logistical aspects of working with the agency. The nurse in this case demonstrated autonomy by making independent clinical and other decisions, as well as seeking referrals to other health care professionals in the patient's care independently.
>
> *(Continued)*

Stage 2: The professional in this stage will demonstrate more comfort in dealing with health care issues and the complexity of the home care environment. There is still a need to seek the experience of other health professionals to problem solve and negotiate the care needs of the patient. The nurse may be aware of MRSA but may be unaware of how it is treated in the home health arena. The nurse may be unaware of the resources available in home health and the community.

Stage 1: The clinician in this stage will assess the patient and recognize the need for assistance with the case but may be unsure as to how to proceed in the home setting. The nurse will need to interact with a more experienced nurse to ask questions and require assistance in managing the patient's care and treatment plan. The nurse may not recognize that the "spider bite" is actually a MRSA infection and may delay proper diagnosis and treatment.

? CRITICAL THINKING

1. What is another goal that would be reasonable for the nurse and patient to set?
Answer: There is a knowledge deficit displayed by the patient's elevated daily blood sugars and the behavior of covering her ingestion of candies with insulin in an unplanned manner. A reasonable goal would be for the patient to demonstrate adequate knowledge of diabetes management to incorporate her preferred food choices (candy, but sugar free) within her food plan on a daily basis. Another alternative would be to replace this refined sugar with another food option like fresh or dried fruit

2. What is the priority for care for Mrs. H?
Answer: The priority of care in this case is infection control. The patient has an open wound that is being packed in a wet-to-dry method. This type of wound has a high risk of infection. Good aseptic technique for dressing changes is needed. Additionally, the patient has diabetes, which is a known risk factor that affects wound healing. This patient also has blood sugars in a range that is higher than desired in well-managed diabetes. All of these factors combine to make infection control a priority of care.

BACK TO THE CASE

The nurse comes every morning to complete the dressing change on the right-toe amputation. The wound edges are pink, and there is minimal thin, reddish-yellow, non-odiferous drainage. On day 3 of the nursing visits, the patient calls the nurse's attention to the "spider bite" on her posterior left calf. The nurse notes that the red area is now the size of a quarter. There appears to be a cluster of pustules in the center. There is some drainage noted.

CRITICAL THINKING

1. What action should be taken by the nurse concerning this new area of concern on the left calf?
Answer: The nurse should notify the physician from the home during the nursing visit about the reddened area, the drainage, and the pustules.

2. What order by the physician should the nurse anticipate?
Answer: The nurse should anticipate an order for a wound culture to be obtained.

BACK TO THE CASE

As anticipated, the nurse received an order for a wound culture. Forty-eight hours later, the results confirm that the left posterior calf wound is community-associated MRSA.

CRITICAL THINKING

1. What are the risk factors for community-acquired MRSA in this patient?
Answer: This patient reported a spider bite, which is a frequently reported description of an initial presentation of the infection. The patient's nephew's football team had a recent outbreak of MRSA related to the use of sports equipment that is exchanged by the players. Although not showing signs of MRSA himself, the nephew may act as a carrier for the disease.

2. **What signs and symptoms of community-associated MRSA might be present in this patient?**
Answer: The patient may believe they have been "bitten by a spider." The most commonly reported symptoms are related to skin and soft tissue. The lesion may occur as single or multiple pustular, open areas ranging from 1 cm to 10 cm in size. They can be located on areas of the body such as arms, legs, buttocks, groin, or face.

3. **What is the current treatment for community-associated MRSA?**
Answer: Currently, treatment includes antibiotic therapy. Antibiotics such as sulfamethoxazole-trimethoprim and some of the tetracyclines are known to be effective against most strains of community-associated MRSA. It may also be necessary for the physician to incise and drain the wound during an office visit. Additionally, a culture taken during the incision and drainage may be obtained to further establish the MRSA infection and allow for tracking by public health officials. Due to possible colonization, the physician may also order intranasal and topical decolonization.

BACK TO THE CASE

Although the right-toe wound is healing well, the left-calf wound has now added more time to the recuperation phase. During this nursing visit, the patient states that she is worried about her finances and her job. She had used her two-week vacation time to recover from the right-toe amputation; but with the additional healing time needed for the left-calf wound infected with MRSA, she is worried that she may be fired if she does not return to work. She asks the nurse if she can help her.

CRITICAL THINKING

1. **What other health professionals should the nurse request to assist in this case?**
Answer: The nurse should contact a medical social worker (MSW) to meet with the patient regarding her financial needs. The MSW can educate the patient on the Family Medical Leave Act (FMLA). The MSW will work with Mrs. H to find other resources to help until she is able to return to work. The nurse should also contact the certified diabetes educator available through the home health agency to provide education related to dietary intake. The patient's blood sugars are not within the optimum range to prevent long-term effects of diabetes such as neuropathy and retinopathy. The patient has also reported that she has a desire consume candy daily, and this may be one of the reasons that she has not maintained good diabetic control. Once the diabetic educa-

tor has met with the patient and a change to the diabetic routine has been made, the physician may need to be contacted to adjust the insulin regimen.

BACK TO THE CASE

The diabetes educator has met with the patient and collaborated with the patient to make several changes in the diabetic regimen. These changes have allowed for the daily blood sugars to range from 120 to 150. The patient's right-toe wound is healing without infection. The patient's left-calf wound pustules are drying with no new pustules noted, and the wound appears to be responding to the antibiotic therapy. The nurse is preparing the patient for discharge by the end of the week.

? CRITICAL THINKING

1. What further action should the nurse initiate in the prevention of MRSA in this home?
Answer: A key component is to prevent the reinfection of all members of the family. These prevention strategies include:

- Keep any draining wounds covered.
- Perform good hand hygiene.
- Family members should not share items that may have had contact with the wound.
- Launder clothing that may become soiled with drainage from the wound.
- Clean surfaces that family members share with an appropriate environmental cleaner effective against the MRSA organism.

Interdisciplinary Care Plan

Problem	Plan	Interventions	Evaluation
Potential for infection at right fifth digit toe amputation site and left-calf site	Patient's right fifth digit amputation site heals without infection in 2 weeks. Patient's left-calf site heals without infection in 2 weeks.	Use sterile technique for right fifth toe amputation site. Use clean technique for dressing change to left calf. Avoid cross contamination of both wounds.	The right foot fifth digit amputation healed without infection. The left-calf open area did not heal and was colonized with MRSA.

(Continued)

Problem	Plan	Interventions	Evaluation
Knowledge deficit: Diabetes management Optimum wound healing	Patient will verbalize correct understanding of her diabetes and its connection to dietary intake in 2 visits. Patient's wounds will heal with good hygiene practice, adequate nutrition, and wound care.	Educate patient concerning the consequences of eating refined sugars on diabetes. Educate the patient concerning Hgb A1c and its relationship to optimum diabetes management. Refer to a diabetes educator for more information on dietary exchanges. Educate patient to keep wounds clean and dry. Educate patient to elevate legs as much as possible.	Patient removed candy from home and substituted fresh fruit in the dietary plan. Patient's right fifth digit amputation healed without infection.
Alteration in skin integrity	Patient's open area on left calf heals without infection in 2 weeks.	Educate patient to cover site at all times and make dressing changes as ordered by physician. Educated patient in antibiotic therapy ordered for left-calf wound.	Patient's open area was diagnosed as MRSA by culture.
Inability to perform ADL/IADL independently	Patient will manage ADL/IADL in 3 weeks.	Home health aide for bathing to assist patient 2 times a week until patient resumes self-care for ADL.	Patient is able to remain in her home with support of agency personnel.
Anxiety	Patient will verbalize a decrease in anxiety level (2–3/10) with regard to finances and employment in 1 week.	Refer to MSW to educate patient with regard to financial needs and the federal Family Medical Leave Act (FMLA) for this crisis.	Patient contacts her employer for the FMLA (and keeps her job for 12 weeks). MSW assists patient in receiving temporary financial assistance to remain in her home.

REFERENCES & RESOURCES

[1] M. Mendyk, "Community-associated MRSA: Coming to a patient near you? *The Nurse Practitioner*, 33(3):27–32, 2008.

[2] G. Moran et al., "Methicillin-resistant *S. aureus* infections among patients in the emergency department," *New England Journal of Medicine*, 355(7):666–674, 2006.

[3] Sanofi Aventis U. S. LLC, "Lantus®Home," Retrieved from http://www.lantus.com/default.aspx, Nov 2009

Case 13.3 Influenza

By Sharon D. Martin, RN, MSN, PhD(c)

This case study illustrates how the home health nurse works with the patient, the patient's family, with public health, and with health care providers in the community to care for a patient with a highly communicable disease. The patient, Mrs. P, is a full-time bank teller, wife, and mother of a 3-year-old girl. She has no chronic disease and takes no medications except birth control pills. She was well until yesterday when she started complaining of a cough, general malaise, and body aches in the morning before going to work. She has no paid sick leave, so she went to work hoping to feel better as the day wore on. When she returned home in the evening her symptoms were worse; she had chills, sweats, severe muscle and body aches, productive cough, headache, and fatigue. She went to bed, leaving her husband to prepare supper and care for their child. The next morning she was no better and reluctantly called in sick. She is currently bedfast. Her husband is concerned but hesitant to stay home to care for her as he has only been employed as a maintenance man for 8 months. He has paid sick leave for himself but no paid vacation or personal time accrued. He does have employer-provided health insurance for the family. As no family members live close by he asked a neighbor to drive his wife to the doctor that morning. He dropped his daughter at her usual day care on his way to work. Coordination with family, primary care provider (PCP), and public health agency is key to the management of this case.

Clinical Case Studies in Home Health Care, First Edition. Edited by Leslie Neal-Boylan.
© 2011 John Wiley & Sons, Inc. Published 2011 by John Wiley & Sons, Inc.

Reimbursement Considerations

The patient is too young for Medicare and not financially eligible for Medicaid. The private insurance provided by the husband's employer will be called to determine home care benefits and for preauthorization of visits. The public health department should be contacted to determine their involvement in terms of the nasal swab test for influenza as well as for nursing follow-up visits to the patient, family, and any followup deemed necessary with the places of employment or the day care of the child.

ORDERS FOR HOME CARE

Patient: 28-year-old Caucasian female
Diagnosis: Potential influenza
Current medications: Oral birth control
Relevant past medical history:
- Previously healthy with no chronic diseases
- No smoking history
- Hospitalized only for delivery of daughter

RN: Assess and evaluate.

THE HOME VISIT

The home health nurse serves a rural area with limited public health nursing. Therefore, the home health agency received a request from the patient's PCP for a home visit to evaluate the situation and report findings. The patient had called the doctor in the morning for an appointment; but was unable to get to his office because the neighbor had been unable to drive. Mrs. P was too sick to drive herself and was unwilling to call an ambulance. The home health nurse phoned the patient to confirm the information provided by the doctor and to schedule the visit. The patient said that she was weak and in bed and that the nurse should enter through the unlocked back door.

Relevant Community Resources

Public health services

The PCP instructed the nurse to take respiratory precautions in view of the patient's symptoms. In addition, the nurse called the public health office in the next county to inquire about outbreaks of communicable respiratory disease and discovered that there was an outbreak of influenza in the county where the patient worked, but not in the county where she lived.

The nurse donned her fit-tested, N-95 mask before entering the home. She left her home health bag in the car, bringing only those tools necessary for the visit. She saw no evidence of pets or environmental hazards as she walked toward the home. Walking through the home, she noted it was a small ranch that was neat, clean, and fresh smelling; that there was hot and cold running water and a full bathroom in the hallway to the bedrooms; and that there was a modern kitchen. The usual evidence of a child was seen around the home. No pills or medications were seen. No evidence of smoking, illegal substances, or weapons was observed.

The patient, Mrs. P, was home alone lying in a small bedroom in a twin bed with the shades pulled. She was weak but could speak coherently, was a good historian, and showed no confusion. She frequently coughed thick, white sputum into tissues and then disposed of the tissues into a paper bag set near the bed. A small, half-empty bottle of sports drink sat on the bedside table next to a bottle of acetaminophen.

After introducing herself, explaining the need for the mask, and performing hand hygiene, the nurse began the assessment. Mrs. P complained of severe body aches, extreme fatigue, and loss of appetite. "I feel like I got hit by a truck," she said. A sports drink, 250 mL, was the only fluid consumed since her husband left for work 4 hours prior. She had not urinated since before her husband left for work. "Good thing," she says, "I don't think I could make it to the bathroom. I'm so weak." She had had no solid food for 24 hours and could not provide an estimate of her fluid intake for the past 24 hours. She had taken 1000 mg of acetaminophen 4 hours earlier which, she said, helped control the muscle aches, chills, and sweats. She had not taken her oral birth control medication since becoming ill.

She was of the Christian faith but did not regularly attend church. She explained that she was in the guest bedroom rather than in her own bed to avoid coughing on her husband or keeping him up. She worried about making her child sick. No one at her workplace, at her husband's workplace, or at her child's day care was sick to her knowledge.

During the physical exam, the nurse gathered the following data:

- Temperature 101.8 degrees Fahrenheit
- Rhonchi on inspiration, clear with cough
- Frequent cough with white sputum production

Cultural Competence

Mrs. P is a young Caucasian wife and mother from a rural area who has no family support nearby. The nurse will need to provide encouragement for the husband who will need to provide care for his wife while protecting the health and well-being of himself, his daughter, and members of the community. Financial stressors need to be recognized.

- Respiratory rate 24, unlabored
- Skin pink, dry, flushed, poor turgor
- Heart rate 103, regular rhythm
- BP 90/50
- Throat slightly reddened, no pus or drainage
- Abdomen soft, pain free on palpation, with bowel sounds in all four quadrants
- O^2 via portable pulse oximetry 95%
- Denies nausea, vomiting, diarrhea, difficulty breathing or shortness of breath, pain or pressure in the chest, or dizziness

The primary concerns Mrs. P expressed to the nurse during the assessment were:

- Being out of work with no paid sick leave
- Care of her child as she is the primary childcare provider when the child is not in day care and her husband sometimes must work overtime
- Being able to pay for any medicine prescribed, as the family's health insurance does not cover prescription medications

---

Neal Theory Implications

Stage 3: The nurse in this stage collaborates effectively with the patient, family, PCP, health insurance provider, and public health department and is autonomous with the clinical aspects of the case and logistical aspects of working within the agency.

Stage 2: The nurse in this stage may not feel comfortable collaborating with the public health department or PCP or working with the patient's family to develop a plan of care for the patient, family, and community.

Stage 1: The nurse in this stage can assess the patient and recognize abnormal findings that require intervention but may be unsure how to manage a case involving a public health agency.

?	**CRITICAL THINKING**

1. **The nurse was instructed by the PCP to follow respiratory precautions in view of the patient's symptoms. What constitutes "respiratory precautions" according to the Centers for Disease Control (CDC)?**

Answer: The CDC has several types of precautions that relate to respiratory precautions, and the PCP's instructions were unclear as to which the nurse was expected to use. The best way to get the latest precautions that relate to respiratory precautions from the CDC is to go to http://www.cdc.gov and search for respiratory precautions. Another helpful site is http://www.cdc.gov/flu/professionals/infectioncontrol/resphygiene.htm [1].

Generally, for influenza-like–illness (ILI) and known influenza (flu), one is required to follow respiratory hygiene/cough etiquette, droplet precautions, and at times airborne precautions, all of which might relate to respiratory precautions. Flu is also known to be transmitted via contact, so contact precautions should also be in place for the nurse entering the home. These recommendations change over time and are based on the epidemiology of the flu involved; therefore, it is best to retrieve the latest recommendations from the CDC when seeing a patient with a communicable disease.

2. **The nurse had discovered from the public health department that there was an outbreak of influenza in the county where the patient worked. According to the CDC, what infection control precautions should the nurse have used when entering the home of a patient with potential influenza?**

Answer: This can be answered using the information the nurse already gathered from the http://www.cdc.gov or http://www.cdc.gov/flu/professionals/infectioncontrol/resphygiene.htm web pages [1]. There is nothing in this case study to suggest that this is pandemic flu, so the nurse should explore the recommendations for seasonal flu.

3. **While the nurse was walking to the door and through the home, she assessed the patient's environment. Why would she do that?**

Answer: The nurse gathers important data through the observation of the patient's environment. The nurse uses all senses while approaching and walking through the home environment, especially on the first visit. Safety is always important, so the nurse watches for any items, such as guns, or behaviors, such as street-drug use. The nurse also watches for pets or other living creatures that might pose a hazard to the nurse or patient, as pets and other living creatures can be vectors of disease. Finally, in view of the patient's respiratory illness, it is useful to note any other obvious risk factors, such as evidence of smoking, mold, or mildew in the home.

4. The nurse left her bag in the car and brought in only what she needed for the visit. Why would she do that, and what tools would she need for the visit?

Answer: The bag can become a vector of disease when contaminated and then carried from home to home and back to the agency. In this case the nurse needs the following tools for the visit: hand hygiene supplies, solution to disinfect tools, a stethoscope that can be disinfected, a means to take the patient's temperature that can be disposed of or disinfected, a pen light that can be disinfected, disposable tongue blade, nonsterile gloves, portable pulse oximeter that can be disinfected, and a BP cuff that can be disinfected.

5. One of the goals of the home health nurse is to intervene in order to avoid unnecessary patient hospitalization. After assessing the patient, what was the nurse's first priority of care for Mrs. P?

Answer: Though it is common to focus on the respiratory problems of the patient, fluid and electrolyte balance are crucial priorities and common problems for people afflicted with ILI. The lack of adequate fluid over the past 24 hours created the potential for dehydration. The likelihood of dehydration was supported by other physical findings. An immediately increased by-mouth fluid intake and a plan for ongoing increased fluid intake were needed in order to prevent Mrs. P from potentially needing hospitalization for intravenous rehydration. Oral rehydration will also help to control her temperature, increase her BP, decrease her heart rate, decrease her feeling of malaise, and increase her strength. Lack of food is not a problem for several days as long as she gets some calories via the sports drink. She has no chronic diseases that need attention. (For example, diabetes would complicate the case.)

6. What problem would rehydration create that the nurse should plan for with Mrs. P?

Answer: Mrs. P will have to make frequent trips to the bathroom, something she does not want to do because she feels weak and is in pain. This should be discussed with Mrs. P so that she understands the critical need for rehydration. In addition, the nurse may have some suggestions for addressing the need for frequent bathroom trips.

7. What is the nurse's priority of care for herself and for other people with whom the nurse will interact that day?

Answer: Though it is unknown whether the patient has the flu, it is wise to follow the guidelines recommended by the state or local health department or the CDC for infection control of flu until flu is ruled out, especially in view of the symptoms and the known outbreak in the county where the patient works. A primary concern of the nurse should always be to prevent infection transmission both from the patient to herself and, thereafter, from the nurse to others, including patients, staff of the home care agency, and the nurse's family. The nurse may have contaminated her clothing by failing to observe contact and droplet precautions. In view of that, it would be wise to use the change of clothes that home health nurses carry with them in the car. It would be useful to consult with the public health department or CDC to determine the proper barrier precautions when reentering the home.

8. What is the nurse's priority for the patient's family?
Answer: Infection control is crucial for home care of the patient with flu. The husband must be taught the basics of caring for his wife at home so that she can recover without infecting either himself or their child.

9. What is the nurse's priority in terms of public health?
Answer: If the patient does have flu, it must be contained to the home in order to protect the community from infection. In addition, if flu is present, the public health department may want to be involved to evaluate any additional cases in Mr. and Mrs. P's workplaces or in the day care of their child. Generally, the flu patient is cared for at home unless hospitalization is necessary.

 BACK TO THE CASE

The nurse explains to Mrs. P that she will call the PCP from the home to provide a report of her findings and to receive any additional orders. Since the PCP is with another patient, the nurse leaves a report with the PCP's office nurse but asks for a callback on her cell phone as soon as possible. Returning to Mrs. P, the nurse finds Mrs. P willing and able to consume the rest of the sports drink and agreeing to increase her fluid intake to drinking every 15 to 30 minutes while awake until she starts urinating in good quantities. She says she has plenty of sports drink and water in the refrigerator; the nurse confirms that. The nurse discovers that the master bedroom has a small toilet with a sink close to the bed.

During the discussion, the cell phone rings and the PCP's office nurse reports the following to the home health nurse on behalf of the PCP:

- The patient should be treated empirically, as if she has influenza with appropriate precautions.
- No antiviral medications are ordered at this time.
- The family is to be taught appropriate infection control and care of the influenza patient at home.
- A nasal swab should be obtained and sent to the lab to determine if it is influenza and to determine the subtype and strain.
- The patient is to remain out of work until she has been fever free for at least 24 hours without the aid of antipyretic medication.

- The patient should increase her fluid intake and take acetaminophen as needed to control the fever and malaise.
- The patient should be seen by the PCP if certain problems arise.

The nurse explains all this to Mrs. P who replies, "I can't be out of work that long! We can't afford it."

? CRITICAL THINKING

1. What should the nurse discuss with Mrs. P first?
Answer: Mrs. P is upset about the financial pressure her illness will create in the family. Therefore, the nurse should encourage her to discuss this first. Then she should discuss the other concerns she had expressed—the lack of paid sick leave and the care of her child (as the patient is the primary childcare provider when the child is not in day care and her husband sometimes must work overtime). Mrs. P is unlikely to be able to focus on other information or teaching from the nurse while she is upset about these issues.

2. How can the nurse help the patient to get adequate fluid in view of the fact she is alone and unable to walk to the refrigerator frequently?
Answer: Fluid can be left in a cooler near the bedside.

3. What is a simple solution to the problem of having to walk a long way to the bathroom?
Answer: Move the patient to the master bedroom which has a toilet and sink near the bed. Ask the husband to change the guest-room bedding and then move into the guest room.

4. The nurse did not anticipate having to take a nasal swab and did not bring it to the visit. In view of the other orders just received, how can she make the return visit most efficient?
Answer: Arrange to return after the husband is home from work so the family teaching can take place at the same time the nasal swab is done.

5. Reimbursement is always a critical issue in home health. What is the likely source of funding for the visits made to Mrs. P?
Answer: Many private insurance plans cover home health care. The insurance company should be called to determine coverage, how many visits will be authorized, and any co-pay if applicable. The public health department may be willing to provide the nasal swab kit and cover the cost of the lab analysis or they may want to do the lab analysis themselves to determine if it is flu, as many labs do not have the capability of identifying flu subtypes and strains. In addition, the public

health department may wish to continue visits using public health nurses as flu cases may fall under their jurisdiction.

6. The PCP said Mrs. P must be seen in the office if certain problems arise. What problems would the PCP most likely have listed as reasons for Mrs. P to be seen in the office immediately?
Answer: Emergency warning signs requiring PCP evaluation are currently found at http://www.cdc.gov/flu/takingcare.htm#howlong [2] but these can change over time so the nurse should explore http://www.cdc.gov and http://www.flu.gov to determine if more recent warning signs have been posted. They are: difficulty breathing or shortness of breath, pain or pressure in the chest or abdomen, sudden dizziness, confusion, severe or persistent vomiting, flu-like symptoms that improve but then return with fever and worse cough.

7. What problem must the nurse address in view of the fact Mrs. P did not take her birth control pill yesterday?
Answer: She should take 2 birth control pills today and resume her normal medications. Additional forms of birth control may be needed if she engages in sex and has not been taking her oral birth control medication.

8. What are the principles of caring for the influenza patient at home that will be taught to the husband that evening?
Answer: The CDC recommendations for care of the influenza patient at home change over time and based upon the epidemiology of the virus, so the nurse should find this information at http://www.cdc.gov when it is needed. The current information is found at http://www.cdc.gov/flu/takingcare.htm#howlong [2] and http://www.flu.gov/individualfamily/caregivers/index.html [3] but these may change. However, the basic principles of care of the flu patient at home are to separate the sick from the well with a closed door when possible, have a bathroom assigned to the sick person when possible, keep pets and children away from the sick person as they are unable to understand or follow infection control strategies, assign one reliable caregiver to the sick person who is able to understand and follow infection control strategies as taught by the nurse. Care should be taken when changing bedding of the sick to avoid sending the virus into the air; normal clothes washing technique kills the virus. Flu patients do not need separate utensils or dishes; normal soap and hot water hand washing of dishes or dishwasher use kills the virus. If the husband and daughter are asymptomatic and able to get flu immunization they should do so despite the fact that it won't prevent them from getting the disease if they have already been exposed and infection has already begun. Immunization may prevent or decrease the severity of disease if they have not yet been exposed but the vaccine will only cover certain subtypes and strains each year.

Interdisciplinary Care Plan

Problem	Goal/Plan	Intervention	Evaluation
Knowledge deficit disease process	Patient and family will verbalize understanding of disease process by end of second visit Nasal swab to lab on day 1.	Teach patient and family about flu, infection control, care of flu patient at home, and signs and symptoms requiring a PCP visit.	Patient and family verbalize and demonstrate infection control, care of patient at home, and signs and symptoms requiring a PCP visit.
Dehydration	Oral rehydration immediately and ongoing every 15 minutes until urinating at least 30 mL/hour.	Oral sports drink or water as tolerated immediately and ongoing every 15 minutes.	Pt is urinating at least 30 mL per hr; other signs and symptoms of dehydration subside.
Social stressors: lack of social supports; financial pressures	Patient and family will care for patient at home with husband continuing to work and daughter continuing in day care.	Assist patient and husband in development of strategies for the patient's safety while alone, as well as access to fluid, bathroom, telephone, medication, and food as desired.	Patient is safe alone at home. Husband is caring for the child.
Personal care deficit	Ineligible for home health aide assistance. Husband to provide assistance with bathing in the evening.	Husband providing care outside of work hours.	Patient is clean and dry. Bedding is clean and dry.
Altered respiratory function	Cough and deep breathe as needed and hourly.	Demonstrate cough and deep breathing.	Lungs are clear bilaterally.
Fever, malaise, muscle pain	Acetaminophen 1000 mg every 6 hours by mouth as needed	Patient is to self-medicate every 6 hours as needed,	Temperature is within normal range Malaise and myalgia are minimal.

Problem	Goal/Plan	Intervention	Evaluation
Public health infection control	Visitors to home limited to those absolutely necessary. Interaction with patient is limited to 1 designated caregiver: the husband. Nurse visits only as needed and in PPE as recommended by public health/CDC. Nursing tools should be disposable or disinfected before reuse. Patient is out of work until temperature returns to normal for 24 hours without antipyretics.	Teach the patient and family public health restrictions.	Visitors are limited or avoided with the husband serving as primary caregiver. Patient is out of work as recommended.
Potential unplanned pregnancy	Patient resumes oral birth control.	Patient is instructed to resume oral birth control and/or use an additional method.	Patient and husband maintain a plan for fertility.

📖 **REFERENCES & RESOURCES**

[1] Centers for Disease Control and Prevention, "Respiratory Hygiene/Cough Etiquette in Healthcare Settings," http://www.cdc.gov/flu/professionals/infectioncontrol/resphygiene.htm

[2] Centers for Disease Control and Prevention, "The Flu: What to Do If You Get Sick," http://www.cdc.gov/flu/takingcare.htm#howlong

[3] FLU.GOV, "Caregivers," http://www.flu.gov/individualfamily/caregivers/index.html

[4] A. Knebel and S.J. Phillips (eds.), *Home Health Care during an Influenza Pandemic: ISSUES and Resources*, AHRQ Publication No. 08-0018, Agency for Healthcare Research and Quality, July 2008.

Section 14

Endocrine

Case 14.1 Diabetes Mellitus Type 1

By Caryl Ann O'Reilly, CNS, CDE, MBA

Type 1 diabetes mellitus (DM) presents very different challenges from type 2 diabetes, both to the patient and to the home health nurse. While the preponderance of home health patients with diabetes will have type 2 DM, it is important to understand the unique needs of persons with type 1 DM. This case is presented to illustrate the needs of a person with newly diagnosed type 1 DM. Although the patient is an adolescent, the clinical issues are relevant in other age groups.

John is a 16-year-old high school student who was recently admitted to the hospital following a bout of severe nausea, vomiting, and weakness. He was diagnosed with new-onset type 1 diabetes and diabetic ketoacidosis. During the 3-day stay in the hospital, John and his parents were given instructions in blood glucose monitoring, insulin administration, and nutrition. He was seen by an endocrinologist who ordered Lantus insulin 14 units daily and Humalog insulin 5 units before each meal. No other medications were ordered. Blood pressure was within normal range. John had an 8-pound weight loss in the past 2 weeks, now weighing 165 pounds. His height is 5 feet, 11 inches. While in the hospital, John self-injected his insulin using prefilled insulin pens, for both Lantus and Humalog.

John is a sophomore in high school and plays basketball for the junior varsity. He is the eldest of 3 children and lives at home with his parents and siblings. John's grandfather lives with the family and has diabetes and limited vision and has lost 3 toes on his left foot. John will be seeing a pediatric endocrinologist the week following discharge.

Clinical Case Studies in Home Health Care, First Edition. Edited by Leslie Neal-Boylan.
© 2011 John Wiley & Sons, Inc. Published 2011 by John Wiley & Sons, Inc.

> **Cultural Competence**
>
> John is a teenager and, as such, is a member of a culture that holds peer acceptance in the highest value. It will be challenging for John to learn how he can manage his DM and still do everything his peers do.

ORDERS FOR HOME CARE

Diagnosis: Diabetes mellitus type 1
Medications:
- Lantus insulin 14 units once a day in the a.m.
- Humalog insulin 5 units before each meal

Relevant past medical history:
- Healthy up until this point
- No acute or chronic illnesses or injuries

RN: Teach diabetes management skills, including insulin administration and glucose monitoring. Notify physician if blood glucose <60 or >240 mg/dL. The managed care insurer has authorized one visit for evaluation.

? CRITICAL THINKING

1. Before contacting the family to set up an appointment for the initial visit, what are some issues that the nurse should consider?
Answer: Assessing the health literacy of the patient and family is a first step in determining the best approach to help them successfully manage newly-diagnosed diabetes. The nurse should review and assess the patient's and family's understanding of survival skills and provide strategies that reduce risk while the patient is learning to self-manage his diabetes. Look for age-appropriate involvement in self-management. Parents should be overseeing activities but John should be coached and supported to take on the tasks of daily diabetes management.

Insulin is a *high risk* medication. It is essential that the patient and family understand the timing, action, and duration of the different types of insulin being used. Both Lantus and Humalog are colorless. Confusing them would be dangerous.

Regarding blood glucose monitoring, it is important that the patient and family understand when to measure blood glucose and what the numbers mean. They need to understand what to do based on the glucometer readings.

Meal planning and the symptoms and treatments for hypoglycemia should be discussed. Meal planning is always a significant concern of persons newly diagnosed with diabetes. In this case, the patient is of normal weight and is an active, healthy teenager. Recommend that it is best to have regular meals and snacks with attention to blood glucose readings around those meals and snacks. This information will help to determine if meals are appropriate and if the insulin regimen is working. Concentrated sweets should be limited and sugared drinks should be avoided unless a patient is treating low blood glucose. "Sugar-free" foods are not recommended since many have large amounts of carbohydrates. The patient may be willing to keep a food journal, along with the blood glucose monitoring information. A more detailed meal planning session can be held at a later date.

The patient and family should be taught that mild symptoms of hypoglycemia should be treated with 15 grams of carbohydrate, followed by waiting 15 minutes and then retesting the blood sugar. If necessary, retreat with 15 grams of carbohydrates. If low blood glucose is severe and the patient is unresponsive or unable to take food by mouth, 911 should be called and then glucagon administered.

While generally not as sudden as hypoglycemia, hyperglycemia can present risks, so the nurse needs to instruct the patient and family accordingly. Hyperglycemia should be addressed with emphasis on when to use ketone sticks and when to call the physician or seek emergency assistance.

Reimbursement Considerations

The patient's family is enrolled in managed care and requires authorizations for visits followed by timed reports. Overutilization is scrutinized, as is underutilization. Where there is appropriate need for additional services, such as social work, it is expected to be documented and provided.

THE HOME VISIT

The nurse arranges the initial home visit with John's mother and arrives to find John and both of his parents present for the visit. John's grandfather is not in the room during the visit. John and his parents appear somewhat nervous, exhausted, and overwhelmed with the new diagnosis and the hospital experience.

The nurse assesses the patient and notes the following:

• John and his parents seem willing to learn.
• John has led a normal teenage life up until his hospitalization.

- John's parents appear interested in and supportive of John's care.
- John and his parents have several misconceptions about diabetes based on the grandfather's experiences with DM.

The nurse, John, and his parents outline the goals for this and subsequent visits:

- To learn dietary management of DM type 1
- To learn how and when to measure blood glucose and what the test results mean in terms of DM management
- To learn how to manage medication in relation to the timing of meals, activities, and a normal adolescent life
- To learn self-management of DM during unstructured times such as weekends, holidays, and athletic and after school activities

The home health nurse also realizes that there could be a psychosocial impact on John as a result of his illness. She makes a mental note to request an order for medical social work (MSW) to assess John's risk for depression and high-risk behaviors.

> **Relevant Community Resources**
>
> Local support groups for parents and teenagers with diabetes
> Insulin pump support groups
> Local chapters of national diabetes organizations

During the first visit, the nurse reviews and observes insulin dosing and administration skills. This is an opportunity to discuss the timing and action of the different insulins and stress the importance of avoiding medication errors. The nurse suggests that it may be useful to put a rubber band around the rapid-acting insulin (Humalog). ("R" for "rubber" band and "R" for "rapid"-acting insulin.)

The nurse asks the patient to demonstrate how to monitor blood glucose. Does the patient know how to check the monitor for accuracy, care for the strips, and perform meter coding, if necessary? The nurse reviews the blood glucose record stored in the glucometer and discusses plans for sharps disposal. The patient is encouraged to keep a record of blood glucose readings according to date, time, before and / or after meals, bedtime, and so forth.

The nurse asks the patient and family if they have any questions about the insulin, insulin pens, or glucometer. Each of these has a customer service 800# that can provide ongoing support and information. An emergency or sick-day box should always be available. This should contain emergency phone numbers, ketone sticks, glucagon, regular soda, can or packet of broth, extra pen needles, lancet, and meter strips.

Everyone in the family should know where these emergency supplies are kept and when and how to use them.

Before leaving the home the home health nurse communicates with the referring health care provider, reconciling medications, reporting findings, and making appropriate recommendations. The nurse discusses the need for communication with school and the school nurse to help John transition back to classes and to discuss a medical management plan with the patient, family, and referring provider.

Neal Theory Implications

Stage 3: The professional in this stage collaborates with other disciplines to provide quality care for the patient. This nurse recognizes the potential for a significant psychosocial impact on the patient and family due to the DM 1 diagnosis. This nurse enlists a number of resources both from within the agency and in the community to assist this family through this transition. This nurse also looks to the future for this teenage boy and plans care and teaching to help the family anticipate John's future needs and concerns.

Stage 2: The professional in this stage is likely to be more focused on the patient's disease and on assisting the family to adjust to the diagnosis and is less likely to be aware of or recommend various community and national resources that might assist this family. This nurse will focus on teaching and interventions that are necessary for the initial needs of the patient and family.

Stage 1: The clinician in this stage may not consider the impact of an adolescent's life on his diabetes management.

? CRITICAL THINKING

1. When newly diagnosed with a chronic illness, there are many concerns and fears that patients may face. When a child is diagnosed, there are likely fears, anger, and depression experienced by the whole family. "Will my child have a normal life?" "Am I going to go blind like my grandfather?" "How did this happen to my child? What could I have done to prevent it?" How should the nurse address these questions?
Answer: Family support is important right from the time of diagnosis. Would the family benefit from social work intervention? Are there

religious or cultural factors or beliefs that may interfere with clinically accurate thinking? It is likely that John and his parents are concerned about how diabetes will affect John given the complications his grandfather has experienced from DM. It is important, with the help of the MSW, to address these concerns. The nurse should coach and support both the patient and family in self-care management strategies to give John more control over his diabetes. Reassure them that with new treatment paradigms and advanced knowledge about how to maintain blood glucose control, John can take control of his diabetes. With planning, he is able to continue to play sports, drive a car, go to college, and pursue all of the plans and dreams he and his family may have for John. The family may express concern about the other children in the household. While type 1 DM is not highly genetic, there are studies being done to track family members of newly diagnosed type 2 diabetics. The nurse will refer the family to their health care provider for information.

BACK TO THE CASE

Earlier in the visit, the nurse encouraged John and his parents to identify long-term goals for their visits. However, before leaving, the nurse asks the patient if there is one short-term goal he would like to work on for the next week. John agrees that he will not drink regular soda for this week. On a scale of 1–10 how confident does he feel about being successful with his goal? John says, "About 8!"

CRITICAL THINKING

1. When goal setting with a patient, it is important that the goal be the patient's choice, not the clinician's. The nurse can and should help the patient refine his goals. For example, if John had said, "I won't eat anything with sugar from now on," the nurse might help him narrow the time line and be more specific about one particular food or drink. It would also be a good opportunity to introduce the role of carbohydrates as fuel for energy.

When goal setting, if the confidence level stated is less than 7 on a scale of 1–10, the goal will probably not be successful. The nurse will coach the patient to change or refine the goal to one about which he can be more confident. This can help to avoid feelings of frustration and failure.

Table 14.1.1. The patient's record.

Date	Before Breakfast	After Breakfast	Before Lunch	After Lunch	Before Dinner	After Dinner
11/9	116	145	89	288	202	312
11/10	124	68	243	289	112	242
11/11	119					

 BACK TO CASE

The nurse requests and receives authorization from the insurer and the physician to continue visiting the patient. She contacts the family to schedule another visit. The patient will be returning to school in 2 days. John's mother indicates that the blood glucose readings have been erratic, and she is concerned about her son returning to school. The nurse asks John to show her his blood glucose log, meter, and any other record keeping he may have so they can review them.

The patient has good documentation of his blood glucose readings both before and after meals for the 2 days since the last visit (Table 14.1.1).

? **CRITICAL THINKING**

1. What factors are influencing the blood glucose readings? Remember the insulin regimen is Lantus 14 units daily with 5 units of Humalog before each meal. A review of the patient's meals reveals the following:

Day 1   Breakfast: Bowl of cereal, milk, toast with butter
Lunch: Meatball hero sandwich with diet soda, banana
Dinner: Grilled chicken with rice and vegetables, apple, milk

There are a number of factors that influence glucose control; but, for this patient with type 1 diabetes, the insulin regimen may require adjusting. Lantus insulin, basal insulin, is usually titrated up or down until fasting morning glucose is approximately 100 mg/dL. Based on John's record, we can conclude that the Lantus dose of 14 units is providing the basal coverage. However, the mealtime readings are concerning. What conversation might you have with the family and health care provider to improve the glucose control?

Answer: The insulin regimen that has been ordered is most suitable for persons with insulin-requiring type 2 diabetes. These are generally older persons who do not vary their activity or diet very much. John is an active adolescent whose activity and meal schedules may not be predictable. He would probably benefit from a more flexible regimen. On day 1 of the glucose log entry sheet, he had a large lunch, perhaps as much as 80–90 grams of carbohydrates. On day 2, he was not hungry in the morning and had some toast for breakfast, perhaps 15–20 grams of carbohydrate. The set dose of 5 units of Humalog before each meal did not provide satisfactory individualized prandial coverage.

John should continue to keep his log, including food entries, so that the pediatric endocrinologist will have the information necessary to determine John's insulin sensitivity and his insulin-to-carbohydrate ratio. With this information, a more suitable insulin regimen can be initiated.

2. What other factors will have to be considered to provide John with an individualized diabetes regime?
Answer: There is no set answer, especially when someone is newly diagnosed. The goal should be to keep within a safe target range while gathering data about what does affect the blood glucose. On basketball practice days, John should include extra carbohydrates before, during, and after practice to provide the energy needed to carry out the activity without having a hypoglycemic episode. He should be coached to inject his insulin in his abdomen, not in his arms or legs. His limbs are actively involved in the exercise; and insulin absorption may be increased, leading to an increased risk for hypoglycemia.

On weekends, John's activity level may be very different from his activity level during the week. By keeping a detailed journal, he will be able to look for patterns that will give him and his health care team the necessary information for insulin and carbohydrate adjustments. John needs to become a "detective!"

3. What is *insulin sensitivity factor*? What is *insulin-to-carbohydrate ratio*?
Answer: *Insulin sensitivity factor* (sometimes called *correction factor*) is the amount of mg/dl blood glucose is lowered with 1 unit of regular insulin. A starting point that is often used is that 1 unit of insulin lowers blood glucose 30 mg/dL. This is dependent on age, weight, insulin resistance, duration of diabetes, other medications, and other factors.

Insulin-to-carbohydrate ratio is the number of grams of carbohydrates metabolized by 1 unit of regular insulin. A starting point for this ratio is 1 unit of insulin for 15 grams of carbohydrate. This, too, has to be adjusted based on weight, body mass index, activity, and so forth. Both of these formulae are used for setting the rates in insulin pump therapy. It is likely that John will be able to use pump therapy once he and his endocrinologist feel he is ready.

4. What other considerations might be brought to this family and adolescent before discharge?

Answer: Chronic illness is always a difficult diagnosis to hear, but when it involves a child there can be a sense of guilt, grief, fear, accusation, and shame by parents and child. It is helpful to bring these feelings to the surface, acknowledge them and let the family know that this is a normal response. Help them to find support through the social work referral, Juvenile Diabetes Association, and the American Diabetes Association. There are a number of web sites that are helpful.

It is not useful to discuss the long term complications of diabetes at this point. Long term complications of diabetes do not usually present until at least 5 years after diagnosis. It is helpful to remind the patient and family that all of those complications are a result of prolonged hyperglycemia and poor management.

5. How will members of the interdisciplinary team communicate with one another?

Answer: Team members will communicate through the agency's documentation system where available, telephone and face-to-face meetings, and case conferences when warranted. Multi-discipline care plans are kept up to date and provide sufficient information to link interventions in a meaningful and professional manner.

Interdisciplinary Care Plan

Problem	Goal/Plan	Intervention	Evaluation
Knowledge deficit regarding disease process	Patient and family will verbalize understanding of type 1 diabetes within 1 week.	Teach patient and family about type I diabetes. Coach family and patient about the importance of learning self-management skills and developing confidence.	Patient will participate more fully in self-management of his diabetes, and parents will be available as coaches and support.
Knowledge deficit regarding insulin therapy	Patient will understand the importance of taking his insulin as ordered in 2 days. Patient will understand the action, timing, and peak of his insulin in 1 week.	Coach and support the patient in his understanding of what insulin is, what role it plays in metabolism, and why he needs to provide it on a regular basis.	Patient will gain skill and confidence in managing his insulin regime successfully and will not hesitate to ask for help when he is not sure about timing or doses of insulin.

(Continued)

Problem	Goal/Plan	Intervention	Evaluation
Deficit in knowledge regarding blood glucose monitoring and patterns	Patient will verbalize understanding of both hyper- and hypoglycemia, what the signs are, and how to treat within 2 weeks.	Coach patient about diabetes self-management, how the medications work, and the importance of monitoring blood glucose. Work toward the patient-stated goal.	Patient is able to verbalize how to recognize abnormal blood glucose patterns, how to treat them, and when to call the physician, nurse, or 911.
Ineffective coping of family system	Patient and son are more able to understand and cope with sequelae of diabetes process within 3 weeks.	Nurse will provide information about community resources and diabetes self-management programs in their area.	Nurse will evaluate and document the patient's and family's moods in addition to allowing the patient and family to express their feelings, fears, and concerns.
Sharing the onset of chronic illness with those persons who are in a need-to-know position	Information will be shared with those who need to know within 1 week.	Discuss with family the need to inform school, athletic coach, and anyone who may need to know about John's newly diagnosed DM in 1 week.	Successful collaboration with health care team including school nurse

REFERENCES & RESOURCES

[1] American Association of Diabetic Educators, *A Core Curriculum for Diabetes Educators* (5th ed.), American Association of Diabetes Educators, 2003.
[2] B. Childs, M. Cypress and G. Spollett (eds.), *Complete Nurse's Guide to Diabetes Care*, American Diabetes Association, 2008.

Case 14.2 Diabetes Mellitus Type 2

By Caryl Ann O'Reilly, CNS, CDE, MBA

Many home care cases involve a diagnosis of diabetes, occasionally as the initiating diagnosis, but more frequently as a comorbid condition that affects the overall well-being of the patient. This case demonstrates the challenge of identifying barriers to self-managing diabetes in an elderly patient who has the effects of long-term diabetes and persistent exposure to hyperglycemia. Mrs. J is a 75-year-old widow and lives alone. She has been independent in her diabetes care since the diagnosis of type 2 diabetes 22 years ago. She has been referred to home health services following a recent hospitalization as a result of a fall in the home.

Following the fall, Mrs. J used an emergency response unit to summon help. Her blood glucose was 43 mg/dL when emergency medical services (EMS) arrived. The patient was belligerent, refusing to be transported to the emergency room (ER). She was given intravenous dextrose and emergency treatment for a heavily bleeding cut on the forearm. She ultimately agreed to go to the hospital. Mrs. J brought her current list of medications with her to the ER.

Current medications:
- Lantus insulin 30 units at bedtime
- Apidra insulin sliding scale three times a day; before meals
- Aspirin 81 mg once a day
- Folic Acid 1 mg once a day
- Glyburide 10 mg twice a day
- Labetalol 200 mg twice a day
- Metoclopramide 10 mg once a day

Clinical Case Studies in Home Health Care, First Edition. Edited by Leslie Neal-Boylan.
© 2011 John Wiley & Sons, Inc. Published 2011 by John Wiley & Sons, Inc.

- Metoprolol tartrate 25 mg twice a day
- Plavix 75 mg once a day
- Simvastin 40 mg at bedtime

Diagnoses at time of admission:

- Type 2 diabetes, controlled
- Depression
- Hypertension
- Anemia
- Dyslipidemia

ORDERS FOR HOME CARE

- Resume prior medications.
- Teach diabetes management skills, including insulin administration and glucose monitoring.
- Assess cardiac status.
- Teach nutrition.
- Notify primary health care provider if blood glucose is >240 or <80 mg/dL.

Reimbursement Considerations

The patient is enrolled in Medicare managed care and requires authorizations for visits, followed by timed reports. Overutilization is scrutinized, as is underutilization. Where there is an appropriate need for OT, PT, and social work, it is expected to be documented and provided.

The home care nurse places a phone call to the patient's primary care physician (PCP) to let her know she will be making an initial visit the next morning. The PCP is unaware of the patient's recent hospitalization and the precipitating events and expresses annoyance that she had not been notified by the hospital or family. The visiting nurse will need signed orders from the PCP.

Neal Theory Implications

Stage 3: The professional in this stage is not intimidated by the annoyance of the physician and recognizes her own value as a health care team member.

Stage 2: The professional in this stage may not feel comfortable collaborating with the physician regarding orders for other disciplines, case managing, or working within the patient's environment to manage care.

Stage 1: The clinician in this stage may be very knowledgeable about diabetes mellitus but does not understand the significance of the home setting in diabetic management.

? CRITICAL THINKING

1. Before even visiting the patient, what concerns might the nurse have when reviewing the available information?
Answer: There are a number of questions about the medications to consider:
- Both types of insulin are clear and therefore may be difficult to differentiate.
- The combination of aspirin and Plavix needs to be addressed.
- There is a diagnosis of depression with no antidepressant medication.
- Is glyburide necessary when insulin therapy for both basal and prandial effect is prescribed?
- Metoclopramide is generally used for gastric reflux and/or gastroparesis. If this is the reason the patient is taking it, then it should be taken 30 minutes before the meal. Does the patient have gastroparesis; and if so, should the timing of mealtime insulin be adjusted?
- There is a diagnosis of renal failure. This is a significant complication of prolonged exposure to hyperglycemia. Should diet therapy include any protein or fluid restrictions? The nurse will need to request the latest lab values to determine the patient's renal status.
- Who are the members of this patient's health care team? Does the patient see a nephrologist, cardiologist, endocrinologist, or dietician? All of these questions need to be considered in order to optimize patient outcomes.

THE HOME VISIT

During the initial visit, the nurse asks the patient to read the information from the prescription medication vials and let her know when she takes each medication, what dose she takes, what the medication is for, and how often she forgets to take the medications. These questions are asked in a matter-of-fact manner, without being judgmental. The nurse discovers that the patient has a significant visual deficit and is unable to read the print on the prescription bottles. The patient acknowledges that she has "some difficulty," but "I do just fine." The patient's son is present and is surprised by the finding. The nurse discovers a number of pills on the floor where the patient probably dropped them when pouring her medications.

Cultural Competence

The patient is fiercely independent and wants little or no help from others. She may benefit from a senior center or group of peers who can support each other.

? CRITICAL THINKING

1. What barriers to patient's medication safety has the nurse identified?

Answer: Visual deficits may prevent the patient from taking medications as ordered. Additionally, although the patient is using insulin-prefilled pen devices to dose and administer the Lantus and Apidra, the combination of visual deficits and limited manual dexterity may be preventing her from dosing correctly. She may also have mistaken the Apidra pen for the Lantus pen on the day of the fall and dosed the 30 units of Apidra instead of Lantus. One possible solution to overcome this barrier is to ask the patient's son to put rubber bands around the rapid-acting insulin pens right from the pharmacy. This should alert the patient to only use those rubber-banded pens for premeal injections. Because of the patient's diminished manual dexterity, the patient drops pills without being aware of it; and she has difficulty opening some of the containers.

The patient does not want to be a burden to her son, so she has not shared these issues with the family; she has chosen to manage on her own. Because she is comfortable in her own surroundings, she has been able to mask her deficits quite successfully. She has also not shared this information with her primary care physician. She has not been to her ophthalmologist in more than 18 months. Asking the patient to make an appointment while the nurse is present is an option. It is important that the nurse document the outcome.

Relevant Community Resources

The patient may benefit from an organization that provides low-vision services such as Lighthouse, Commission for the Blind, and Jewish Guild for the Blind.

↻ BACK TO THE CASE

The nurse asks the patient if she would mind testing her blood glucose while the nurse is there. The patient responds that she has been doing it so long that she has no problems. The nurse acknowledges that the patient is capable of monitoring, but she asks her to do it so that they can both see the current blood glucose value. It is approximately 2 hours after breakfast.

? CRITICAL THINKING

1. What can the nurse learn from having the patient self-monitor her blood glucose?
Answer: Because the patient is administering rapid-acting insulin premeal, it is important that the patient be able to accurately assess blood glucose. Do the visual deficits present a problem for successfully monitoring blood glucose? The patient may also not realize that she is using strips that are outdated or improperly coded. The patient does not close the cap on the monitoring strips tightly because of her difficulties with dexterity. This can cause faulty results. If the screen is not large enough, the patient may not accurately read the results. Having completed the testing, the nurse reviews the events. She asks the patient to read the last few entries in the glucometer memory to assess how accurately she sees them. It is no surprise that the patient struggles with the task.

2. What steps might the nurse consider to overcome these barriers?
Answer: Depending on the severity of the deficits, several options are available. Having an occupational therapy (OT) assessment for fine motor training and/or adaptive equipment is an appropriate choice. Not only can OTs assess the patient's capacity to perform diabetes tasks that need to be done, but they can also address some of the activities of daily living skills that require fine motor skills. OT assessment and intervention may give the patient the training and adaptive equipment necessary to carry out the diabetes self-management tasks with the independence that she desires.

If vision is so limited that further intervention is required, a voice-activated glucose meter, a free-standing magnifier, and stronger lighting might be considered.

BACK TO THE CASE

It is important to check the patient's blood pressure both sitting and then standing. One of the autonomic neuropathies of prolonged diabetes is orthostatic hypotension. When the patient fell prior to hospitalization, what was the precipitating factor? Several of the medications she is taking also have orthostatic hypotension as potential side effects including labetalol, metoclopramide, and metoprolol tartrate. Obtaining the sitting/standing blood pressure can provide important information.

CRITICAL THINKING

1. What information regarding the medication regime needs to be communicated to the patient's PCP?
Answer: All findings are relevant, but it is important to prioritize. If the patient has difficulty with a sliding-scale insulin regime, the nurse should let the PCP know of the barriers and risks. There should be a discussion with the PCP about medications that do not have accompanying diagnoses and the conversation should be documented. Verification of the use of aspirin and Plavix should be obtained and documented. Recommending a change to prefilled, premixed insulin might be an answer. If the same dose is ordered for both before breakfast and before dinner, an error in dosing will be avoided. If the patient is found to have orthostatic hypotension, a discussion about medications that may contribute should occur and be documented. A simplified medication regime reduces the risks of medication errors. The nurse should recommend the use of a home monitor for ongoing assessment of blood pressure. Use of weekly pill boxes that the patient's son might be willing to fill could be helpful.

BACK TO THE CASE

The nurse next asks the patient if she would lead the nurse to the bathroom or bedroom so that the patient can be weighed. It is important for the nurse to assess the patient's ability to get up out of the chair and walk to the scale. Does she struggle to get up from a sitting position? How is her gait? Does she use an adaptive device, such as a cane? Are there urine stains on the chair, the back of her clothing, or her footwear? Is the footwear appropriate for a person with diabetes? All of these things can be assessed in the few moments it takes to get from point A to point B.

? CRITICAL THINKING

1. How can the nurse use the information gained from observing the patient move from one place to the next?
Answer: Gait abnormality is a common complication of diabetes. Peripheral neuropathy can cause loss of sensation in the lower extremities preventing the person from knowing where their feet are in relation to the floor. Vascular compromise may cause numbness, pain, or other limiting side effects. Deformities are a result of small muscle atrophy associated with diabetes, resulting in an unsteady gait. Referral to physical therapy (PT) for assessment and intervention should occur. Fall prevention measures should be instituted, evaluated, and documented.

By observing the patient's clothing for any urine or feces stains, incontinence can be detected. Patients are often embarrassed to acknowledge that they have an incontinence problem. Urinary incontinence is a frequent consequence of long-term diabetes. Patients lose the ability to fully empty their bladder, with resultant residual urine and chronic urinary tract infections. This can be the forerunner of "dribbling" or frank incontinence. Another potential complication is "diabetic diarrhea." This can be caused by gastroparesis, or slowing of the gastrointestinal tract. Constipation may occur followed by an overgrowth of bacteria in the gut. The results are bouts of explosive diarrhea. Mrs. J is taking medication generally prescribed for gastroparesis, so this is a potential problem to be considered.

↺ BACK TO THE CASE

Once all assessments are completed, a telephone call to the PCP should be made. The home care nurse describes the situation found in the home, provides the relevant background, prioritizes and delivers information, and makes recommendations. This includes requesting orders for assessment by the OT and PT. If, during the initial or subsequent visits, the nurse administers a depression scale, the results should be shared with the PCP with followup as indicated by the results.

Rehabilitation Needs

Occupational therapy
Physical therapy
Social work consideration for future

| ? | CRITICAL THINKING |

1. How will members of the interdisciplinary team communicate with one another?
Answer: Team members will communicate through the agency's documentation system where available, via telephone and face-to-face meetings, and in case conferences when warranted. Multi-disciplinary care plans should be kept up to date and provide sufficient information to link interventions in a meaningful and professional manner.

Interdisciplinary Care Plan

Problem	Goal/Plan	Intervention	Evaluation
Medication reconciliation and knowledge deficit regarding medications	Medications will be reconciled within 48 hours. Patient will be able to discuss medications and when to take them within 3 weeks of medication reconciliation.	Contact PCP for medication reconciliation and simplification. Coach and support patient's understanding of her medications and when and how to take them.	Patient will have fewer daily doses of medications without compromise in health status. Risk of medication error will be diminished.
Knowledge deficit regarding disease process	Patient and son will verbalize understanding of diseases processes and the recent changes in the patient's condition within 3 weeks.	Teach patient and son about diabetes and the importance of participating in self-management.	Patient will more fully participate in her care; she will have one patient-stated goal to improve status. Son will verbalize understanding of his mother's condition.

Problem	Goal/Plan	Intervention	Evaluation
History of falls	Patient will have assessment for gait abnormality and insensate foot within 1 week.	Contact PCP for authorization for PT and OT for further assessments and make recommendations. Medications will be assessed for orthostatic hypotension side effects.	Patient will have appropriate adaptive devices to assist with ambulation and will use these devices. The son will be the coach and support for process. Medications will be adjusted as needed.
Reduced dexterity	Assessment by PT and OT for assistance with ADLs	Nurse will provide ongoing assessment of patient's ability to self-manage her diabetes equipment, pill containers, etc. and will keep PCP informed.	Patient will have more confidence in managing her health and her ADLs.
Ineffective coping of family system	Patient and family are able to cope with sequelae of disease process with 3 weeks.	Provide information about community resources, support groups and services, and diabetes educations programs in the area.	Patient and son have resources for emotional support and are using them.

REFERENCES & RESOURCES

[1] American Association of Diabetes Educators, *A Core Curriculum for Diabetes Educators* (5th ed.), American Association of Diabetes Educators, 2003.
[2] B. Childs, M. Cypress and G. Spollett (eds.), *Complete Nurse's Guide to Diabetes Care*, American Diabetes Association, 2008.

Section 15

End-of-Life Care

Case 15.1 Grief

By Debra Riendeau, MN, APRN, BC, PMHNP-BC

This case study illustrates the complexity of providing end-of-life nursing care to individuals. This patient was a school teacher, Ms. T who left teaching to care for her 3 children when they were young, and she never returned to the workforce. She has remained socially active, volunteering in her community for such causes as raising money for needy families who have children with cancer and for those who have lost everything in a fire. She is married to her husband of 35 years. She has 3 adult children who live nearby raising their families. They meet regularly for family dinners. Everyone is supportive of the grandchildren who play sports. Subsequently, the usual Friday night activity is attending the local high school football games to watch the grandchildren play.

One year ago, after seeing her family physician for her annual physical, Ms. T was given "a clean bill of health." She is careful with her family's diet, drinks only socially and within limits, and likes to golf with a group of ladies in the community. She has been a 1-pack-per-day smoker since her mid 20s. She has tried to quit many times, but she has been unsuccessful due to concerns about subsequent weight gain. Over the past year, she developed a cough that seemed more severe than it used to be. She also noted that starting very recently, she gets very anxious and her heart races at night when she rolls over in bed.

Ms. T presented to her primary care physician with these last two symptoms. At the visit, the physician had lab work drawn and took a chest x-ray that revealed a small mass in her left lung. She was given alprazolam (Xanax) for the anxiety and was sent to the oncologist for

Clinical Case Studies in Home Health Care, First Edition. Edited by Leslie Neal-Boylan.
© 2011 John Wiley & Sons, Inc. Published 2011 by John Wiley & Sons, Inc.

a consult. A lung biopsy was performed, which revealed that she had small cell lung cancer, which grows quickly and often metastasizes to other organs before diagnosis.

She was admitted to the hospital for a course of chemotherapy with palliative radiation therapy. A triple lumen Hickman catheter was inserted for the chemotherapy and other fluids. After the course of therapy, it was initially felt that she was in remission. However, about 15 months after diagnosis, her symptoms returned and the severe level of anxiety or "panic attacks" seemed more frequent throughout the day. After a return visit to the oncologist and more tests, the decision was made that a referral for palliative home health care was the best option for her.

Application of the understanding of the process of loss and grief within the diagnosis of a terminal illness is the key to supporting this patient and her family. Additionally, knowledge of the services offered within the framework of palliative end-of-life care, for both the patient and the family, is critical to bringing a peaceful resolution for those involved in this process.

Cultural Competence

The patient is of Italian descent. She has a large extended family that lives in close proximity of one another. The nurse may need to incorporate significant members of this family into the care of this patient and adapt to changes within the family structure.

 ORDERS FOR HOME CARE

Patient: 56-year-old married female of Italian descent
Diagnosis: Small cell lung cancer with metastasis to the adrenal glands
Current medications:
- MS Contin 80 mg by mouth twice a day
- Morphine Sulfate IR 15 mg by mouth as needed for breakthrough pain
- Alprazolam (Xanax) 0.25 mg by mouth 4 times a day as needed for anxiety
- 10 mL prefilled syringe with 3 mL Heparin 100 units intravenously once a day to flush the Hickman catheter
- Supplemental oxygen via nasal cannula to keep saturations above 90%

Relevant past medical history:
- Has no other comorbid medical conditions
- Is a 1-pack-per-day smoker for 30 years

Durable Medical Equipment: Oxygen concentrator and portable oxygen
RN: Skilled nursing assessment and evaluation. Skilled procedure: Due
to the weakened immune state of this patient, the insurance company
authorized weekly sterile Hickman catheter dressing changes.
Respiratory therapist: Initiate oxygen therapy and provide education
to the patient and family in safe use of oxygen in the home. Provide
initial oxygen saturation assessment on room air and on supplemental oxygen to keep blood oxygen saturation above 90%.

Rehabilitation Needs

Respiratory therapist
Potential for Durable Medical Equipment (commode and hospital
bed)
Monthly delivery of sterile all-inclusive central line dressing kits

THE HOME VISIT

On a Monday afternoon in the fall, the patient was admitted to home
health services after a visit to her oncologist. The patient has just been
told that her cancer is no longer in remission and that she is terminal.
She is being placed into the home health palliative care program. As
part of the admission process, the nurse performs a basic skilled nursing
assessment, monitors for side effects from the medications that the
patient is taking, assists with pain control, assists with anxiety control,
and schedules the weekly sterile dressing changes of the Hickman
catheter. The nurse also educates the patient about the best practice for
cleansing the port on the Hickman catheter before each use to prevent
infection.

The patient is alone, since her husband has returned to work as the
town clerk in this small community. The admission takes approximately 2 hours. During the conversation, the patient shares that her
bone pain is currently being managed with her pain medications, but
the anxiety level seems to "skyrocket" at times. She shares that sometimes her heart will just race when she is sitting and not upset about
anything. During the admission, the respiratory therapist arrives with
the oxygen concentrator and the portable oxygen tanks. Education
concerning safe use of oxygen is provided with the emphasis on the
fact that no one should smoke while oxygen is being used in the
home. Ms. T shares that she no longer smokes but that her husband
still does.

Relevant Community Resources

American Cancer Society: http://www.cancer.org/docroot/home/
   index.asp1-800-ACS-2345
Notification of the fire department and police department that she
   is homebound, unable to drive, and has oxygen in her home

Before leaving, the nurse instructs the patient in the process of flushing the Hickman catheter daily to maintain patency and sterility. As the nursing visit is coming to an end, the patient is teary making statements such as, "My youngest daughter is getting married next summer, and I may not see her get married" and "My daughter-in-law is expecting our first grandchild."

Neal Theory Implications

Stage 3: The nurse in this case demonstrated autonomy by independently making clinical and other decisions based on a thorough knowledge of the grieving process that she has learned while caring for other patients during the end-of-life process. Additionally, the nurse was aware of community resources available for people with terminal illnesses.

Stage 2: The professional in this stage will demonstrate more comfort in dealing with health care issues and the complexity of the home care environment. There is still a need to seek the experience of other health professionals to problem solve and negotiate the care needs of the patient. For this case, the nurse may understand the medical care needs of the patient, but may be unfamiliar with the emotional and spiritual toll the terminal process requires. The community resources may not be part of the awareness of the nurse, and the referral process to outside professionals may not be utilized.

Stage 1: The nurse will need to ask questions and require assistance in managing the patient's care and treatment plan. The complexity of the terminal illness in all areas of the patient's life may be overwhelming. Being a primary support for the patient in this case may be difficult.

| ? | **CRITICAL THINKING** |

1. Based on the patient's statements, what is the nurse's priority goal for the care of this patient?

Answer: Initially, the nurse would focus on establishing trust and building a therapeutic working relationship with the patient. A therapeutic relationship provides the foundation for a collaborative agreement with the patient to establish reasonable goals for care.

2. What factors can interfere with achieving these goals?

Answer: This patient has received a terminal diagnosis after a period of remission from cancer. The patient and family will require support through the dying process, which is new for them. The manner in which a person grieves is very individualized, but it can follow some predictable patterns which vary in length and intensity.

3. What is the best evidence-based practice for cleansing the hub of the catheter to prevent catheter-related bloodstream infections?

Answer: Scrubbing the hub of the catheter port vigorously for 15 seconds with either alcohol alone or chlorhexidine/alcohol was deemed to be effective in reducing catheter-related bloodstream infections.

4. Regarding the medications, what education is important for the nurse to reinforce during this initial visit?

Answer: The nurse should review the reason that the patient is taking the opioid, the prescribed dose, and the possible adverse effects. The nurse should educate the patient on the safe use of MsContin. This includes that the patient should be counseled not to drive while on this narcotic. Additionally, care should be taken, while she is on the MsContin, since she is also on alprazolam (Xanax), a benzodiazepine from the sedative-hypnotic class, as there is a high risk of oversedation with the use of both medications. She should also be instructed in the use of the instant release formula of the opioid. Some of the expected side effects of opioids include dry mouth, constipation, and respiratory depression if too much is taken.

Common side effects of the alprazolam (Xanax) include drowsiness, dizziness, decreased alertness, and decreased ability to focus and concentrate. As benzodiazepines may cause dependence, the patient should not stop taking the medication without notifying her physician due to withdrawal symptoms. The patient should watch for paradoxical effects of excitement, hostility, and angry outbursts and call the physician if they occur.

5. The patient's statements about her daughter's marriage and the upcoming birth of her grandchild are indicative of what process?

Answer: The patient is experiencing preparatory grief. When a patient learns that they have a terminal illness, they must begin to adjust to the fact that their life, as they had hoped and planned, has just changed. This patient is beginning to see that she may not survive long enough to participate in her daughter's wedding or greet the new baby. The idea of her own death coming sooner than she expected can precipitate a crisis that may overwhelm her usual coping skills. The patient must readjust her values, goals, beliefs, and life to incorporate this realization.

BACK TO THE CASE

The nurse returns to the patient's home the following week to assess the patient and perform the sterile dressing change of the Hickman catheter. The nurse begins with a general systems assessment. The patient's vital signs, including her temperature, are within normal limits. Ms. T states that during the past week, her pain has been managed with her medications. She has had a "couple" of episodes of her heart racing that required the use of the alprazolam, but not more than once a day. She states she is experiencing some constipation and has not had a bowel movement in 4 days. She also states that she has a very poor appetite and has been eating mostly bland foods like mashed potatoes and gravy, and toast.

After proper hand hygiene, the nurse removes the old Hickman dressing noting that the insertion site is slightly pink, but it has no drainage or odor. Using sterile technique, the nurse performs the dressing change according to the policy of the home health agency. The nurse instructs the patient in the correct way to cleanse the hub of each port of the catheter. As this technical skill is completed, the nurse asks the patient how she is "doing with all of this." The patient emphatically states, "It wasn't supposed to be this way; I am too young to die!"

Reimbursement Considerations

The patient is too young to be eligible for Medicare and has had too much income to qualify for Medicaid.

The private insurance company has authorized payment for a specific number of weekly visits that incorporate skilled nursing visits and allows sterile central line dressing changes. The insurance company also authorized 1–2 emergency skilled nursing visits.

CRITICAL THINKING

1. What interventions should the nurse offer to combat the side effect of constipation in this patient?
Answer: The nurse could suggest adding more bran fiber or prunes to the patient's diet. However, since the patient has a poor appetite, the nurse should call the physician from the home to report the constipation and no bowel movement for 4 days. The patient may need a stool softener or perhaps a laxative to aide in gastrointestinal motility.

2. What could account for the patient's emphatic statement that she is "too young to die?"
Answer: According to the Kubler–Ross theory, there are 5 stages of grief. These include denial, anger, bargaining, depression, and acceptance. The stages were once thought to be linear, occurring one after another. The current thinking (which echoes that of Kubler-Ross in later years) is that these stages, rather than being definable and sequential, may actually overlap or occur simultaneously. In that case, the patient may be reflecting some anger and/or denial.

BACK TO THE CASE

The nurse returns the following week to find a patient who is sullen and withdrawn. She reports that her family members are not visiting as much. She states that her husband seems uncomfortable around her. He is talking less and won't look her in the eye. He has been attending to all of his outside volunteer commitments in the evenings, leaving her alone. She asks the nurse what all of this means.

CRITICAL THINKING

1. What stage of Kubler-Ross's stages of loss might the patient be experiencing by being sullen and withdrawn?
Answer: The patient may be in the depression stage. Although the family was initially very supportive and frequently available, the patient is now alone much of the time while her husband is at work and at his volunteer activities. The children have now been visiting only on Sunday rather than daily.

2. What other theory related to grief could explain the behaviors of the patient's husband and family?
Answer: Rather than using a stage theory to describe grief, the Awareness of Dying theory (Glaser and Strauss, 1965) may still be applicable and reflect evidence-based practice. In this theory, there are

4 different awareness contexts, which are: closed awareness, suspected awareness, mutual pretense awareness, and open awareness. Closed awareness refers to the situation in which patients are unaware of their own impending death. Suspicion awareness includes patients who do not know they are dying, but they suspect that they are. Both of these do not apply to this case. Mutual pretense occurs when individuals know that the patient is dying but pretend otherwise. This does apply in this case. The husband is aware of the fact that his wife is terminal, but is continuing to live as though nothing has happened. The fourth, open awareness, is when the family and patient all know and acknowledge the terminal illness. Although the patient is already in this type of awareness, the husband and family have not yet reached it.

By applying this theory, nurses may better understand the actions of the people surrounding the patient. It also allows the nurse to envision predictable processes experienced by their patients, thereby, allowing the nurse to alter their interventions when dealing with their particular patient. With this knowledge, nurses can assist their patients and their families in adapting through the transition phases.

BACK TO THE CASE

When the nurse arrives for the next weekly visit, the patient states that her daughter has been in to visit and plans have been made to move the wedding up to 2 weeks from now. The patient's daughter wants her to be part of the ceremony. The patient is tired and is now on continuous oxygen at 2 liters by nasal cannula. She states that her bowels are slow but working "okay" since the addition of the stool softener. She states that she is still using the alprazolam, but now 2–3 times a day. Her pain is not being controlled as well, and she has been using more of the instant release formula. She states that she is still not sleeping well and is frequently up at night 2–3 times. The nurse notes that the Hickman catheter site is still without signs and symptoms of infection, and it is still patent. At the end of the visit, the patient states that she promised God that she would make a charitable donation to a local homeless shelter if God will allow her to see her daughter get married and live long enough to hold her new grandchild.

CRITICAL THINKING

1. What is the best course of action by the nurse to assist the patient with attaining better pain control?
Answer: The nurse should contact the doctor for an increase in the patient's morphine routine dose. The use of increasingly frequent

breakthrough pain is an indication that the patient's pain is increasing and the round-the-clock dose is not high enough.

2. According to Kubler-Ross, which stage is best reflected by her promise of a gift to a charity in exchange for more time to live?
Answer: This promise would reflect the stage known as "bargaining." She is still working through the process of grief and is making some peace with the inevitability of her death. She is attempting to complete the 2 tasks (watching her daughter marry and seeing the new grandchild) that she has verbalized as most important to her.

BACK TO THE CASE

A few weeks later, before one of the next scheduled nursing visits, the patient calls to inform the nurse that the next visit will take place at her lake home and gives the nurse directions to the home. She has relocated there as the house has a great view of the water from her windows. She can watch the deer and the birds. She states it is her favorite place to be and that it is "so peaceful." She states that her husband is going to stay in town to live where he can work and continue with his evening activities. Upon arrival, the nurse notes that the house is large and well kept. The patient has a bedroom and bathroom on the main floor in close proximity of one another. The patient's oxygen concentrator is there as well as all of her supplies. She states that her family will be coming in and out and will get her groceries and whatever else she needs. She is peaceful and content. Both the nurse and the patient sit down to talk at the window looking out over the lake. The patient tells the nurse that her daughter's wedding was small and had only a few of their closest friends and family, but it was still wonderful to have lived to see her get married. The patient cries softly and states that she is sad that she won't live long enough to see her first grandchild. She also states that "watching me die" was too hard on her husband and that she understands that his way of coping was to work and stay busy to keep his mind off of the fact that he was losing her. She states that she is grateful for the life she had even though it was shorter than she had hoped. She gives the nurse the name of the funeral home and shows her where she has a list of her final wishes, including the songs to play at her funeral.

CRITICAL THINKING

1. What is the best action for the nurse to take during this visit?
Answer: Using active listening is the best way to respond. Nurses who are sensitive and open to dying patients may be better able to assist

patients to conclude their lives with proper rituals (such as planning funerals). This attitude allows the patient to openly express their thoughts and feelings as they process thorough grief and the loss of the plans they had for the remainder of their lives.

2. What stage of the process of dying is best reflected by the statements of the patient in this visit?
Answer: The patient is demonstrating a transition into acceptance of her death. Since her admission into the palliative home care program, she has actively transitioned from her initial feelings of denial and anger of having to die at such a young age. The family altered their wedding plans in order for her to see her daughter get married. She continued to work through depression and bargaining. She has chosen to accept her husband's way of grieving his loss for her. She is now at peace with the fact that she is dying and is residing in a place of peace and serenity at her lake house. She has remained active in the dying process and has made plans to honor her own life after she has gone with the funeral arrangements.

Interdisciplinary Care Plan

Problem	Goal/Plan	Interventions	Evaluation
Potential for infection (Hickman catheter)	Patient's insertion site will remain without signs or symptoms of infection. Sterility of the Hickman catheter will be maintained.	Educate the patient related to the signs or symptoms of infection at the insertion site (redness, swelling, tenderness, heat and drainage). Teach patient to take and record temperature daily. Teach the patient the correct technique for cleansing the hub of the catheter before and after each use.	Patient's insertion site does not become infected. Patient demonstrates no signs or symptoms of systemic infection (especially fever) related to the use of the Hickman catheter.

Problem	Goal/Plan	Interventions	Evaluation
Alteration in comfort: pain	Patient reports pain is managed to a level of 2–3/10.	Teach patient to use the pain scale 1–10 to rate pain daily and record for the nurse. Teach patient to call the nurse if pain is not controlled to the 2–3/10 level. Nurse will contact the physician to report any increase in pain and obtain changes in pain medication per physician.	Patient's pain is routinely controlled to 2–3/10 level. Patient's instant relief formula of pain medication manages her breakthrough pain.
Anxiety	Patient's anxiety is controlled to a level of 2–3/10 with the use of her antianxiety medication.	Assess patient's anxiety level using the 1–10 scale. Teach patient safety information and potential side effects related to benzodiazepines.	Patient reports that her anxiety is managed by her antianxiety medication.
Alteration in gastrointestinal motility: constipation	Patient will have a formed bowel movement every 1–3 days.	Educate the patient in the correct use of the stool softener and/or laxative ordered by the physician. Educate the patient related to foods that will assist in bowel regularity (prunes, prune juice, and bran fiber).	Patient reports a bowel movement every 1–3 days.
Grieving	Patient will readjust the values, goals, beliefs, and life to the impending death. Patient will successfully navigate through the stages of grief and into acceptance of death.	Nurse is fully present during the process with the patient. Employ active listening and support of the patient as she verbalizes and demonstrate the stages of grief. Contact the agency social worker to provide in-home support for grief work.	Patient verbalizes adjustments in life values, goals, beliefs to assist in movement toward adjustment to death. Patient navigated through the stages of grief to come to acceptance.

(Continued)

Problem	Goal/Plan	Interventions	Evaluation
Alteration in mood: depression	Patient will verbalize a decrease in level of depression to 1–2/10 in 1 month.	Teach patient the 1–10 scale for rating depression. Nurse uses active listening and support during each patient interaction. Educate patient in alternative/complementary methods of decreasing depression (i.e., massage, spiritual support, support groups, music). Nurse contacts the physician about a possible antidepressant.	Patient verbalizes a decrease in level of depression to 1–2/10 with the use of available support services nurse, social worker, etc.).
Spiritual distress	Patient will verbalize purpose and find meaning with the remainder of her life in 3 months. Patient will find strength within her spiritual beliefs within 1 month. Patient will verbalize acceptance and peace in 3 months.	Nurse actively listens to patient related to what has given meaning and comfort to her. Support patient as she accesses her spiritual leaders and expands her spiritual connections.	Patient verbalizes meaning and new purpose for the remainder of her lifespan. Patient verbalizes inner strength as she copes with changes in hopes, dreams, and lifespan expectations. Patient finds acceptance and peace before she expires.
Ineffective coping of family systems	Patient and family are able to successfully cope with the process of the terminal illness process in 1 month.	Nurse provides information concerning community resources (American Cancer Society), support services, and support and groups.	Patient and family utilize resources as needed to alleviate distress and assist with resolution of the terminal illness process.

REFERENCES & RESOURCES

[1] T. Andrews and A. Nathaniel, "Awareness of dying revisited," *Journal of Nursing Care Quality*, 24(3):189–193, 2009.

[2] Y. D'Arcy, "Avoid the dangers of opioid therapy," *American Nurse Today*, 4(5):18–22, 2009.

[3] K. Dunne, "Grief and its manifestations," *Nursing Standard*, 18(45):45–51, 2004.

[4] C. Hatler, J. Hebden, W. Kaler and J. Zack, "Walk the walk to reduce catheter-related bloodstream infections," *American Nurse Today*, 5(1):26–30, 2010.

[5] Hospice and Palliative Nurses Association, Retrieved from http://www.hpna.org/

[6] K. Mystakidou, E. Tsilika, E. Parpa, A. Galanos and L. Vlahos, "Screening for preparatory grief in advanced cancer patients," *Cancer Nursing*, 31(4):326–332, 2008.

[7] L. Neal, "Neal theory of home health nursing practice," *Journal of nursing scholarship*, 31(3):251, 1999.

[8] M.C. Stoppler, "Lung Cancer," *Emedicinehealth*. Retrieved from http://www.emedicinehealth.com/lung_cancer/article_em.htm February 13, 2008.

[9] United States. National Institutes of Health, "Managing Your Tunneled Catheter: Hickman, Neostar, Broviac, Leonard," Retrieved from http://www.cc.nih.gov/ccc/patient_education/pepubs/hickman.pdf September, 2003.

[10] E. Kubler-Ross and D. Kessler. On grief and grieving: Finding the meaning of grief through the five stages of loss. Scribner, 2005.

[11] B. L. Glaser and A. L. Strauss. "Dying on time. Arranging the final hours of life in a hospital." *Hospital Topics*, 43:28, 1965.

Case 15.2 Palliative Care

By Susan Breakwell, APHN-BC, DNP

The case of Mrs. C illustrates a shift in the focus of care that occurs when a patient has chronic disease that is advancing. The degree to which a palliative approach to care is implemented with Mrs. C is based greatly on her goals and wishes and what she defines as quality of life. It does not mean the discontinuation of other restorative/ curative focused aspects of care; the aim is rather for a balance among all aspects of care.

Mrs. C is an 85-year-old woman with a history of congestive heart failure (CHF), recently hospitalized for an exacerbation of the problem with fluid retention, shortness of breath and reduced endurance. During her hospitalization, her ejection fraction was 40%. She has a history of coronary artery disease with angioplasty and hypertension. She was diuresed, and her medications were adjusted during the brief stay. In discussions at that time about her goals of care, Mrs. C stated that she wanted to feel better and wanted to be as active and symptom free as possible, but without having to undergo more surgery or at-home intravenous therapy. She was referred by the hospital discharge coordinator/case manager for home health followup. Consults with social work and the dietician are available if needed. She has been a home health patient off and on for several years, primarily for

Clinical Case Studies in Home Health Care, First Edition. Edited by Leslie Neal-Boylan.
© 2011 John Wiley & Sons, Inc. Published 2011 by John Wiley & Sons, Inc.

exacerbations of her CHF and associated problems. Mrs. C has typically been followed by the same home health team members, including the nurse case manager for her home health care. The time between her CHF exacerbations is lessening over time, and this is her second admission to home health in 5 months.

Reimbursement Considerations

While there is a shift in the focus of care for the patient at this point, home health is still covered under Medicare. The patient's needs are still for part time, skilled, intermittent services and based on orders of the physician.

ORDERS FOR HOME CARE

Patient: 85-year-old female with congestive heart failure (CHF)
Diagnoses: Exacerbation of CHF; past history of coronary artery disease with angioplasty and hypertension
Current medications:
- Lisinopril (Beta blocker) once a day
- Carvedilol (ACE inhibitor) once a day
- Furosemide (diuretic) once a day and as needed for increased fluid retention/edema
- Norco (hydrocodone 5 mg + acetaminophen 325 mg) as needed for pain
- Oxygen, 2 liters per minute by nasal cannula as needed

Services needed: RN, home health aide (HHA), physical therapy (PT) (short term), occupational therapy (OT) (short term), medical social worker (MSW) for consult and services

THE HOME VISIT

Mrs. C lives with her husband of 60 years, but his health is frail and his activities of daily living (ADL) and instrumental ADL (IADL) are limited. The C's have limited finances and have Medicare. They have lived in their 1-story home for many years. They have a small circle of aging friends and value their connection with their local church. Their daughter and her family live close by, but they have busy lives and visit on a weekly basis.

> **Relevant Community Resources**
>
> Possible need for chaplain or church pastor
> Community services for housekeeping and home maintenance
> Community services to assist patient and husband with personal
>   care in light of patient's advancing disease

At the time of admission to home care, Mrs. C states that she feels better than before going to the hospital. Now, 2 weeks later, she is distressed over her continued fatigue, limited endurance, and periodic breathlessness. She needs to rest after walking more than 30 feet (i.e., from the front door to the back door in the house). Her weight fluctuates and she has a corresponding range of lower extremity edema and crackles in her lungs. Her blood pressure ranges from 140/80 to 160/90.

Cognitively, Mrs. C manages her own medications and the household checkbook. The visiting nurse notes that there is a growing stack of unopened mail and that Mrs. C's medications are not as meticulously organized as in the past. She admits to having some difficulties with her new medication regimen, having forgotten to take them "about once a week or so" and sometimes foregoing her diuretic because "I get tired out just having to run to the bathroom so often."

Mrs. C's goals include:

- To remain at home with her husband and not go back to the hospital
- To resume as much of a daily routine as possible
- To not be a burden to her family
- To enjoy her favorite foods in moderation
- To get some assistance with things she can no longer manage (i.e., home maintenance)
- To have enough energy to enjoy time with family and friends
- To not be in pain or short of breath

> **Rehabilitations Needs**
>
> Registered nurse
> Home health aide
> Physical therapy
> Occupational therapy
> Social worker
> Chaplain or pastor

The nurse collects the following data:

- Mrs. C's levels of endurance and activity are lower than before the hospital admission.
- Mrs. C has not been getting any help with personal care, chores, or home maintenance up to this point in time.
- Mrs. C has limited endurance, does not sleep well at night, and is distressed over her constant fatigue.
- Mrs. C's lungs are clear to auscultation.
- Mrs. C has trace lower extremity edema.
- Mrs. C's advance directives have not been recently updated.

Neal Theory Implications

Stage 3: The professional in this stage recognizes that the patient's cardiac disease is advanced. This professional can work with the patient and family and collaborate with others (within and outside of the home care team) to identify the patient's goals/wishes and focus adjustments to the plan of care. A palliative care consult may be beneficial for management of complex symptoms with further advancement of the patient's disease.

Stage 2: The professional in this stage may recognize that the cycle of exacerbations is typical for this diagnosis, but only partly recognize that a shift in goals of care is appropriate and that a palliative approach can be incorporated into this patient's care. This professional will benefit from collaborating with others within the team and outside of the team about the patient's cardiac and palliative care related needs. Such collaboration may include a request for a palliative care consult if management of the patient's symptoms becomes increasingly complex.

Stage 1: The professional in this stage recognizes signs and symptoms of exacerbation of CHF and is comfortable reporting changes in the patient's status and updating the care plan to a degree. However, the nurse at this stage benefits from assistance/guidance in managing the bigger picture of the patient's care as a shift toward incorporating more elements of palliative care occurs. This nurse may benefit from encouragement or assistance in obtaining orders for and pursuing consultation with a palliative care clinician and support in preparing to talk with the patient about delicate issues such as advance directives.

CRITICAL THINKING

1. What elements of palliative care can be incorporated into the care of Mrs. C at this point? Can palliative and restorative/curative care be provided together?

Answer: As a philosophy and an organized system of care, palliative care can be provided in conjunction with curative/restorative focused care. It is care that extends across health care settings from inpatient to home and across the health-illness continuum. Palliative care is patient centered and family focused care that aims to be proactive and aggressive in addressing the physical, psychological, social and spiritual needs of a patient. There is a balance between the restorative and palliative aspects of care that will likely shift with time and as the patient experiences increased or new cardiac symptoms. Working with the patient to ascertain her wishes and goals of care is an ongoing process and is crucial to attaining the most meaningful balance of care for the patient.

2. How should the nurse address the issue of advance directives with Mrs. C?

Answer: The nurse should find out if she has advance directives in place, and if so, what type (health care power of attorney, living will, do-not-attempt-to-resuscitate form, or others). The nurse might ask something like, "If you were not able to speak for yourself, is there someone else who could speak for you about your health care wishes?" If she has made some decisions, who knows about them? It is important to find out if her loved ones know about her wishes and whether they are current and accessible. If her wishes are now different than they were in the past, it is important to communicate the changes to her family and health care team.

3. Mrs. C states, "I know the Norco has helped my pain, but I don't want to take it and become a drug addict." What key things about Norco are important for Mrs. C to understand?

Answer: Barriers to effective use of opioids in treating chronic pain such as Mrs. C's remain prevalent among the public and health care workers. Yet opioids such as Norco can be very effective. In addition to pain relief, the medication can also help relieve shortness of breath with exertion. In talking with Mrs. C, it will be important to dispel myths about addiction with her and her family to assure that they understand the purpose and actions of the medication in relieving distressing pain and respiratory symptoms. It will also be important to evaluate the use and effectiveness of the medication.

Table 15.2.1. Palliative Performance Scale (PPS).

%	Ambulation	Activity Level Evidence of Disease	Self-Care	Intake	Level of Consciousness	Estimated Median Survival in Days (a) (b) (c)		
						(a)	(b)	(c)
100	Full	Normal / *No Disease*	Full	Normal	Full	N/A	N/A	108
90	Full	Normal / *Some Disease*	Full	Normal	Full			
80	Full	Normal with Effort / *Some Disease*	Full	Normal or Reduced	Full			
70	Reduced	Can't do normal job or work / *Some Disease*	Full	As above	Full	145		
60	Reduced	Can't do hobbies or housework / *Significant Disease*	Occasional Assistance Needed	As above	Full or Confusion	29	4	
50	Mainly sit/lie	Can't do any work / *Extensive Disease*	Considerable Assistance Needed	As above	Full or Confusion	30	11	41
40	Mainly in Bed	As above	Mainly Assistance	As above	Full or Drowsy or Confusion	18	8	
30	Bed Bound	As above	Total Care	Reduced	As above	8	5	
20	Bed Bound	As above	As above	Minimal	As above	4	2	
10	Bed Bound	As above	As above	Mouth Care Only	Drowsy or Coma	1	1	6
0	Death	—	—	—	—			

a. Survival post-admission to an inpatient palliative unit, all diagnoses (Virik 2002).
b. Days until inpatient death following admission to an acute hospice unit, diagnoses not specified (Anderson 1996).
c. Survival post admission to an inpatient palliative unit, cancer patients only (Morita 1999).
Source: Authors: L. Scott Wilner MD and Robert Arnold MD. Courtesy of the End of Life/Palliative Education Resource Center.
References: [6], [7], [8], and [9].

Interdisciplinary Care Plan

Problem	Goal/Plan	Intervention	Evaluation
Knowledge deficit regarding advanced disease process	Patient and family will verbalize understanding of recent changes in patient's condition within 1 week. Patient and family will demonstrate increased understanding about advanced cardiac disease within 3 weeks.	Teach patient and family about advanced CHF. Teach patient about new medications. Teach patient and family to identify and report any new symptoms or changes early on so they can be managed effectively.	Patient and family will identify and implement adaptations to environment that are based on patient's changing level of endurance, mobility, and symptoms.
Knowledge deficit regarding palliative care	Patient and family will articulate their goals/wishes about the focus of care for the patient within 2 weeks and when other changes are warranted. Patient and family can identify the focus of palliative care on quality of life and that it can be provided in conjunction with management of her CHF within 2 weeks. Patient will communicate her advanced directives with family and team members within 2 weeks.	Foster trusting relationship between patient and family and health care team for early and ongoing dialogue about their questions, worries, and wishes. Arrange family meeting, team meeting, and/or consultation with primary care provider to review, revise, and coordinate goals of care in conjunction with patient's and family's wishes. Teach patient and family about how palliative care can be provided in conjunction with other care measures. Provide information and resources to patient and family about palliative care. Provide information about advance directives. Reinforce that advance directives can be changed/revised. Provide appropriate resources for patient to make new or changed decisions about her advance directives	Patient and family will discuss their goals/wishes for care with home health nurse and team members. Plan of care will be revised as needed over time to include patient and family wishes for the goals of care. Advance directives are in place and communicated to team members and family.

(Continued)

Problem	Goal/Plan	Intervention	Evaluation
Limited endurance and fatigue related to disease process	Attain a balance between rest and activity, as well as independence and assistance with daily activities to foster patient's quality of life within 4 weeks.	Therapy (PT, OT) to work with patient and family on adaptations to the home, daily routine, and patient activity level for effective management of fatigue. Assess sleep patterns. Nurse to instruct on use of oxygen as needed. Nurse to teach/reinforce about balancing periods of rest and activity. Nurse to help patient prioritize activities she wants to continue to do and those that she wants to delegate to others (family and/or outside resources). Home health aide to assist with personal care short term. Social worker to link patient and family with longer term assistance in light of her reduced endurance and mobility.	Patient will access resources (home health aide, outside resources) as needed. Patient will be able to participate in activities meaningful to her (i.e., church, family). Source of long-range assistance for patient and husband's personal care will be identified. Additional help for chores such as shopping and cleaning will be obtained.
Fluid retention as evidenced by lower extremity edema, adventitious lung sounds, weight gain, and self-reported difficulties with medication effects/side effects.	Patient will work with home health nurse and team to balance quality of life and CHF management.	Teach self-management of fluid retention (self-monitoring of symptoms, timely reporting, and making changes in regimen). Review medication and specialty diet restrictions with patient and identify appropriate ways of improving patient's perception of quality of life in balance with CHF management issues.	Patient will routinely weigh herself and report changes of +2 pounds, increased shortness of breath, edema, or chest pain to home health nurse. Patient and health care team will identify the most and least important medications and diet restrictions in managing her CHF and promoting best quality of life for her.

Problem	Goal/Plan	Intervention	Evaluation
Pain	Patient's chronic pain will be controlled in a range acceptable to the patient (i.e., a range of 1–3) by the end of 1 week. Patient will maintain regular bowel regimen.	Patient to report episodes of pain, action taken, and response by contacting the home health nurse and/or use of a log. Nurse to review pain record regularly for any changes in pain or response to medications. Nurse will instruct patient on pain medications. Nurse will allay patient's and family's fears or misconceptions about use of Norco for chronic pain. Nurse will instruct about potential for constipation while on Norco and measures to minimize its occurrence.	Patient reports pain does not exceed 3/10. Patient will report effective bowel regimen, including use of appropriate medication (stool softener plus stimulant) in conjunction with Norco. Patient will report incidences of constipation in a timely manner so bowel regimen can be adjusted as needed.
Risk for depression related to advanced disease	Patient will implement coping strategies to manage depressive mood.	Assess patient using established tool such as the Geriatric Depression Scale-Short Form (GDS-SF). Provide emotional support and active listening. Encourage patient to access resources and accept help when needed. Collaborate with other services as needed. Instruct patient and family that depression can occur in conjunction with advanced disease. Integrate instruction about coping strategies and/or use of medications for management of depression as the need arises.	Patient will maintain open communication with family and health care team regarding how she feels she is coping and depressive symptoms.

REFERENCES & RESOURCES

[1] R. Arnold, "Why patients do not take their opioids," *Fast Facts and Concepts* (2nd ed.). Retrieved at: http://www.eperc.mcw.edu/fast/ff_083.htm, 2007, October.

[2] S.J. Goodlin, "Palliative care in congestive heart failure," *Journal of the American College of Cardiology*, 54(5):386–396, 2009.

[3] National Consensus Project for Quality Palliative Care, *Clinical Practice Guidelines for Quality Palliative Care* (2nd ed.). Retrieved at: http://www.nationalconsensusproject.org, 2009.

[4] National Healthcare Decisions Day, *Get an Advance Directive*, Author. Retrieved at: http://www.nationalhealthcaredecisionsday.org/resources.htm (n.d.).

[5] National Institute of Nursing Research, *Palliative Care: The Relief You Need When You're Experiencing the Symptoms of Serious Illness*, Author. Retrieved at: http://www.ninr.nih.gov/NR/rdonlyres/01CC45F1-048B-468A-BD9F-3AB727A381D2/0/NINR_PalliativeCare_Brochure_508C.pdf, 2009, November.

[6] Virik, K., Glare, P. "Validation of the Palliative Performance Scale for Inpatients Admitted to a Palliative Care Unit in Sydney, Australia." *Journal of Pain Symptom Management*, 23(6):455–457, 2002.

[7] Anderson, F, Downing, GM, Hill, J. "Palliative Performance Scale (PPS): A new tool." *Journal of Palliative Care*, 1996, 12(1), 5–11.

[8] Morita, T., Tsunoda, J., Inoue, S., et al. "Validity of the Palliative Performance Scale from a Survival Perspective. *Journal of Pain and Symptom Management*, 18(1):2–3, 1999.

[9] L.S. Wilner, R. Arnold. The Palliative Performance Scale. Fast facts and concepts, 125. End of life/Palliative Education Resource Center (EPERC). Medical College of Wisconsin. Retrieved at: http://www.epercmcw.edu/fastfact/ff_125.htm

Case 15.3 Hospice

By Susan Breakwell, APHN-BC, DNP

Mr. O is a 75-year-old male who was diagnosed several years ago with colorectal cancer. He had a colostomy and underwent aggressive chemotherapy and radiation therapy. He did well for a year. Home health followed him at that time as he was learning his ostomy care. It was then that he established a bond with the agency and its staff. Now, a year later, Mr. O has been diagnosed with metastasis to his liver and bone; his prognosis is likely limited. He says he is "all done" with aggressive treatments. The nurse recognizes that his goals and wishes need to be revisited. His advance directives have not been updated since his first round of chemotherapy and radiation. Mr. O saw his physician yesterday. In a follow-up conversation with the doctor, the nurse is told that Mr. O is not a candidate for further aggressive curative treatments as his prognosis is likely "months." The physician has talked briefly with Mr. O about hospice; the nurse is to talk further with him and his family.

A widower, Mr. O lives in an apartment building with family. He is on the first floor and they are on the second. His son and daughter-in-law are spending increasing hours assisting Mr. O to appointments and treatments in light of his growing care needs. Of Mexican heritage, Mr. O prides himself on taking care of his family and is respected as head of the household. He is Catholic; and, though he only

Clinical Case Studies in Home Health Care, First Edition. Edited by Leslie Neal-Boylan.
© 2011 John Wiley & Sons, Inc. Published 2011 by John Wiley & Sons, Inc.

occasionally goes to church services, he has known the parish priest for a long time.

Reluctantly, he has turned over responsibility for household and yard chores to the family. They now bring meals down to him. He says to the nurse, "I feel like one of their kids; I need help with so many things now." He struggles with his activities of daily living (ADL) and instrumental ADL (IADL) and has not let his family help him with personal care or colostomy care. He rates his pain as 3 (on a scale of 0 to 10 with 10 being the most pain), but the nurse wonders what this means to him. He winces with movement, walks in a stooped position, and seems to be guarding his abdomen. The nurse decides to apply the Palliative Performance Scale (PPS) and assesses him to be 50–60%. From past visits, the nurse knows that Mr. O is concerned about being a burden to his family—physically or financially. He has tried to stretch his medications to make them last longer and has been fearful of becoming addicted to pain medications.

Cultural Competence

The patient is of Mexican heritage. He clearly feels concern regarding his role as head of his family and whether his illness will result in some loss of control. It is important to discuss cultural, ethnic, and religious practices with Mr. O to discover what is important to him. He, his family, and the hospice team can try to accommodate his beliefs as much as possible.

 ## ORDERS FOR HOME CARE

Patient: 75-year-old Mexican male
Diagnosis: Colorectal cancer with metastasis to liver and bone
Current medications:
- Furosemide once a day as needed for increased fluid retention/edema
- Fentanyl transdermal patch every 12 hours
- Reglan before meals and at bedtime for nausea

Services (for provision of hospice at home): RN, home health aide (HHA), physical therapy (PT) (short term), occupational therapy (OT) (short term), medical social work (MSW) for consult and services, wound-ostomy nurse (for consult about ostomy care as needed), pharmacy

Reimbursement Considerations

In cases where there is an advanced illness, a limited prognosis (likely 6 months or less), and no desire to pursue aggressive treatment, hospice services are appropriate. Hospice under Medicare is an elected benefit, so this needs to be discussed in detail with any patient thinking of switching their Medicare. Hospice is responsible for providing all care and services that are part of the patient's terminal disease including medications, supplies, and equipment. Hospice coverage under Medicaid and other health care plans varies, and there are some areas of the country without hospice providers. So it is important to verify coverage and accessibility of hospice before pursuing the option with a patient.

THE HOME VISIT

Mr. O's goals include:

- To remain as independent and maintain as much of his role as possible (i.e., as a contributor to the family)
- To be "at peace with God"
- To minimize being a burden to family by having his affairs in order
- To maintain his self-rated pain at 3 or less on a scale of 0–10
- To have less nausea
- To regulate his bowel and ostomy regimen

Rehabilitation Needs

Registered nurse
Physician
Home health aide
Physical therapy
Occupational therapy
Social worker
Chaplain or pastor
Volunteer
Medications associated with terminal diagnosis
Supplies associated with terminal diagnosis
Support services for family (including bereavement services)
Respite services (short term)

The nurse gathers the following data:

- Mr. O's role in the family is as respected patriarch.
- Mr. O refers regularly to his spiritual/religious beliefs.
- Mr. O's abdomen is large with ascites.
- Mr. O has diminished bowel sounds.
- Mr. O has limited endurance.
- Mr. O's appetite fluctuates from poor to fair.
- Mr. O complains of nausea which increases with some odors and foods.
- Mr. O's last bowel movement was yesterday.
- Mr. O rates his pain at 5 (on a 0–10 scale) and reports that he is taking his Fentanyl once per day (instead of every 12 hours).

Neal Theory Implications

Stage 3: The professional in this stage recognizes that the patient is appropriate for hospice due to the extent of his disease and is effective in working with increasingly complex symptoms. This professional is prepared and confident in talking with the patient and family about changing goals of care and hospice services. This nurse embodies the hospice and palliative care philosophies when working with patients whose illnesses are advanced. The nurse is proactive in seeking resources and information when needed about more complex issues related to the advanced illness, symptom management, and cultural considerations.

Stage 2: The professional in this stage understands the advanced state of the patient's disease. This nurse recognizes that the goals of care will change and is willing to talk this through with patient and family, but may benefit from input or guidance from another team member with expertise. This nurse may need guidance and assistance with the complexities of transitioning a patient from home health to hospice. Collaboration with other team members (active services and case/team manager) is an essential part of this nurse's role. This nurse has the skills to discharge the patient to hospice or to follow the patient in hospice as the primary nurse. This nurse has experience and skill providing culturally congruent care, but may benefit from input about research findings about differences in end-of-life care preferences of various cultural and ethnic groups.

Stage 1: The professional in this stage recognizes that the patient's disease is advanced and that they meet hospice criteria for coverage under Medicare, but she may have limited or no experience talking with someone about hospice. Additionally the Stage 1 nurse may have a limited understanding of what hospice can provide to a patient and their family and limited experience in managing the increasing number and complexity of symptoms that occur during the last months of life. This nurse may be unsure how to engage in dialogue with the patient and family about whether to revise advance directives. This nurse may have some misconceptions about hospice, thinking that a patient must have a do-not-resuscitate order to receive hospice services. Additional guidance will benefit the Stage 1 nurse in managing increasingly complex symptoms that often occur with advanced illness. This nurse may identify a limited range of resources and have little prior experience serve as a guide to providing culturally congruent care.

? CRITICAL THINKING

1. **How is Mr. O an appropriate candidate for hospice? If Mr. O goes on hospice services, does that mean he cannot have treatment for something like an infection if he should develop one? Can a person receive hospice services if they have not signed a "do-not-resuscitate" form?**

Answer: Mr. O meets the criteria for hospice. He has an advanced illness, has a likely prognosis of 6 months or less, and the physician is involved and will order the services.

Individuals receiving hospice can still receive treatment for problems that occur, such as an infection; the extent to which it would be treated is individualized in accordance with the patient's condition, wishes, and goals of care. Signing a do-not-resuscitate form is not a requirement for receiving hospice services. When this is one of the patient's wishes, however, it is crucial that everyone—the patient, family, and health care team—have a clear understanding about the patient's care.

Relevant Community Resources

Community services for housekeeping and home maintenance
Legal assistance to plan provisions for loved ones after death

2. What are some things a nurse can do to prepare for having a conversation about hospice services and patient goals for care?

Answer: Some of the groundwork has already been laid in the case of Mr. O. His physician has talked with him about his advancing disease and has introduced the idea of hospice. Finding out more from the physician about how the conversation went would be beneficial. If needed, the nurse should review information about the patient's disease process in advance. Reviewing the agency's policies related to transitioning to hospice care is also important. In preparing for the visit, the nurse should schedule enough time for the visit and find out if the patient wants any other family members to be present. Once at the visit, the nurse will find out what the patient understands about the present illness and what to expect in the foreseeable future. By also assessing what the patient and family want to know and what their wishes are, the nurse can better meet their needs.

3. What is different about the focus, intensity, and schedule of hospice services in comparison to home health services?

Answer: The focus on hospice services is on the quality of life remaining including comfort measures. Unlike home health (where the visits and services diminish as the patient becomes more independent), hospice visits and services are more likely to increase as the patient's disease advances, as symptoms become more difficult to manage, and as the need for assistance and guidance with care becomes greater. In hospice there is tremendous focus on the family *and* the patient; volunteer services and access to limited respite services can benefit both the patient and their loved ones. A hallmark of hospice is its bereavement services, which can be provided to the family for approximately 1 year after the death of a patient.

Interdisciplinary Care Plan

Problem	Goal/Plan	Intervention	Evaluation
Knowledge deficit about metastatic cancer of the colon	Patient and family will demonstrate understanding of patient's diagnosis and the extent of his disease.	Nurse, physician, and other team members are to review patient's status and discuss likely prognosis ("likely to be months"). Nurse to facilitate open discussion with patient and family as followup after physician has discussed prognosis with patient.	Effective, open, ongoing communication between patient and family and the health care team about diagnosis, treatment options, prognosis and goals of care.

Problem	Goal/Plan	Intervention	Evaluation
Knowledge deficit about hospice benefit	Patient and family will verbalize understanding of hospice services. Patient will elect hospice. Transition to hospice care	Provide information to patient and family about hospice services and the process of electing the benefit. Collaborate with hospice admission team (typically nursing and social work or chaplain) to meet with patient and family about hospice services. Implement hospice services. If patient wishes and if it is possible, some home health team members may be part of the hospice care team.	Patient/family makes decision about initiating hospice services. Patient and family utilize hospice services. Patient and family are satisfied with hospice.
Knowledge deficit and limited self-efficacy (level of confidence in self-management) regarding advanced disease	Patient and family will verbalize understanding of recent changes in patient's condition within 1 week. Patient and family have increased understanding about advanced gastro-intestinal and metastatic disease within 2 weeks.	Teach patient and family about advanced disease trajectory. Teach patient about new medications. Teach patient and family about reporting and managing new symptoms. Collaborate with other team members such as pharmacy and wound-ostomy nurse to address complex disease and symptom issues. Provide information, encouragement, and positive reinforcement to patient and family. Engage patient as an active partner in planning his care.	Patient and family will report new or increasing symptoms in a timely manner. Patient and family describe actions to take to manage symptoms. Patient and family will identify resources to contact if problems or new/exacerbated symptoms occur. Patient, with assistance from family as needed, will manage routine medications and ostomy care with minimal cueing from health care team.

(Continued)

Problem	Goal/Plan	Intervention	Evaluation
Spiritual distress, altered coping mechanisms, and role change related to advanced illness with limited prognosis	Patient will verbalize existential concerns about illness, meaning of own existence, and quality of life. Support patient role as family patriarch.	Nurse will conduct a spiritual assessment. Interdisciplinary team will demonstrate respect for patient's cultural beliefs and preferences. Provide spiritual support through referral to chaplain and/or spiritual guide (i.e., patient's and family's clergy). Present an open, accepting, and listening approach when working with patient and family. Provide referral/resource information for community-based legal aid per patient wishes.	Patient and family will report sense of spiritual well-being. Patient and family are satisfied with legal aid planning referral.
Fatigue and limited endurance related to disease process	Attain a balance between rest and activity, independence, and assistance with daily activities to foster patient's quality of life within 4 weeks.	Therapy (PT and OT) to work with patient and family on adaptations to the home, daily routine, and patient activity level for effective management of fatigue. Assess sleep patterns. Nurse to instruct on use of oxygen as needed. Nurse to teach/reinforce about balancing periods of rest and activity. Nurse to help patient prioritize activities he wants to continue to do and those that he wants to delegate to others (family and/or outside resources). Home health aide to assist with personal care short term. Social worker to link patient and family with longer-term assistance in light of his reduced endurance and mobility.	Patient will access resources (home health aide, outside resources) as needed. Patient will be able to participate in activities meaningful to him (i.e., religion and family). Source of long-range assistance for patient's personal care will be identified. Additional help for chores such as shopping and cleaning will be obtained.

Problem	Goal/Plan	Intervention	Evaluation
Abdominal distention with fluid retention as evidenced by weight gain, increased abdominal girth, dyspnea, decreased endurance and limited mobility effects/side effects	Promote maximum comfort and mobility.	Teach patient self-management of fluid retention (self-monitoring of symptoms, reporting timely, and making changes in regimen).	Patient will be independent in managing abdominal distension through prn medications and adjustments in dietary/fluid intake. Patient will report increases in distension not responsive to interventions.
Alterations in elimination (bowel) related to advanced disease/ treatment and colostomy At risk for constipation related to disease process and medications	Promote effective bowel regimen and prevent constipation. New symptoms of change in bowel regimen will be addressed timely.	Teach bowel regimen, including use of stool softener and motility agent. Encourage adequate fluid and fiber intake. Teach patient and family that alterations in appetite and eating patterns are common.	Evaluate bowel regimen, nutrition, and symptoms (nausea) using assessment and patient self-report regularly (every nursing visit). Patient report of regular bowel regimen Bowel regimen is adjusted when changes warrant it.
Alterations in nutrition (nausea) related to disease process	Nausea will be managed to a degree that is acceptable by the patient within 1 week. Patient and family will adjust meal patterns within 2 weeks and as needed.	Teach measures to promote maximum enjoyment of foods including smaller more frequent meals, allowing patient to select foods that sound appealing, avoiding extreme spices and temperatures. Obtain order for and teach use of appetite stimulant if needed (Megace). Teach complementary/ alternative strategies for controlling nausea including use of ginger, chamomile, and mint.	Patient report of satisfaction with measures to enhance appetite and reduce nausea Patient and family satisfaction that he is able to participate in most family meals

(Continued)

Problem	Goal/Plan	Intervention	Evaluation
		Confer with physician as needed about changes in medication regimen to manage symptoms. Teach adaptations to ostomy care (use of different techniques, supplies) if difficulties with appliance arise. Ostomy nurse consultation as needed to address complex bowel regimen or ostomy care concerns.	
Pain	Patient's chronic pain will be controlled in a range acceptable to the patient (not to exceed 3) by the end of 1 week.	Patient to report episodes of pain, action taken and response by contacting the home health nurse and or use of a log. Nurse to review pain record regularly for any changes in pain or response to medications. Nurse will instruct patient about pain and prescribed pain medications. Nurse will allay patient and family fears or misconceptions about use of pain medications on a regular schedule (instead of "as needed"). Nurse will instruct on potential for constipation and measures to minimize its occurrence. Health care team will collaborate to revise pain management regimen as needed. Consultation with pharmacist as needed to address complex, undermanaged pain	Patient's pain not to exceed 3/10. Patient will take prescribed pain medications regularly. When changes in medication regimen occur, evaluate for effectiveness.

REFERENCES & RESOURCES

[1] R. Arnold, "Why patients do not take their opioids," *Fast Facts and Concepts* (2nd ed.), p. 83, Retrieved at: http://www.eperc.mcw.edu/fast/ff_083.htm 2007, Oct.

[2] Center for Medicare and Medicaid Services, *Medicare Hospice Benefits*, Author, Retrieved at: http://www.medicare.gov/publications/pubs/pdf/02154.pdf (n.d.).

[3] Intercultural Cancer Council, *Cancer Fact Sheets: Hispanics/Latinos, and Cancer*, Author, Retrieved at: http://www.iccnetwork.org/cancerfacts/ICC-CFS4.pdf (n.d.).

[4] National Consensus Project for Quality Palliative Care, *Clinical Practice Guidelines for Quality Palliative Care* (2nd ed.), Retrieved at: http://www.nationalconsensusproject.org 2009.

[5] National Healthcare Decisions Day, *Get an Advance Directive*, Author, Retrieved at: http://www.nationalhealthcaredecisionsday.org/resources.htm (n.d.).

[6] National Institute of Nursing Research, *Palliative Care: The Relief You Need When You're Experiencing the Symptoms of Serious Illness*, Author, Retrieved at: http://www.ninr.nih.gov/NR/rdonlyres/01CC45F1-048B-468A-BD9F-3AB727A381D2/0/NINR_PalliativeCare_Brochure_508C.pdf 2009, November.

[7] S.M. Parker et al., "A systematic review of prognostic/end-of-life communication with adults in the advanced stages of a life-limiting illness: Patient/caregiver preferences for the content, style, and timing of information," *Journal of Pain and Symptom Management*, 34(1):81–93, 2007. doi:10.1016/j.jpainsymman.2006.09.035

[8] D.E. Weissman, "Determining prognosis in advanced cancer," *Fast Facts and Concepts* (2nd ed.), p. 13, Retrieved at: http://www.eperc.mcw.edu/fastFact/ff_13.htm 2005, July.

[9] L.S. Wilner and R. Arnold, "The palliative performance scale," *Fast Facts and Concepts* (ed.), p. 125, End of Life/Palliative Education Resource Center (EPERC), Medical College of Wisconsin. Retrieved at: http://www.eperc.mcw.edu/fastfact/ff_125.htm 2004, November.

Case 15.4 Amyotrophic Lateral Sclerosis

By Susan Breakwell, APHN-BC, DNP

This case focuses on working with a patient and their family in the final hours and at the end of life. It also looks at the nurse's role in prioritizing and coordinating care.

Mr. A is a 65-year-old male with advanced amyotrophic lateral sclerosis (Lou Gehrig disease) (ALS). The home health agency, which provides both home health and hospice services, has followed him throughout the progression of his symptoms. When he elected the hospice benefit 2 months ago, he and his family asked if the nurse who had seen them in the past could continue on with him in conjunction with the other hospice staff.

Reimbursement Considerations

One hallmark of hospice is the inclusion of bereavement services. Upon the death of a patient, bereavement services can be provided to the family for approximately one year.

Complementary/alternative medicine (CAM), such as music therapy, can be covered as part of the hospice benefit under Medicare when they are part of a hospice program's services.

Clinical Case Studies in Home Health Care, First Edition. Edited by Leslie Neal-Boylan.
© 2011 John Wiley & Sons, Inc. Published 2011 by John Wiley & Sons, Inc.

ORDERS FOR END-OF-LIFE CARE

Patient: 65-year-old male
Diagnosis: ALS
Current medications: Oxygen 2 liters/min. by concentrator and nasal
   cannula as needed
Services needed: RN, HHA, MSW for consult and services, chaplain,
   volunteer and bereavement services, music therapy consult

THE HOME VISIT

The patient and his wife identified goals early on in hospice care:

- To be surrounded by loved ones
- To have a peaceful death
- To be at home
- To be comfortable

Additional data by the nurse from observation and the history and physical examination are:

- Mr. A is anuric.
- Mr. A's respirations and heart rate are irregular.
- Mr. A is not exhibiting signs of pain.
- Mr. A has mottled, blue, and cold extremities.
- Mr. A's unresponsiveness diminished over the past day. He seemed to briefly recognize his children when they arrived at the house.
- Mr. A's respirations have become less noisy and more shallow and irregular over the past day.
- Mr. A's wife needs support, information, and reassurance.
- Mr. A's children also need support and information.

Mr. A gets nutrition via his feeding tube and is bedbound. He is finding it more difficult to use his communication device, relying more and more on facial expressions and his wife's intuition. He and his wife have worked with the hospice team to ensure, as much as possible, that he remain at home until the end of life. They have also worked with hospice to make funeral arrangements. In accordance with their Jewish faith traditions and practices, there is to be a service within 24 hours of Mr. A's death. This was difficult for both of them; they had so many things they hoped to do together after Mr. A's retirement and struggled to identify new hopes and wishes for his time remaining. Mrs. A has been primary caregiver and is exhausted. The nurse has worked closely with her, teaching her how to care for someone who is bedbound and dependent on others for all his needs and how to manage his symptoms. She states she has never seen a person who was near death and is "not sure what to expect—or if I can handle it."

At the joint nurse and aide visit 2 days ago, Mr. A was awake and aware, lying in bed. Though nonverbal, he communicated by blinking his eyes. His urine output was low and concentrated. His wife reported that he spent much of his time sleeping. He did not seem to want to be moved, furrowing his eyebrows when he was repositioned.

A short while ago, Mrs. A called, tearfully stating, "My husband's hands and feet are bluish and cold, and his breathing isn't right. It's not regular, and he's making gurgling sounds. Can our nurse come see him, or should I call 911?" This sounds like a definite change in his status. At the house for this visit, the nurse sees that Mr. A is propped up in his hospital bed. His color is pale, extremities blue and cool to touch. Yesterday, even with his oxygen on, his respirations were agonal (rate and depth) and noisy. They are now becoming more shallow and infrequent. He is not exhibiting facial grimace or furrowed brow. He has not had any urine output for 24 hours. Mrs. A is concerned that she needs to turn him because she has not repositioned him since last evening. The nurse assesses that he is at 10% on the Palliative Performance Scale (PPS).

Rehabilitation Needs

Registered nurse
Physician
Home health aide
Social worker
Chaplain or rabbi
Volunteer
Medications associated with terminal diagnosis
Supplies associated with terminal diagnosis
Support services for family
Funeral home
Bereavement services for family

The nurse spends time listening to Mrs. A's questions and reminds her of things that were discussed at earlier visits, for example that Mr. A is exhibiting signs that he has limited time before death. The nurse reflects back on the many things Mrs. A has done to care for her husband and promises to stay with Mr. A while she calls the children and asks them to come home to say goodbye to their father. The nurse contacts the office to ask if the rabbi can come to the house per the family's request. The nurse calls the physician to report the patient's changes; the wife wants to talk with the physician, too.

Neal Theory Implications

Stage 3: The professional in this stage is confident and skilled in working with patients and families at the end of life and knows what needs to be done before and after the death of a patient. Documentation is thorough and timely. The nurse can effectively reprioritize care in response to changes in the patient and the needs of the family. The stage 3 nurse is familiar with CAM, is confident in collaborating with the team, and seeks their input in order to incorporate aspects of music into the care of the patient and comfort of the family. She demonstrates genuine human caring in balance with a professional rapport. This nurse also recognizes when she or other team members may be having a difficult time with the death of a patient and is proactive in seeking support or offering it to others. This nurse may benefit from reminders about individualizing care of each patient and family in accordance with their cultural or religious practices.

Stage 2: The professional in this stage recognizes that this patient is near the end of life. The nurse may be independent in providing the end of life and postmortem care, she but may need some assistance with prioritizing things and with completing required documentation. The stage 2 nurse understands that music therapy and other CAM is available through hospice. She may not be as familiar with ways that nursing can coordinate with music therapy to incorporate use of music into her work with the patient. This nurse is familiar with most agency policies and procedures, but she may need to review them to ensure that everything is addressed. The nurse can identify resources to access for providing culturally appropriate care. This nurse may recognize her own needs for support to deal with the death of a patient, but may not as readily recognize similar needs of other team members.

Stage 1: The professional at this stage may not be quite certain that the patient is near the end of life and his prognosis is likely "hours," and have cared for few if any patients at home near the time of death. This nurse will benefit from the expertise of other team members for assistance in following agency policies and procedures and prioritizing care, as well as for guidance and support while with the patient and family. This nurse may not be familiar with the hospice's use of CAM, such as music therapy. Additionally, the nurse will need information and guidance for completing required documentation. This nurse may also need assistance and guidance for contacting the physician at the time of death and for postmortem care. The nurse may welcome an opportunity for debriefing afterward, through an individual or team meeting. The stage 1 nurse is less certain of her professional boundaries, among other things wondering if it is okay to display emotion to the family or what to do if the family asks about praying with them.

CRITICAL THINKING

1. Who is the focus of care at this time?
Answer: The focus of care continues to be the patient and the family. Recognizing that the patient's signs and symptoms are consistent with being in the final hours of life and that the patient expressly wanted to be surrounded by loved ones, it is important to allow time for the patient and family to be together.

2. Should the nurse remain in the home or leave?
Answer: It is important to assess the situation thoroughly to arrive at a good decision. Remembering back to some of the wife's comments, she may need and welcome the nurse's presence at this time. An equally appropriate decision may be for the nurse to wait until the rabbi arrives, reassess if the wife has adequate support and that the patient is comfortable, then leave with a plan to return in a couple of hours.

3. If the nurse stays at the home, what arrangements should be made for any remaining patient visits for the day?
Answer: The nurse will need to contact others on the team (case manager, supervisor, or other designated person) to coordinate schedule changes. Some of the remaining patients might be rescheduled for another day or be seen by another nurse. The handoff and communication with other staff and patients need to occur in a timely fashion.

 ## BACK TO THE CASE

The nurse has remained with Mr. A and family. When his children arrive, he seems to recognize them for a moment. After everyone is gathered around Mr. A's bedside, they play some of his favorite music as the music therapist had recommended. Soon after, his respirations gradually decrease, he appears quiet and is unresponsive. His pulse and respirations cease while he is surrounded by his wife, children, rabbi, and the nurse. The nurse remains quietly in the room as the family prays with the rabbi. The nurse contacts the physician who will sign the death certificate, then calls the funeral home. The nurse prepares Mr. A's body for the family to say their goodbyes in the home and for the subsequent transport to the funeral home. The nurse notifies the agency of the death. The nurse finishes up with remaining tasks before leaving the home and going back to the office to talk with the manager of the team.

Relevant Community Resources

Funeral home; Jewish burial society
Local support groups and programs
Legal assistance

? CRITICAL THINKING

1. What relevance does a family's culture have on the care of a patient upon their death?
Answer: Just as with all other care, the care at the time of death needs to be individualized in accordance with patient and family wishes, cultural beliefs, and practices. Assessment data about this aspect of care is collected throughout earlier encounters, such as during earlier discussions about final wishes, funeral planning, and related issues. Whether the family wants the hospice staff (nurse, hospice aide) to bathe the body will be very individualized. Some will be unable or uncomfortable bathing and dressing their loved one, while other families will be distressed if a person from outside the family attempts to provide care of the body after death.

2. Who pronounces the patient's death and determines time of death?
Answer: The nurse at the patient's home will have a role upon the death of a patient; however, regulations and agency policies and procedures vary. It is vital that the nurse be familiar with applicable policies beforehand and that she contact the appropriate manager with any questions as they arise.

3. What is the nurse's responsibility for disposal of medications?
Answer: Extra care, attention, and documentation are called for, particularly in the handling of the patient's remaining narcotics. Again, the nurse must be familiar with regulations and turn to agency policies and procedures and managers for guidance.

Interdisciplinary Care Plan

Problem	Goal/Plan	Intervention	Evaluation
Knowledge deficit about signs of end of life Limited self-efficacy about caring for someone at the end of life	Patient family will recognize changes indicating the end of life is near. Family will be confident in providing comfort care measures for the patient.	Nurse, physician, and other team members to reinforce patient's status and discuss likely prognosis (likely to be "hours"). Nurse to provide information to family about signs of the end of life. Nurse and other team members to demonstrate comfort care measures. Nurse and/or other team members to be present with family in accordance with their wishes.	Nurse and/or team members observe family and their interaction with the patient. Family appears confident in providing comfort measures. Patient's wish to be surrounded by family is honored.
Caregiver role strain Altered family coping Potential for spiritual distress Grief	Support wife and family Respect spiritual and cultural preferences Family will be supported as they work through the grief process.	Provide services, care, and assistance with tasks so family can be present with patient and say their goodbyes. Provide reassurance and information to the family about signs that death is imminent. Schedule an adequate block of time to be with patient and family. Communicate with hospice volunteer and bereavement services about patient's changing status and family's upcoming need for additional services. The interdisciplinary team will demonstrate respect for the patient's cultural beliefs and preferences. Provide spiritual support through referral to chaplain and/or spiritual guide (i.e., patient's and family's priest). Assure the presence of team members during the patient's end of life.	Services are available when the family needs them: chaplain, nurse's aide, and nursing. The patient and family will report a sense of spiritual well-being. Patient's wish of a peaceful death surrounded by loved ones is met.

(Continued)

Problem	Goal/Plan	Intervention	Evaluation
		Incorporate use of complementary/alternative medicine that fits patient's needs (i.e., music therapy). Communicate with hospice bereavement program about the family's needs upon death of the patient.	

REFERENCES & RESOURCES

[1] Center for Medicare and Medicaid Services, *Medicare Hospice Benefits*, Author, (n.d.). Retrieved at: http://www.medicare.gov/publications/pubs/pdf/02154.pdf

[2] B. Ferrell and N. Coyle (eds.), *Textbook of Palliative Nursing*, Oxford University Press, 2006.

[3] R.E. Hilliard, "Music therapy in hospice and palliative care: A review of empirical data," *Evidence-Based Complementary and Alternative Medicine*, 2(2):173–178, 2005. Doi. 10.1093/ecam/neh076.

[4] B. Karnes, *Gone from My Sight: The Dying Experience*, Author, 1986.

[5] National Consensus Project for Quality Palliative Care, "Clinical practice guidelines for quality palliative care (Second edition)," Retrieved at: http://www.nationalconsensusproject.org, 2009.

[6] National Quality Forum, "A National Framework and Preferred Practices for Palliative and Hospice Quality Care," Consensus Report. Author. Retrieved at: http://www.qualityforum.org/Publications/2006/12/A_National_Framework_and_Preferred_Practices_for_Palliative_and_Hospice_Care_Quality.aspx, 2006, December.

[7] L.S. Wilner and R. Arnold, "The Palliative Performance Scale," Fast Facts and Concepts, 125. End of Life/Palliative Education Resource Center (EPERC), Medical College of Wisconsin. Retrieved at: http://www.eperc.mcw.edu/fastfact/ff_125.htm, 2004, November.

Index

Clinical Case Studies in Home Health Care, First Edition. Edited by Leslie Neal-Boylan.
© 2011 John Wiley & Sons, Inc. Published 2011 by John Wiley & Sons, Inc.

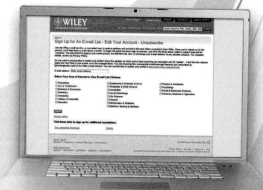
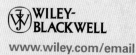